Linear Models and Design

Jay H. Beder

Linear Models and Design

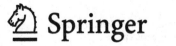

Jay H. Beder
University of Wisconsin–Milwaukee
Milwaukee, WI, USA

ISBN 978-3-031-08178-1   ISBN 978-3-031-08176-7 (eBook)
https://doi.org/10.1007/978-3-031-08176-7

This Springer imprint is published by the registered company Springer Nature Switzerland AG
The registered company address is: Gewerbestrasse 11, 6330 Cham, Switzerland

To my parents

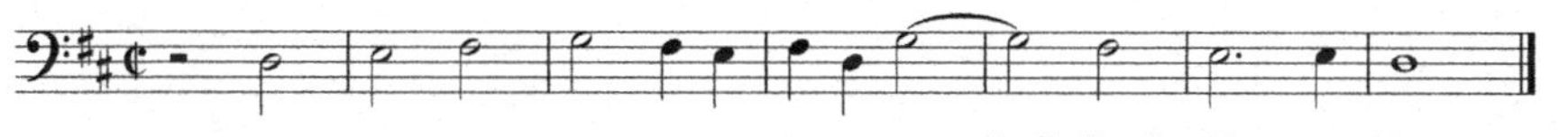

– J. S. Bach, Cantata 29, mvt. 2

Preface

This book is intended to give a graduate-level introduction to the theory of linear models and to basic concepts and results in the design of experiments. It takes a distinctly different approach to its subject from other texts, and the purpose of this preface is to alert the reader and provide a road map into the material.

Linear models encompass both regression models and factorial models. Ideally, the reader will thus have some familiarity with regression and the analysis of variance, along with a solid grounding in linear algebra and general mathematical sophistication. Chapters 5 and 6 make significant but elementary use of finite fields and commutative groups. An extensive mathematical appendix provides background for the topics covered, and the reader is encouraged to consult it as well as the comprehensive index, as needed. That said, everything is developed from scratch, with examples to help make the material easy to absorb.

The text combines two subjects that, while related, are usually treated separately at this level. Books on linear model theory typically don't go into detail about topics in experimental design, while texts in the latter generally give a relatively brief introduction to linear models, or may even simply assume that material. One goal of this text is to bring out the deep connections between these subjects.

While the reader will find many numerical examples in this book, it is probably not suitable as a main text for an applied statistics course. Rather, it is intended for use in a course emphasizing theory, and as a reference on the foundations of linear models and design of experiments. Chapters 1 through 4 develop the basic, classical results of linear model theory for both regression and factorial (or ANOVA) models, with Chap. 2 concentrating on the latter. The emphasis is on fixed-effects models, and only two sections are devoted to random effects (or variance components). These four chapters form a reasonable one-semester course on linear models.

The design part of the book is in Chaps. 5 and 6. Chapter 5 deals with the general theory of factorial designs and then develops the theory of confounding with blocks. Chapter 6, which depends heavily on Chap. 5, is devoted to fractional designs, aliasing, and resolution, along with an introduction to relative aberration and other topics. Those two chapters are really the heart of the book, and were my initial motivation for writing it. Excluding the appendix, these two chapters are almost half of the text, and along with Sects. 2.1–2.3 they could be the basis for a special topics course in design.

This book does not by any means cover all topics of interest in linear models and statistical design. My intention is to give the reader enough background to read more advanced literature intelligently and critically. A major goal of the text is to provide complete treatments of topics covered. Numerous references to the literature are provided for students interested in pursuing a topic further.

A particular concern of mine in this field is terminology. I have addressed this by (a) using common, consistent mathematical terminology and (b) explaining, in numerous remarks and in passages such as Sects. 1.2.1 and 6.7, the terminology that one may find in the literature. Hopefully, this book gives the student a helpful lexicon.

Aside from its unusual combination of topics, this text presents the material in a manner that differs in essential ways from other expositions. I want to flag some of these differences now.

- Recall that a linear model is defined by an equation

$$\mathrm{E}(\mathbf{Y}) = \mathbf{X}\boldsymbol{\beta},$$

  where $\mathbf{Y}$ is an $N \times 1$ vector of observations, $\boldsymbol{\beta}$ is a $p \times 1$ vector of parameters ($p \leq N$), and $\mathbf{X}$ is a *design matrix* (in factorial models) or a *regression matrix*. We will frequently view $\mathbf{X}$ not as a matrix but as a *linear transformation* from $\mathbb{R}^p$ (parameter space) to $\mathbb{R}^N$ (observation space). For reasons explained in the text, we will generally assume that $\mathbf{X}$ has full rank, and thus that the transformation is one-to-one.
- As a map, $\mathbf{X}$ has an inverse of sorts, namely a linear transformation from $\mathbb{R}^N$ to $\mathbb{R}^p$ that is indeed an inverse when restricted to the range of $\mathbf{X}$. This is the *Moore-Penrose inverse* of $\mathbf{X}$, and is given by the matrix $\mathbf{T} = (\mathbf{X}'\mathbf{X})^{-1}\mathbf{X}'$. It is introduced in Sect. 3.2, and makes a surprising number of appearances in the text (see the index). Except for a couple of exercises, this is the only "generalized inverse" we use. Generalized inverses typically arise in linear models because of the need to invert $\mathbf{X}'\mathbf{X}$, but that matrix will usually be invertible as $\mathbf{X}$ usually has full rank. I have included a brief discussion of generalized inverses near the end of Sect. 3.1, where I follow Rao [113].
- I have separated the treatment of the *identifiability* of a linear expression $\mathbf{c}'\boldsymbol{\beta}$ [1] from its *estimability*. See Proposition 1.29 and Lemma 3.10.
- A linear hypothesis is often described as a set of equations of the form $\mathbf{c}'\boldsymbol{\beta} = 0$, or as an equation $\mathbf{C}'\boldsymbol{\beta} = \mathbf{0}$ where $\mathbf{C}$ is a matrix. Instead, we view such hypotheses as being statements of the form $\boldsymbol{\beta} \perp U$ or $\boldsymbol{\beta} \in W$, where U and W are subspaces of $\mathbb{R}^p$. This is justified in Sect. 1.7, and I define the term *effect* in Sect. 2.3 simply to be U. This is a basis-free way to describe such hypotheses, and my hope is that

[1] We view vectors as columns, and $'$ denotes transpose, so $\mathbf{c}'\boldsymbol{\beta}$ is the dot product of $\mathbf{c}$ and $\boldsymbol{\beta}$.

the utility of this approach will become clear in later chapters. *The subspaces U and W, together with their images under $\mathbf{X}$, are our main focus of study beginning in Chap. 4. They are the unifying theme of the book, uniting the two main topics of the title.*

- In factorial models, the subspaces U will consist of *contrast vectors* (Definition 1.30). Among these are the spaces $U_{\mathcal{B}}$ where $\mathcal{B}$ is a *partition* (or *blocking*) of the set T of treatment combinations. We define these *block effects* and develop their basic properties in Sect. 5.2. They are fundamental in defining main effects and interaction, and they allow us to express the notion of confounding in a very general setting (Definition 5.40).
- Partially ordered sets, and in particular lattices, pervade the text. They arise rather naturally with regard to linear hypotheses in both regression and factorial models—see Sect. 4.3—and are necessary in any careful discussion of *adjusted* and *sequential sums of squares.*

  The lattice of partitions of a finite set (for us, the set of treatment combinations) is of central interest. The ordering on partitions that we use is actually the opposite of the more common ordering, but more natural; see Theorem 5.5 and Remark A.8.

  Theorem 5.5 introduces one of two lattice maps that play a crucial role. The other map is induced by the linear transformation $\mathbf{X}$; see Proposition 4.15.
- When it comes to factorial models, we follow a *cell-means* approach fairly strictly. This means that rather than writing models such as $\mathrm{E}(Y_{ijk}) = \mu + \alpha_i + \beta_j + \gamma_{ij}$ (which we call a *factor-effects parametrization*), we formulate everything in terms of the *cell means* $\mu_{ij} = \mathrm{E}(Y_{ijk})$ (μ_{ij} is the mean for cell ij). Bose [22] defined main effects and interactions in exactly this way, and the approach we use is essentially his.

  Factor-effects models are discussed in Sect. 2.5 and the cell-means approach in Sect. 2.6. The factor-effects parametrization is very common, and this exposition should give students facility in toggling between that and the cell-means approach.
- If T is the set of cells (treatment combinations) in a factorial experiment, we may denote the mean response in cell t by μ_t (as above) or by $\mu(t)$. Thus, the set of mean responses can be represented as a vector $\boldsymbol{\mu}$ with components indexed by T or as a *function* μ defined on T. Section 5.1 leads the reader to this functional point of view and replaces the parameter space $\mathbb{R}^p$ by the space $\mathbb{R}^T$ consisting of real-valued functions on T. This risks adding a layer of unfamiliarity to the material, but I have found that it is a more natural way to deal with factorial experiments. Each approach has its advantages, and students should feel comfortable with both.

  (This approach is of course necessary in extending linear model theory to functional data, but that is beyond the scope of this book.)
- There are two distinct views of aliasing and resolution in the literature. One common view defines these concepts in terms of estimability and bias. *We emphatically do not follow this view*, which we discuss extensively in Sect. 6.7. The approach we follow springs essentially from Rao's seminal 1947 paper

[111], in which he introduced the fundamental parameter of *strength*. Implicit in his writing is the operation of *restriction*, which we formalize at the beginning of Chap. 6. This allows us to define aliasing in a very general way (Definition 6.4). From this we proceed in two directions.

1. We derive the well-known theory of aliasing and resolution in so-called *regular* fractions (Sects. 6.1 and 6.2). It should be noted that these were originally developed without the use of the results in Rao's 1947 paper: aliasing in 2-level and 3-level designs in a 1945 paper [54] by Finney, and resolution in 2-level designs in a 1961 paper by Box and Hunter [27].[2]
2. We develop the theory of aliasing and resolution in arbitrary fractions (Sect. 6.5). Our general definition of aliasing allows us to interpret Box and Hunter's definition of resolution (Definition 6.25) in this general context, from which we prove a Fundamental Theorem of Aliasing (Theorem 6.43) and a host of related results. It is interesting to note how close Rao came to the concept of resolution in his 1947 paper.

I have paid some attention throughout the text to the history of certain ideas, notably the discovery by Barnard of a useful group structure in so-called 2^k experiments. Her 1936 paper [10] led to generalizations over the next decade using either geometry [23] or group theory [58, 59] and sparked an interest in applications of algebra to design that continues to this day. The beginning of Chap. 5 includes some biographical information about her, and I hope this book helps to spotlight the significance of her contribution.

There are quite a few topics not covered in this text, including robustness, nonnormality, dummy variables, and various designs (BIB and PBIB, split plot, crossover, ...). On the other hand, I have included some topics that are less usual:

Identifiability and its relation to estimability. We include a careful discussion of linear functions of a parameter.

Choice of weights in a two-factor design (Sect. 2.5.2). This analyzes Scheffé's discussion of the factor-effects model [121, pages 93–94].

Three elementary hypotheses (Sect. 2.2.1). These are used to build the usual contrasts that define main effects in a two-factor experiment.

Associated hypotheses (Sect. 4.5.2). These were coined by Searle in [124] in his critique of sequential sums of squares. We prove a general theorem showing that these always exist and giving a method to find them.

The linear parametric function most responsible for rejecting H_0 (Sect. 4.8.2). Scheffé gives a form of this in [121, page 72].

Complex contrast vectors (Sect. 5.6.5). The components of these vectors are sth roots of unity, and yield a generalization of Barnard's original result to p^k factorial designs when $s = p$, a prime. They are studied here primarily to

[2] Box and Hunter include Rao's paper in their bibliography but make no mention of it in their exposition.

lay the groundwork for so-called *generalized wordlength patterns* in nonregular fractions of p^k designs (Sect. 6.8.1).

An unexpected pattern in regular fractions (Sect. 6.4). This arises in "summing contrasts over an alias set" in regular fractions, and offers a basis for the practice of writing expressions such as $A + BC$ for the alias set containing A and BC. The main result (Theorem 6.35) is needed for an alternate approach to aliasing discussed in Sect. 6.7 (see in particular Theorem 6.56).

Projections of regular fractions (Sect. 6.9). Theorem 6.80 (or its corollary) characterizes such projections in arbitrary regular fractions. While the result is generally accepted as known, a complete proof does not (until now) appear to be available in the literature.

Notation

We write vectors and matrices in **boldface**. As mentioned above, vectors are assumed to be column vectors except where explicitly stated otherwise, and $'$ indicates transpose. The notation $|\quad|$ means determinant if the argument is a matrix, and cardinality if the argument is a set. The complement of the set E is denoted by E^c.

"Dot notation" is used to indicate summation: $x_{ij\cdot} = \sum_k x_{ijk}$, $x_{i\cdot\cdot} = \sum_j \sum_k x_{ijk}$, and so on. If the indices have ranges $1 \le i \le I, 1 \le j \le J, 1 \le k \le K$, then we write $\bar{x}_{ij\cdot} = (1/K) \sum_k x_{ijk}$, $\bar{x}_{i\cdot\cdot} = (1/JK) \sum_j \sum_k x_{ijk}$, etc., for averages.

We sometimes use the abbreviation iff for "if and only if." We assume the reader is familiar with the quantifiers $\forall$ ("for all") and $\exists$ ("there exists").

Other notation is introduced in the text, and is referenced in the index.

Acknowledgments

I thank George Seber for a number of helpful discussions over the years concerning the Wald statistic and other topics. This book was partly inspired by his text [128]. I also thank Angela Dean and Dan Voss for sharing their insights. Aside from their publications, Voss's thesis [144] provides a very readable guide to various methods of confounding.

Thanks to Rahul Mukerjee and Boxin Tang for helpful discussions regarding fractional designs. The recent book [98] by Mukerjee and Wu is an excellent introduction to regular designs (and especially to minimum aberration), and influenced some of my presentation of that material.

I am grateful to Terry Speed for alerting me to the survey article [53] containing biographical information about Mildred M. Barnard.

Thanks to John Aldrich and Jeff Miller for help with historical information about identifiability and the Gauss-Markov Theorem. A website on "Earliest Uses of Some Words of Mathematics," originally developed by Jeff, is now maintained at https://mathshistory.st-andrews.ac.uk/Miller/mathword/.

I am indebted to the staff at Springer Nature, and especially to my editor, Dr. Eva Hiripi, for their thoughtful handling of this book as they moved it from manuscript to finished product. I greatly appreciate their responsiveness to my numerous questions.

I am grateful to the Department of Mathematical Sciences and the College of Letters and Science at the University of Wisconsin—Milwaukee for the sabbaticals (more than one!) necessary to see this work to completion. I would also like to thank my students, especially Steffen Domke and Xinran Qi, for comments and questions (and corrections) that led me to tighten my exposition.

Finally, thanks to my family—my wife Dena and our sons Daniel, Jesse, and Naftali—for their love and support. My writing has benefitted both here and elsewhere from Dena's critical reading and keen suggestions. Special thanks to Naftali for the graphics in Fig. 2.2, and to Daniel for the Bach quote above. This book is dedicated to my parents, Bebe and Sy, who gave me my first exposure to math and taught me to value critical thinking.

It has been suggested [133] that "No matter how many times you proofread your book, after publication there will be roughly one typo per page." With that humbling thought in mind, I welcome questions, comments, and corrections, which can be emailed to me at `beder@uwm.edu`. Should it be necessary, I will establish a webpage with comments and corrections (and maybe hints to certain exercises), located at https://sites.uwm.edu/beder/.

Milwaukee, WI, USA Jay H. Beder

Contents

List of Figures

List of Tables

Chapter 1
Linear Models

Abstract This chapter introduces the fundamental concepts and terminology of the text. It includes a discussion of identifiability and, most crucially, a description of the various ways we will describe linear constraints and linear hypotheses. The latter is given in Lemma 1.33. Note especially the use of subspaces of the parameter space to represent hypotheses.

1.1 Random Vectors

A *random vector* is a vector whose components are random variables.[1] Two vectors $\mathbf{X}$ and $\mathbf{Y}$ are *(stochastically) independent* if

$$P(\mathbf{X} \in A, \mathbf{Y} \in B) = P(\mathbf{X} \in A)\, P(\mathbf{Y} \in B) \tag{1.1}$$

for any (Borel[2]) sets A and B. (If $\mathbf{X}$ is $n \times 1$ then this presumes that $A \subset \mathbb{R}^n$, and similarly for $\mathbf{Y}$ and B.) The proof of the following useful remark is an easy exercise.

Theorem 1.1 *If* $\mathbf{X}$ *and* $\mathbf{Y}$ *are independent, then so are* $f(\mathbf{X})$ *and* $g(\mathbf{Y})$ *for any (measurable) functions* f *and* g.

[1] Without loss of generality we may assume that the components are defined on a common probability space, and consequently have a joint distribution.

[2] It is enough to state (1.1) for any open sets A and B, or even just intervals. For this and the measurability requirement in Theorem 1.1, the reader is referred to a measure-theoretic treatment of probability theory such as [30]. The present text makes no direct use of measure theory.

J. H. Beder, *Linear Models and Design*,
https://doi.org/10.1007/978-3-031-08176-7_1

If $\mathbf{Y} = (Y_1, \ldots, Y_N)'$ is an $N \times 1$ random vector, we define its *mean vector* to be the vector

$$\mathrm{E}(\mathbf{Y}) = \begin{pmatrix} \mu_1 \\ \vdots \\ \mu_N \end{pmatrix},$$

where $\mu_i = \mathrm{E}(Y_i)$. We will also use the notation $\boldsymbol{\mu}_{\mathbf{Y}}$ for $\mathrm{E}(\mathbf{Y})$, or simply $\boldsymbol{\mu}$ if there is no chance of confusion.

It is convenient to write a linear combination $\sum_i a_i Y_i$ as $\mathbf{a}'\mathbf{Y}$, where $\mathbf{a} = (a_1, \ldots, a_N)'$. We see immediately that

$$\mathrm{E}(\mathbf{a}'\mathbf{Y}) = \mathbf{a}'\,\mathrm{E}(\mathbf{Y}), \tag{1.2}$$

and more generally that

$$\mathrm{E}(\mathbf{AY}) = \mathbf{A}\,\mathrm{E}(\mathbf{Y}) \tag{1.3}$$

for any N-column matrix $\mathbf{A}$.

The moment-generating function of a random variable Y is the function $M(t) = \mathrm{E}(e^{tY})$. More generally, the *moment-generating function (mgf)* of the random vector $\mathbf{Y}$ is the function

$$M(\mathbf{t}) = \mathrm{E}\left(e^{\mathbf{t}'\mathbf{Y}}\right).$$

When necessary, we will subscript a moment-generating function by its random variable or vector, e.g., $M_Y(t)$. It is always the case that $M(\mathbf{0}) = 1$, of course, but $M(\mathbf{t})$ may not exist for other values of $\mathbf{t}$. When it does, we have this fact:

Theorem 1.2 *If $M_{\mathbf{X}}(\mathbf{t}) = M_{\mathbf{Y}}(\mathbf{t})$ in an open neighborhood of $\mathbf{t} = \mathbf{0}$, then $\mathbf{X}$ and $\mathbf{Y}$ have the same distribution.*

We also recall the following properties of mgfs:

Theorem 1.3

a. If $\mathbf{Y} = \begin{bmatrix} \mathbf{Y}_1 \\ \mathbf{Y}_2 \end{bmatrix}$ and $\mathbf{t}$ is partitioned similarly, then $\mathbf{Y}_1$ and $\mathbf{Y}_2$ are independent if and only if $M_{\mathbf{Y}}(\mathbf{t}) = M_{\mathbf{Y}_1}(\mathbf{t}_1)M_{\mathbf{Y}_2}(\mathbf{t}_2)$ in an open neighborhood of $\mathbf{t} = \mathbf{0}$.
b. $M_{aX}(t) = M_X(at)$.
c. If $X_1, \ldots, X_n$ are independent, then $M_{X_1+\cdots+X_n}(t) = \prod_{i=1}^n M_{X_i}(t)$.

The proof of (b) is elementary. For (a) and (c) as well as Theorem 1.2 in the bivariate case, see [116, Sec. 4.6].

As with random vectors, a *random matrix* $\mathbf{M}$ is a matrix whose entries are random variables, and if M_{ij} is the ijth entry of $\mathbf{M}$ then $\mathrm{E}(M_{ij})$ is the ijth entry of E($\mathbf{M}$). We note in particular that the trace can be interchanged with expectation:

$$\mathrm{E}(\mathrm{tr}(\mathbf{M})) = \mathrm{tr}(\mathrm{E}(\mathbf{M})). \tag{1.4}$$

The symmetric $N \times N$ random matrix $(\mathbf{Y} - \boldsymbol{\mu})(\mathbf{Y} - \boldsymbol{\mu})'$, where $\boldsymbol{\mu} = \boldsymbol{\mu}_{\mathbf{Y}}$, is especially important, as we define the *covariance matrix* of $\mathbf{Y}$ to be

$$\boldsymbol{\Sigma} = \mathrm{Var}(\mathbf{Y}) = \mathrm{E}[(\mathbf{Y} - \boldsymbol{\mu})(\mathbf{Y} - \boldsymbol{\mu})'].$$

We also write $\boldsymbol{\Sigma}_{\mathbf{Y}}$ if necessary. If we let $\sigma_{ij} = \mathrm{Cov}(Y_i, Y_j)$ be the covariance of the random variables Y_i and Y_j, then

$$\boldsymbol{\Sigma} = \begin{bmatrix} \sigma_{11} & \dots & \sigma_{1N} \\ \vdots & \ddots & \vdots \\ \sigma_{N1} & \dots & \sigma_{NN} \end{bmatrix}$$

It is obvious that $\boldsymbol{\Sigma}$ is symmetric, and that the components of $\mathbf{Y}$ are uncorrelated iff $\boldsymbol{\Sigma}$ is diagonal. We have the "computational form"

$$\boldsymbol{\Sigma} = \mathrm{E}(\mathbf{Y}\mathbf{Y}') - \boldsymbol{\mu}\boldsymbol{\mu}', \tag{1.5}$$

the generalization of the formula $\mathrm{Var}(Y) = \mathrm{E}(Y^2) - \mu^2$.

We call two random vectors $\mathbf{X}$ and $\mathbf{Y}$ *uncorrelated* if $\mathrm{Cov}(X_i, Y_j) = 0$ for all i and j. If $\mathbf{X}$ is an $M \times 1$ random vector, we define $\mathrm{Cov}(\mathbf{X}, \mathbf{Y})$ to be the $M \times N$ matrix whose ijth element is $\mathrm{Cov}(X_i, Y_j)$. Thus $\mathbf{X}$ and $\mathbf{Y}$ are uncorrelated if $\mathrm{Cov}(\mathbf{X}, \mathbf{Y}) = 0$.

We moreover have the following useful facts, whose proof we leave as an exercise.

Theorem 1.4 *Let* $\mathbf{Y}$ *be* $N \times 1$ *with* $\boldsymbol{\Sigma} = \mathrm{Var}(\mathbf{Y})$, *let* $\mathbf{a}$ *and* $\mathbf{b}$ *be nonrandom* $N \times 1$ *vectors, and let* $\mathbf{A}$ *and* $\mathbf{B}$ *be nonrandom* N*-column matrices.*

a. $\mathrm{Cov}(\mathbf{a}'\mathbf{Y}, \mathbf{b}'\mathbf{Y}) = \mathbf{a}'\boldsymbol{\Sigma}\mathbf{b}$.
b. $\mathrm{Var}(\mathbf{a}'\mathbf{Y}) = \mathbf{a}'\boldsymbol{\Sigma}\mathbf{a}$.
c. $\mathrm{Cov}(\mathbf{AY}, \mathbf{BY}) = \mathbf{A}\boldsymbol{\Sigma}\mathbf{B}'$. *In particular,* $\mathrm{Var}(\mathbf{Y}) = \mathbf{A}\boldsymbol{\Sigma}\mathbf{A}'$.
d. $\boldsymbol{\Sigma}$ *is positive-semidefinite, and is* non-*definite if and only if there are constants* a_i, *not all zero, and a constant* c *such that* $a_1Y_1 + \cdots + a_NY_N = c$ *with probability 1.*

We note that $\boldsymbol{\Sigma}$ is invertible iff it is positive definite (Theorem A.106).

Expressions of the type $\mathbf{Y}'\mathbf{A}\mathbf{Y}$, called *quadratic forms*, arise in various applications. The proof of the following property is left as an exercise.

Proposition 1.5 *Let* $\mathbf{A}$ *be a (constant) matrix and* $\mathbf{Y}$ *a random vector of the same size having mean* $\boldsymbol{\mu}$ *and covariance matrix* $\boldsymbol{\Sigma}$. *Then* $\mathrm{E}(\mathbf{Y}'\mathbf{A}\mathbf{Y}) = \mathrm{tr}(\mathbf{A}\boldsymbol{\Sigma}) + \boldsymbol{\mu}'\mathbf{A}\boldsymbol{\mu}$.

We say that $\mathbf{Y}$ has a *multivariate normal distribution*, or simply a *normal distribution*, if $\mathbf{a}'\mathbf{Y}$ is normally distributed for every $\mathbf{a} \in \mathbb{R}^N$, and write $\mathbf{Y} \sim N(\boldsymbol{\mu}, \boldsymbol{\Sigma})$. We also say that the components of $\mathbf{Y}$ are *jointly normally distributed.* Two random vectors $\mathbf{X}$ and $\mathbf{Y}$ are jointly normally distributed if the vector $\binom{\mathbf{X}}{\mathbf{Y}}$ has a normal distribution.

Theorem 1.6 *Suppose* $\mathbf{Y}$ *is* $N \times 1$.

a. If $\mathbf{Y}$ *is normally distributed, then so is* $\mathbf{AY}$ *for any matrix* $\mathbf{A}$ *of* N *columns.*
b. $\mathbf{Y} \sim N(\boldsymbol{\mu}, \boldsymbol{\Sigma})$ *iff its moment-generating function is*

$$M(\mathbf{t}) = \exp\left(\boldsymbol{\mu}'\mathbf{t} + \frac{\mathbf{t}'\boldsymbol{\Sigma}\mathbf{t}}{2}\right), \quad \mathbf{t} \in \mathbb{R}^N.$$

c. If $\mathbf{Y} \sim N(\boldsymbol{\mu}, \boldsymbol{\Sigma})$ *and* $\boldsymbol{\Sigma}$ *is positive-definite, then* $\mathbf{Y}$ *has pdf*[3]

$$f(\mathbf{y}) = \frac{1}{(2\pi|\boldsymbol{\Sigma}|)^{N/2}} \exp -\frac{1}{2}(\mathbf{y} - \boldsymbol{\mu})'\boldsymbol{\Sigma}^{-1}(\mathbf{y} - \boldsymbol{\mu}),$$

where $|\boldsymbol{\Sigma}|$ *is the determinant of* $\boldsymbol{\Sigma}$.

Proof Part (a) follows from the definition and the fact that $\mathbf{a}'\mathbf{AY} = (\mathbf{A}'\mathbf{a})'\mathbf{Y}$. The other parts are left as exercises. Note that parts (a) and (b) hold even if $\boldsymbol{\Sigma}$ is semidefinite. □

It is an elementary fact that independent random variables are uncorrelated. With normality, the converse holds:

Corollary 1.7 *Let* $\mathbf{Y} = (Y_1, Y_2)'$ *be normally distributed. If* Y_1 *and* Y_2 *are uncorrelated then they are independent. More generally, if* $\mathbf{X}$ *and* $\mathbf{Y}$ *are jointly normal and if they are uncorrelated, then they are independent.*

Proof Suppose $\mathbf{X} \sim N(\mu_\mathbf{X}, \Sigma_\mathbf{X})$, $\mathbf{Y} \sim N(\mu_\mathbf{Y}, \Sigma_\mathbf{Y})$, and $\Sigma_{\mathbf{XY}} = \mathrm{Cov}(\mathbf{X}, \mathbf{Y})$. Putting

$$\mathbf{Z} = \begin{bmatrix} \mathbf{X} \\ \mathbf{Y} \end{bmatrix}$$

we see that $\mathbf{Z}$ is normally distributed with mean vector

$$\mu_\mathbf{Z} = \begin{bmatrix} \mu_\mathbf{X} \\ \mu_\mathbf{Y} \end{bmatrix}$$

[3] Probability density function.

and covariance matrix

$$\mathbf{\Sigma_Z} = \begin{bmatrix} \mathbf{\Sigma_X} & \mathbf{\Sigma_{XY}} \\ \mathbf{\Sigma'_{XY}} & \mathbf{\Sigma_Y} \end{bmatrix}.$$

Writing out the moment generating function $M_{\mathbf{Z}}(\mathbf{t})$ with $\mathbf{t}$ partitioned in the obvious way, we see that $M_{\mathbf{Z}}(\mathbf{t}) = M_{\mathbf{X}}(\mathbf{t}_1)M_{\mathbf{Y}}(\mathbf{t}_2)$ if and only if $\mathbf{\Sigma_{XY}} = \mathbf{0}$, and an application of of Theorem 1.3(a) gives us what we want. □

Sclove [122] has shown that the above property in some sense characterizes the normal distribution. A particular case of the corollary is this:

Corollary 1.8 *Suppose* $\mathbf{Y} \sim N(\boldsymbol{\mu}, \mathbf{\Sigma})$. *Then* $\mathbf{AY}$ $\mathbf{AY}$ *and* $\mathbf{BY}$ *are independent if and only if* $\mathbf{A\Sigma B'} = \mathbf{0}$.

Proof This is just an application of property (1.4) of Theorem 1.4. □

Theorem 1.9 *Let* $X_1, \ldots, X_n$ *be independent random variables with* $X_i \sim N(\mu_i, 1)$, *and let* $Y = \sum_{i=1}^n X^2$. *Then the mgf of* Y *is*

$$M(t) = \frac{1}{(1-2t)^{n/2}} e^{t\delta/(1-2t)}, \quad t < 1/2, \tag{1.6}$$

where $\delta = \sum_{i=1}^n \mu_i^2$. *In particular, the distribution of* Y *depends only on* n *and* δ.

Sketch of Proof By independence, $M(t)$ is the product of the mgfs of the variables X_i^2. These are evaluated by a standard argument that includes completing the square. □

Definition 1.10 If a random variable Y has mgf of the form (1.6), then we say it has the *noncentral* χ^2 (or *chi-square*) *distribution* with n degrees of freedom and noncentrality parameter δ,[4] and we write $Y \sim \chi^2(n, \delta)$. When $\delta = 0$, we say that Y has the *(central) chi-square distribution* with n degrees of freedom, and write $Y \sim \chi^2(n)$.

In the case of Theorem 1.6, the distribution of $\sum_{i=1}^n X^2$ would be central if (and only if) $\mu_1 = \cdots = \mu_n = 0$. Zero-mean random variables are said to be *centered*, hence the use of the term "central" in the chi-square distribution. "Degrees of freedom" is a term borrowed from physics, and generally represents the dimension of a vector space.

Definition 1.11 Let U and V be independent random variables with $U \sim N(\mu, 1)$ and $V \sim \chi^2(n)$. The distribution of $T = U/\sqrt{V/n}$ is called the *noncentral t distribution* with n degrees of freedom and noncentrality parameter μ. We write

[4] Some authors define the noncentrality parameter to be the square root of ours, or include a factor of $\frac{1}{2}$.

$T \sim t(n, \mu)$. When $\mu = 0$, T has the *(central) t distribution*, and we write $T \sim t(n)$.

This distribution is often called *Student's t* distribution, after W. S. Gosset, who published a derivation of the central t distribution under the pseudonym Student. It is obvious that the distribution of T is determined entirely by the parameters μ and n, thus justifying the definition. We will not need to know the pdf, which may be found in many textbooks.

Definition 1.12 Let U and V be independent random variables with $U \sim \chi^2(m, \delta)$ and $V \sim \chi^2(n)$. The distribution of $F = (U/m)/(V/n)$ is called the *noncentral F distribution* with m and n degrees of freedom and noncentrality parameter δ. We write $F \sim F(m, n, \delta)$. When $\delta = 0$, F has the *(central) F distribution*, and we write $F \sim F(m, n)$. The numbers m and n are sometimes called the *numerator and denominator degrees of freedom*, respectively.

We note the following:

Proposition 1.13 *If* $T \sim t(n)$ *then* $T^2 \sim F(1, n)$. *More generally, if* $T \sim t(n, \mu)$ *then* $T^2 \sim F(1, n, \mu^2)$.

Proof Write $X \sim Y$ to mean that X and Y have the same distribution. Since $T \sim U/\sqrt{V/n}$, with U and V as in Definition 1.11, we have $T^2 \sim U^2/(V/n)$. By Theorem 1.9, $U^2 \sim \chi^2(1, \mu^2)$, and so the result follows from Definition 1.12. □

Note that the assumption $T \sim t(n, \mu)$ does not imply that $T = U/\sqrt{V/n}$ for appropriate U and V, but merely that T has the same distribution as such a quotient. Similar remarks hold for the χ^2 and F distributions. The proof is stated carefully to take this into account. We have also made use of the following fact, whose proof is an exercise.

Lemma 1.14 *If* $X \sim Y$ *and* f *is any (measurable) function, then* $f(X) \sim f(Y)$.

As is customary, we use the notation D_α for the $(1 - \alpha)$-quantile of the distribution D—in particular:

z_α	if D is the $N(0, 1)$ distribution
$\chi^2_{n,\alpha}$	if D is the $\chi^2(n)$ distribution
$t_{n,\alpha}$	if D is the $t(n)$ distribution
$F_{m,n,\alpha}$	if D is the $F(m, n)$ distribution

For example, if $Z \sim N(0, 1)$ then $\mathrm{P}(Z > z_\alpha) = \alpha$.

1.2 Some Statistical Concepts

Let $\mathcal{P}$ be a family of probability distributions[5]. If we can write $\mathcal{P} = \{\mathrm{P}_\theta \colon \theta \in \Theta\}$, the index θ is said to be a *parameter* of the distribution, and may be univariate, vector-valued, or even more general. For example, $(\boldsymbol{\mu}, \boldsymbol{\Sigma})$ is the parameter of the $N(\boldsymbol{\mu}, \boldsymbol{\Sigma})$ distribution. The components $\boldsymbol{\mu}$, $\boldsymbol{\Sigma}$, μ_i and σ_{ij} are also called parameters.

A distribution P_θ determines many other things, for example the cumulative distribution function and the expected value. We will often index these by P, or by the parameter θ: for example, $\mathrm{E}_{\mathrm{P}}(X)$ is the expected value of X with respect to the distribution P, and $\mathrm{E}_\theta(X)$ is the expected value of X with respect to the distribution P_θ.

In writing P_θ, we often intend the value of θ to determine the probability distribution P_θ completely. However, when θ is a multiparameter we often abuse this notation. For example, if $\theta = (\mu, \sigma^2)$ we will often write P_μ, say, if it is only necessary to specify μ in a particular application, even though μ does not completely determine the distribution if σ is unknown. The context will make clear what we mean by the subscript.

1.2.1 Identifiability

Definition 1.15 Let $\mathcal{P} = \{\mathrm{P}_\theta \colon \theta \in \Theta\}$ be a family of probability distributions, and assume that θ completely determines P_θ. The parameter θ is said to be *identifiable* if the correspondence $\theta \mapsto \mathrm{P}_\theta$ is one-to-one.

Thus if $\mathbf{Y} \sim N(\boldsymbol{\mu}, \boldsymbol{\Sigma})$, the parameter $\theta = (\boldsymbol{\mu}, \boldsymbol{\Sigma})$ is identifiable. We will see examples of non-identifiability in linear models in Sect. 2.5.

Since we will deal with parameters that do not completely determine a distribution, we extend the concept of identifiability. We leave it as an exercise to show that the following generalizes Definition 1.15.

Definition 1.16 Let $\mathcal{P}$ be a family of probability distributions, and suppose that for each $\psi \in \Psi$ there is a subfamily $\mathcal{P}_\psi$ of distributions such that $\mathcal{P} = \cup_\psi \mathcal{P}_\psi$. Then we say that the parameter ψ is *identifiable* if $\psi_1 \neq \psi_2$ implies $\mathcal{P}_{\psi_1} \cap \mathcal{P}_{\psi_2} = \emptyset$.

It is sometimes useful to state the implication in Definition 1.16 in the contrapositive: $\mathcal{P}_{\psi_1} \cap \mathcal{P}_{\psi_2} \neq \emptyset$ implies $\psi_1 = \psi_2$.

Example 1.17 Let $\mathbf{X}$ have a distribution in some family $\mathcal{P}$ such that $\mathrm{E}_{\mathrm{P}}(\mathbf{X})$ is finite for all $\mathrm{P} \in \mathcal{P}$. Then $\boldsymbol{\psi} = \mathrm{E}_{\mathrm{P}}(\mathbf{X})$ is identifiable. Here, for each value of $\boldsymbol{\psi}$ the set $\mathcal{P}_{\boldsymbol{\psi}}$ contains all the distributions in $\mathcal{P}$ giving $\mathbf{X}$ the same mean $\boldsymbol{\psi}$. To show identifiability,

[5] Or probability measures on a sample space.

let $\mathrm{P} \in \mathcal{P}_{\psi_1} \cap \mathcal{P}_{\psi_2}$ (where we assume that the intersection is nonempty). Then $\psi_1 = \mathrm{E}_\mathrm{P}(\mathbf{X})$ and also $\psi_2 = \mathrm{E}_\mathrm{P}(\mathbf{X})$, so $\psi_1 = \psi_2$.

Thus identifiability implies that the same distribution P cannot give two different values of $\mathrm{E}_\mathrm{P}(\mathbf{X})$.

The problem with non-identifiable parameters is that there is no way to make statistical inference about them. Even if we could perfectly determine the probability distribution P that gave rise to a set of data, we would not be able to distinguish between two values of θ if both of them index that distribution. Grenander [66, page 470] takes identifiability as an automatic assumption. Lehmann and Casella [88, page 24] call non-identifiable parameters "statistically meaningless", and point out (page 57) that a "parameter that is unidentifiable cannot be estimated consistently". We might state this more strongly: *a parameter that is not identifiable cannot be estimated.* We will come back to this question briefly in Chap. 3.

Remark 1.18 The term "identifiability" is due to Koopmans and Reiersøl [80, page 169], although they refer to the identifiability of a "structure". Our Definition 1.16 follows Neyman [102, page 499].

1.2.2 Estimation

We distinguish between an *estimate* and an *estimator*. If θ is a parameter, an *estimator* of θ is a random variable, often denoted $\hat{\theta}$. Given some data, the resulting value of $\hat{\theta}$ is an *estimate* of θ. We assume that $\hat{\theta}$ takes values in the same set as θ: for example, both are real, or both are vectors of the same dimension.

Definition 1.19 Let $\mathcal{P} = \{\mathrm{P}_\theta \colon \theta \in \Theta\}$ be a family of probability distributions. We say that $\hat{\theta}$ is *unbiased for* θ if $\mathrm{E}_\theta(\hat{\theta}) = \theta$ for all $\theta \in \Theta$.

Definition 1.20 Suppose Y has probability density function $f_\theta(y)$, $\theta \in \Theta$. The *likelihood function of* θ, given $Y = y$, is $L(\theta) = f_\theta(y)$. The *maximum likelihood estimate* of θ, given $Y = y$, is the value $\hat{\theta} = \hat{\theta}(y)$ that maximizes L. The random variable $\hat{\theta} = \hat{\theta}(Y)$ is the *maximum likelihood estimator* of θ. We use the abbreviation MLE for both the estimate and the estimator.

In general, the MLE need not be unique, but it will be in the applications we have in mind.

1.2.3 Testing: Confidence Sets

Let $\mathcal{P} = \{\mathrm{P}_\theta : \theta \in \Theta\}$ be a family of probability distributions. A *statistical hypothesis* is a statement of the form

$$H \colon \theta \in \Theta'$$

where Θ' is a subset of Θ. If θ has components, say $\theta = (\theta_1, \theta_2)$, then the statement $\theta_1 = 3$ is understood to mean that θ_2 is unrestricted. A hypothesis of the form $\theta_1 = 3$ is called a *point hypothesis*. A hypothesis is *simple* if it completely determines a probability distribution; otherwise it is *composite*. Note that point hypotheses need not be simple. A hypothesis is *empty* if Θ' is empty.

In hypothesis testing we are presented with two disjoint hypotheses, H_0 and H_1, the *null* and *alternate hypotheses*. In classical (frequentist) theory, the former gets the benefit of doubt and the latter bears the burden of proof. Typically H_1 is the negation of H_0. A test consists of a random quantity X (possibly vector-valued or even more general), the *test statistic*, and a *rejection region* R, such that we reject H_0 if $X \in R$, and don't reject H_0 if not.[6] A *type I error* is the rejection of H_0 when H_0 is true, and a *type II error* is the failure to reject it when it is false.

Definition 1.21 Consider a test of $H_0 : \theta \in \Theta_0$ *vs.* $H_1 : \theta \in \Theta_1$ with rejection region R. The *power* of the test *at* θ is $\mathrm{P}_\theta(X \in R)$. The function $k(\theta) = \mathrm{P}_\theta(X \in R)$ is the *power function* of the test.

The *size* of the test is $\sup_{\theta \in \Theta_0} k(\theta)$. A test is said to have *level* α if its size is at most α.

If $k_1(\theta)$ and $k_2(\theta)$ are the power functions of two tests of H_0 *vs.* H_1 of level α, we say that the first test is *more conservative* if it has smaller size.

The *p-value* of a test, given a set of data, is the smallest[7] size at which H_0 would be rejected.

Thus the size of a test is the probability of a type I error. Note that we distinguish between *size* and *level*. One sometimes refers to the level as the *nominal significance level*, so that the size is the *actual* significance level. Informally, a test is conservative if its size is a lot less than its (nominal) level.

In practice, most tests have the property that the lower the significance level, the lower the power overall. Thus lowering the significance level of the test (i.e., requiring more significant data) makes the test more conservative.

The distributions P_θ, $\theta \in \Theta_0$, are often called *null distributions*, and those for $\theta \in \Theta_1$, *alternative distributions*.

Definition 1.22 Let θ be a parameter of a distribution. A *confidence set* for θ with *confidence level* γ is a random set S such that $\mathrm{P}_\theta(\theta \in S) \geq \gamma$ for all θ. The quantity $\inf_\theta \mathrm{P}_\theta(\theta \in S)$ is called the *confidence coefficient* of S. If θ is real-valued and S is an interval, we call S a *confidence interval*.

If two procedures yield confidence sets with the same confidence level, the procedure with the larger confidence coefficient is said to be *more conservative*.

---

[6] Technically we are dealing with a so-called *non-randomized* test; see [89]. They are the only ones we shall encounter.

[7] More precisely, the p-value is the infimum of those sizes at which H_0 would be rejected.

Generally, the larger the confidence coefficient, the larger the confidence set. Thus, roughly speaking, a conservative confidence set is one that is "larger than it needs to be" in order to attain a given confidence level.

Let $R(\theta_0)$ be the rejection region for a test of H_0: $\theta = \theta_0$, and let $A(\theta) = R(\theta)^c$ (so $A(\theta_0)$ is the non-rejection region of the test). Define the random set $S(X)$ by

$$\theta \in S(x) \text{ iff } x \in A(\theta). \tag{1.7}$$

That is, $S(x)$ consists of all values of θ that would *not* have been rejected, based on the observation $X = x$. We see that

$$\begin{aligned} \mathrm{P}(\theta \in S(X)) &= \mathrm{P}(X \in A(\theta)) \\ &= 1 - \mathrm{P}(X \in R(\theta)), \end{aligned}$$

so that if the test has significance level α then the set $S(x)$ has confidence level $1-\alpha$. We say that we have *inverted the test* to create the confidence set.

Conversely, any confidence set procedure produces a hypothesis test by the equivalence (1.7), and if the interval has confidence level γ then the test has significance level $1 - \gamma$. Of course, it is traditional to denote significance levels by α and confidence levels by $1 - \alpha$. The relationship (1.7) is known as the *duality* between hypothesis tests and confidence intervals.

1.3 Linear Models

In an experiment, whether in nature or in the laboratory, we are interested in measuring a random *response variable* Y under various conditions. Typically we will measure several responses, say $Y_1, \ldots, Y_N$. We are interested in modeling the random vector $\mathbf{Y} = (Y_1, \ldots, Y_N)'$.

We say that $\mathbf{Y}$ satisfies a *linear model* if there is a matrix $\mathbf{X}$ and a vector $\boldsymbol{\beta}$ such that

$$\mathrm{E}(\mathbf{Y}) = \mathbf{X}\boldsymbol{\beta}. \tag{1.8}$$

In applications, $\mathbf{X}$ is known, while the vector $\boldsymbol{\beta}$ consists of unknown parameters. We will usually denote the length of $\boldsymbol{\beta}$ by p, so that $\mathbf{X}$ is $N \times p$. **Unless otherwise noted, we will assume that** $N \geq p$. Data sets for which $p > N$ have become more common due to advances in technology; see, for example, [131].

In many cases the components of $\boldsymbol{\beta}$ are expected values. In such situations, we will often write $\boldsymbol{\mu}$ instead of $\boldsymbol{\beta}$, so that the linear model is

$$\mathrm{E}(\mathbf{Y}) = \mathbf{X}\boldsymbol{\mu}.$$

Unless we impose some constraints on the model, we assume that $\boldsymbol{\beta}$ (or $\boldsymbol{\mu}$) can take any value in $\mathbb{R}^p$. It is natural to refer to $\mathbb{R}^p$ as the *parameter space* of the model, and $\mathbb{R}^N$ as its *observation space*. The link between these two spaces is $\mathbf{X}$, viewed as a linear transformation from $\mathbb{R}^p$ to $\mathbb{R}^N$. Constraints are discussed in Sect. 1.7.

We will define the *rank* of a linear model (1.8) to be rank($\mathbf{X}$). Thus the rank is at most p. If rank($\mathbf{X}$) $= p$, we will say that the model has *full rank*. If a model does not have full rank then $\boldsymbol{\beta}$ is not identifiable, since then one may have distinct $\boldsymbol{\beta}_1$ and $\boldsymbol{\beta}_2$ for which $\mathbf{X}\boldsymbol{\beta}_1 = \mathbf{X}\boldsymbol{\beta}_2$. In this case $\boldsymbol{\beta}_1$ and $\boldsymbol{\beta}_2$ index the same probability distribution, and therefore give rise to the same expected value: $\mathrm{E}_{\boldsymbol{\beta}_1} = \mathrm{E}_{\boldsymbol{\beta}_2}$. With this understanding, the statement $\mathrm{E}(\mathbf{Y}) = \mathbf{X}\boldsymbol{\beta}$ still makes sense. We will take up the issue of identifiability further in Sects. 1.6 and 2.5.

Linear models occur in two contexts, as illustrated by the following examples, in both of which $p = 3$.

Example 1.23 Suppose a response variable Y is to be measured at various settings of two independent variables x_1 and x_2. For example, Y might be the output of a chemical process that depends on temperature and pressure. Assume that the expected response is a linear function of x_1 and x_2, that is,

$$\mathrm{E}(Y) = \beta_0 + \beta_1 x_1 + \beta_2 x_2.$$

If Y_i is the response to the values x_{i1}, x_{i2}, $i = 1, \ldots, N$, then

$$\mathrm{E}(Y_i) = \beta_0 + \beta_1 x_{i1} + \beta_2 x_{i2},$$

and so

$$\mathrm{E}\begin{pmatrix} Y_1 \\ \vdots \\ Y_N \end{pmatrix} = \begin{pmatrix} 1 & x_{11} & x_{12} \\ \vdots & \vdots & \vdots \\ 1 & x_{N1} & x_{N2} \end{pmatrix} \begin{pmatrix} \beta_0 \\ \beta_1 \\ \beta_2 \end{pmatrix},$$

which is of the form (1.8) with the obvious choices of $\mathbf{Y}$, $\mathbf{X}$ and $\boldsymbol{\beta}$. This is called a *regression model*, and $\mathbf{X}$ is called the *regression matrix*. The parameters β_i are the *regression coefficients*.

Example 1.24 Suppose Y is a response to a factor, say A, that is measured at three settings, labeled 1, 2, and 3. For example, Y might be yield of a crop, A might be the brand of fertilizer applied. Suppose we observe two responses at each setting of A. The six responses may be labeled Y_{ij}, where $i = 1, 2, 3$ (level) and $j = 1, 2$ (indicating the two responses to a level). We let $\mu_i = \mathrm{E}(Y_{ij})$ be the expected response to level i of the factor. Then

$$\mathrm{E}\begin{pmatrix} Y_{11} \\ Y_{12} \\ Y_{21} \\ Y_{22} \\ Y_{31} \\ Y_{32} \end{pmatrix} = \begin{pmatrix} 1\,0\,0 \\ 1\,0\,0 \\ 0\,1\,0 \\ 0\,1\,0 \\ 0\,0\,1 \\ 0\,0\,1 \end{pmatrix} \begin{pmatrix} \mu_1 \\ \mu_2 \\ \mu_3 \end{pmatrix}, \qquad (1.9)$$

which is again of form (1.8) with $\boldsymbol{\beta} = (\mu_1, \mu_2, \mu_3)'$. Here $\mathbf{X}$ is referred to as the *design matrix*, since it indicates the design of the experiment. We will refer to such models of $\mathbf{Y}$ as *factorial models* or ANOVA models. The term *factorial*, which comes from the presence of *factors*,[8] is also applied to the design and to the experiment. ANOVA refers to the method used to analyze such data, as discussed in Chap. 4.

We will often make further modeling assumptions about $\mathbf{Y}$ beyond (1.8). Most commonly, we assume that $\mathbf{Y}$ has covariance matrix

$$\boldsymbol{\Sigma} = \sigma^2 \mathbf{I}, \qquad (1.10)$$

where $\mathbf{I}$ is the identity matrix of the same size as $\boldsymbol{\Sigma}$–that is, we assume that the components of $\mathbf{Y}$ are uncorrelated and have common variance σ^2, usually unknown. Other models of $\boldsymbol{\Sigma}$ are discussed in Sect. 2.7. For hypothesis testing and related purposes, we usually assume that $\mathbf{Y}$ is normally distributed. This combined with assumption (1.10) means that the components of $\mathbf{Y}$ are independent with equal variance.

Finally, it is common to write a linear model (1.8) in the form

$$\mathbf{Y} = \mathbf{X}\boldsymbol{\beta} + \boldsymbol{\epsilon} \qquad (1.11)$$

where $\boldsymbol{\epsilon}$ is a zero-mean random vector with the same covariance matrix as $\mathbf{Y}$. This may be referred to as a *signal + noise model*, where $\mathbf{X}\,\boldsymbol{\beta}$ is the "signal" and $\boldsymbol{\epsilon}$ represents "noise". We note that $\boldsymbol{\epsilon}$ is a *nonobservable* random vector as long as $\boldsymbol{\beta}$ is unknown, while $\mathbf{Y}$ is *observable*. Because of this, all inferential procedures will be based on the value of $\mathbf{Y}$ and not on that of $\boldsymbol{\epsilon}$.

We have been assuming that in (1.11) (or in (1.8)) the unknown quantity $\boldsymbol{\beta}$ is a vector of constants. There are models in which all or part of $\boldsymbol{\beta}$ is viewed as random. Those in which $\boldsymbol{\beta}$ is random are naturally called *random-effects models*, while those in which $\boldsymbol{\beta}$ has both constant and random components are simply called *mixed models*. These will be discussed briefly in Sects. 2.7 and 4.9. Our main focus

[8] And has nothing to do with $n!$. The term "factorial" was apparently introduced by Yates [153, page 182], such experiments having previously been called "complex".

will be those models in which $\boldsymbol{\beta}$ is constant, and which are thus known as *fixed-effects models*.

If it is necessary to consider several response variables simultaneously, the response Y is replaced by a (row) vector of responses, and $\mathbf{Y}$ and $\boldsymbol{\beta}$ become matrices, still linked by Eq. (1.8). Such models are known as *general linear models* or *MANOVA models* (MANOVA = multivariate ANOVA), and will not be pursued here. The reader is referred to the classic text [5] or to any number of more recent texts in multivariate analysis. Other generalizations, more specific to regression, are discussed briefly in Sect. 1.4.

1.4 Regression Models

The model described in Example 1.23 contains two independent variables (or *regressors*). Generally a *linear regression model* will involve k variables:

$$\mathrm{E}(Y) = \beta_0 + \beta_1 x_1 + \cdots + \beta_k x_k. \tag{1.12}$$

The right-hand side of this equation is called the *regression function*. The model is *simple* if $k = 1$, and otherwise *multiple*. In the latter case there is no restriction on the variables x_i, and in fact one might have $x_2 = \sqrt{x_1}$, $x_4 = x_1 x_3$, etc.

We also note that we may observe the response Y repeatedly at the same settings of one or more regressor variables. Indeed, this is important in making inferences about the parameter σ^2 in (1.10).

When we take N observations on Y based on the model (1.12), the regression matrix $\mathbf{X}$ has the form

$$\mathbf{X} = (\mathbf{1}\, \mathbf{x}_1 \cdots \mathbf{x}_k)$$

where $\mathbf{1}$ is an $N \times 1$ vector of ones and $\mathbf{x}_i$ is the vector of values of regressor x_i at which Y is observed. *Multicollinearity* occurs when the columns $\mathbf{x}_1, \ldots, \mathbf{x}_k$ are nearly linearly dependent, that is, when there is a non-trivial linear combination $c_1\mathbf{x}_1 + \cdots + c_k\mathbf{x}_k$ that is close to zero. This near-linear dependence does occur in practice and has serious computational consequences, as we will see in Sect. 3.1.

Perfect multicollinearity, in which the columns of $\mathbf{X}$ are actually linearly dependent, occurs very rarely in regression models. In fact, a regression model is sometimes simply *defined* to be a full-rank linear model (see, e.g., [37], page 110). (We note that collinearity itself implies that two columns are actually scalar multiples of each other, a very special form of linear dependence. For that reason, the term *multi*collinearity may not be ideal, but its use is now fixed in the literature.)

Polynomial regression models, an important class of regression models, arise when the regressors are themselves monomials in one or more independent variables. In one variable x the model (1.12) would be of the form

$$E(Y) = \beta_0 + \beta_1 x^1 + \cdots + \beta_k x^k, \tag{1.13}$$

and the regression matrix would have the form[9]

$$\mathbf{X} = \begin{pmatrix} 1 & x_1 & x_1^2 & \cdots & x_1^k \\ 1 & x_2 & x_2^2 & \cdots & x_2^k \\ \vdots & \vdots & \vdots & \vdots & \vdots \\ 1 & x_n & x_n^2 & \cdots & x_n^k \end{pmatrix}$$

where $x_1, \ldots, x_n$ are now the specific values at which the variable x is observed. A quadratic polynomial model in two variables would be written

$$E(Y) = \beta_0 + \beta_1 x_1 + \beta_2 x_2 + \beta_3 x_1^2 + \beta_4 x_1 x_2 + \beta_5 x_2^2.$$

The graph of such a model is a *response surface* lying over (or under) the $x_1 x_2$ plane, and is analyzed using response surface methodology (see, for example, [151]).

There are various ways of generalizing regression models.

Nonlinear regression functions: We may replace the regression function with a non-linear function of the variables $x_1, \ldots, x_k$. In certain cases we may recast the model in linear form by a heuristic trick. For example, since

$$E(Y) = \alpha e^{\beta x} \tag{1.14}$$

is equivalent to

$$\ln E(Y) = \ln(\alpha) + \beta x,$$

we may choose to model $\ln(Y)$ by

$$E(\ln(Y)) = \beta_0 + \beta_1 x. \tag{1.15}$$

We must keep in mind, though, that $E(\ln(Y)) \neq \ln(E(Y))$, so that the models (1.14) and (1.15) are not equivalent. (Moreover, the random variables Y and $\ln Y$ can't both be normally distributed!) However, such transformations are often used and frequently yield reasonable and useful results in practice. Of course, the set of regression functions that can be transformed in this way is limited. Treatments of such models can be found in a number of standard texts on regression.

[9] A Vandermonde matrix.

Generalized linear models: In a linear model, each observation Y_j has a mean of form $\mathbf{x}_j\boldsymbol{\beta}$ where x_j is the jth row of the regression or design matrix $\mathbf{X}$. In a generalized linear model (GLM), the mean is $g^{-1}(\mathbf{x}_j\boldsymbol{\beta})$ for a function g called the *link function*, and the observations Y_j are assumed to be distributed according to a family of exponential type. These models were introduced by Nelder and Wedderburn [99] as a unified framework for a number of modeling techniques, including logistic regression, Poisson regression, and probit models, as well as classical linear regression. GLMs are discussed in many texts, such as [1, 49] and [95].

We will concentrate on the classical linear model in the present text.

1.5 Factorial (ANOVA) Models

The model described in Example 1.24 is that of a one-factor model, the factor being measured at three levels, which may represent three treatments. In general, a *factorial experiment* consists of k factors, the ith factor being observed at s_i *levels*. We sometimes refer to this as an $s_1 \times \cdots \times s_k$ experiment. If $s_1 = \cdots = s_k$, we say that the experiment is *symmetric*, or is an s^k experiment, s equalling the common value of $s_1, \ldots, s_k$.

Thus a 2×3 experiment involves two factors, say A and B, observed at 2 and 3 levels respectively. There are 6 *treatment combinations* in this experiment. If we index the levels of factor A by 1 and 2 and those of B by 1, 2, and 3, then the treatment combinations are the ordered pairs (1,1), (1,2), (1,3), (2,1), (2,2), and (2,3), which may also refer to as *cells* due to the obvious diagram:

		B		
		1	2	3
A	1			
	2			

In this experiment we take n_{ij} observations $Y_{ij1}, \ldots, Y_{ijn_{ij}}$ in cell (i, j). We let $\mu_{ij} = \mathrm{E}(Y_{ijk}), k = 1, \ldots, n_{ij}$. If we fix an order of the cells, say lexicographic order (row 1 followed by row 2), then we may write

$$
\mathrm{E}\begin{pmatrix} Y_{111} \\ \vdots \\ Y_{11n_{11}} \\ Y_{121} \\ \vdots \\ Y_{12n_{12}} \\ \vdots \\ Y_{231} \\ \vdots \\ Y_{23n_{23}} \end{pmatrix} = \begin{pmatrix} 1 & & & \\ \vdots & & & \\ 1 & & & \\ & 1 & & \\ & \vdots & & \\ & 1 & & \\ & & \ddots & \\ & & & 1 \\ & & & \vdots \\ & & & 1 \end{pmatrix} \begin{pmatrix} \mu_{11} \\ \mu_{12} \\ \mu_{13} \\ \mu_{21} \\ \mu_{22} \\ \mu_{23} \end{pmatrix}, \tag{1.16}
$$

so that the vector $\mathbf{Y}$ of observations satisfies a linear model. Blank entries of the design matrix are zero, each column corresponds to a cell, and each string of 1's has the same length as the corresponding block of observations in $\mathbf{Y}$.

Remark 1.25 We may allow some n_{ij} to be zero to account for either missing cells or a particular experimental design (for example, a *fractional design*, discussed in Chapter 6). In this case we may still write a linear model for $\mathbf{Y}$, omitting both the parameters μ for the cells not observed and the corresponding entries of $\mathbf{Y}$ and $\mathbf{X}$.

The general set-up for a multifactor experiment is handled analogously. If we let A_i be a set of indices for the levels of factor i, then a treatment combination is a k-tuple whose ith component comes from A_i, and in fact the set T of *treatment combinations* (or *cells*) is the Cartesian product

$$
T = A_1 \times \cdots \times A_k. \tag{1.17}
$$

For each cell $t \in T$ we have n_t observations $Y_{t1}, \ldots, Y_{tn_t}$, all having the same mean $\mu_t = \mathrm{E}(Y_{tj})$. We denote the total sample size by N, so that

$$
N = \sum_{t \in T} n_t.
$$

If the sample sizes n_t are all equal, say $n_t \equiv n$, we say that the data is *balanced*, in which case

$$
N = np,
$$

where $p = |T| = s_1 \cdots s_k$ is the number of cells. An experiment with balanced data is said to follow an *equireplicate design*.

Fixing an order of the cells, say $t_1, \ldots, t_p$, we create a vector of cell means $\boldsymbol{\beta}$. If we stack the observations of each cell into a single vector $\mathbf{Y}$, in the same cell order, then we may write

$$\mathrm{E}(\mathbf{Y}) = \mathbf{X}\boldsymbol{\beta}, \tag{1.18}$$

where $\mathbf{Y}$ is $N \times 1$, $\boldsymbol{\beta}$ is $p \times 1$, and $\mathbf{X}$ is $N \times p$ and consists of p vectors of 1's arrayed "diagonally", as in (1.16), viz.,

$$\mathbf{X} = \begin{pmatrix} \mathbf{1} & & & \\ & \mathbf{1} & & \\ & & \ddots & \\ & & & \mathbf{1} \end{pmatrix}, \tag{1.19}$$

where the vector $\mathbf{1}$ in column t has length n_t.

In this context, the linear model (1.18) is a *factorial model*. The term *ANOVA model* is often used, referring to the method (ANOVA) that is used to analyze such data. This method is discussed in Chap. 4. A very special ANOVA model is the one-factor or *one-way* model, in which there are s treatments, n_i observations Y_{ij} on treatment i, and means $\mu_i = \mathrm{E}(Y_{ij})$, $j = 1, \ldots, n_i$.

The particularly simple form of the design matrix $\mathbf{X}$ is due to the parametrization of the model by the cell means. Models written this way are thus known as *cell-means models*. Other ways of parameterizing such linear models will be taken up in Sect. 2.5.

Remark 1.26 The distinction between the words *experiment*, *design*, and *model* deserves some comment. A *design* is, for us, the allocation of experimental units (plots of land, laboratory animals, etc.) to treatments. A *model* is a mathematical description of the relation of the responses to the treatments in the given design. An *experiment* is the physical realization of a design, which is why *experiment* and *design* are sometimes used interchangeably.

A more precise term for our type of design is *experimental design*, to distinguish it from *combinatorial design*, which is a system of subsets of a given set (usually finite)—for example, a finite geometry consisting of points and lines. Many combinatorial designs began, of course, as experimental designs.

1.6 Linear Parametric Functions

Central to the study of linear models $\mathrm{E}(\mathbf{Y}) = \mathbf{X}\boldsymbol{\beta}$ are linear functions of the parameter vector $\boldsymbol{\beta}$ of the form

$$\mathbf{c}'\boldsymbol{\beta}, \tag{1.20}$$

where $\mathbf{c}$ is a column vector of coefficients.

Example 1.27 In Example 1.23 we may be interested in the expected response Y when x_1 and x_2 are given values of the predictors. This response, namely $\mathrm{E}(Y) = \beta_0 + \beta_1 x_1 + \beta_2 x_2$, may be written in the form (1.20) where $\mathbf{c} = (1, x_1, x_2)$ and $\boldsymbol{\beta} = (\beta_0, \beta_1, \beta_2)$. The values of x_1 and x_2 may be among those originally used in collecting the data, or a pair of new values.

Example 1.28 In Example 1.24 we may be interested in a simple average of mean responses, that is, $(\mu_1+\mu_2+\mu_3)/3$ or in a *weighted average* $w_1\mu_1+w_2\mu_2+w_3\mu_3$, where the weights w_i are nonnegative and sum to 1.

We may also wish to compare mean responses. For example, if we are comparing μ_1 and μ_2, we may consider

$$\mu_1 - \mu_2, \tag{1.21}$$

the statement $\mu_1 = \mu_2$ being equivalent to $\mu_1 - \mu_2 = 0$. In a similar fashion we may use the expression

$$\frac{1}{2}\mu_1 + \frac{1}{2}\mu_2 - \mu_3 \tag{1.22}$$

to group treatments 1 and 2 and contrast them with treatment 3.

1.6.1 Identifiability

We noted in Sect. 1.3 that that if $\mathbf{X}$ does not have full rank p, then $\boldsymbol{\beta}$ is not identifiable. In this case, we need to ask which linear parametric functions $\mathbf{c}'\boldsymbol{\beta}$ are identifiable.

Proposition 1.29 *Given a linear model* $\mathrm{E}(\mathbf{Y}) = \mathbf{X}\boldsymbol{\beta}$ *with* $\boldsymbol{\beta}$ *unrestricted, the linear parametric function* $\mathbf{c}'\boldsymbol{\beta}$ *is identifiable iff* $\mathbf{c} \in R(\mathbf{X}')$.[10] *If* $\mathbf{X}$ *has full rank, all such functions are identifiable.*

Proof Let $\mathcal{P}$ be the family of distributions of $\mathbf{Y}$. Fix $\mathbf{c}$ and let $\psi = \mathbf{c}'\boldsymbol{\beta}$. Each value of ψ defines a subfamily $\mathcal{P}_\psi$ of distributions, namely

$$\mathcal{P}_\psi = \{\mathrm{P} \in \mathcal{P}\colon\ \exists\boldsymbol{\beta} \text{ such that } \mathrm{E}_P(\mathbf{Y}) = \mathbf{X}\boldsymbol{\beta} \text{ and } \mathbf{c}'\boldsymbol{\beta} = \psi\},$$

[10] $R(\mathbf{A})$ is the columnspace of $\mathbf{A}$; $N(\mathbf{A})$ is its nullspace. See Sect. A.4.8, comment after Theorem A.98.

and $\mathcal{P} = \cup_\psi \mathcal{P}_\psi$. According to Definition 1.16, in order for ψ to be identifiable it is necessary and sufficient that the following hold:

$$\psi_1 \neq \psi_2 \text{ implies that } \mathcal{P}_{\psi_1} \cap \mathcal{P}_{\psi_2} = \emptyset. \tag{1.23}$$

We will show that this is equivalent to the condition $\mathbf{c} \in R(\mathbf{X}')$. Since $R(\mathbf{X}') = N(\mathbf{X})^\perp$ (Theorem A.79), we may show that (1.23) holds if and only if

$$\mathbf{c} \perp N(\mathbf{X}).$$

Suppose first that $\mathbf{c} \perp N(\mathbf{X})$, and assume that $\mathcal{P}_{\psi_1} \cap \mathcal{P}_{\psi_2} \neq \emptyset$. We claim that then $\psi_1 = \psi_2$. So let $P \in \mathcal{P}_{\psi_1} \cap \mathcal{P}_{\psi_2}$. Then there are $\boldsymbol{\beta}_1$ and $\boldsymbol{\beta}_2$ such that $\mathrm{E}_P(\mathbf{Y}) = \mathbf{X}\boldsymbol{\beta}_i$, $i = 1, 2$, so $\boldsymbol{\beta}_1 - \boldsymbol{\beta}_2 \in N(\mathbf{X})$. But then $\mathbf{c}'(\boldsymbol{\beta}_1 - \boldsymbol{\beta}_2) = 0$, and multiplying this out shows that $\psi_1 = \psi_2$, as claimed.

Now suppose that $\mathbf{c} \not\perp N(\mathbf{X})$. (This implies that $N(\mathbf{X}) \neq (\mathbf{0})$.) We claim that there are distinct ψ_1 and ψ_2 such that $\mathcal{P}_{\psi_1} \cap \mathcal{P}_{\psi_2} \neq \emptyset$. To this end, let $\boldsymbol{\beta}_1 \in N(\mathbf{X})$ be such that $\mathbf{c} \not\perp \boldsymbol{\beta}_1$. Put $\psi_1 = \mathbf{c}'\boldsymbol{\beta}_1$, so that $\psi_1 \neq 0$. Since $\boldsymbol{\beta}$ is unrestricted, there is a $\mathrm{P} \in \mathcal{P}$ such that $\mathrm{E}_P(\mathbf{Y}) = \mathbf{X}\boldsymbol{\beta}_1$, and in particular $\mathrm{P} \in \mathcal{P}_{\psi_1}$. But $\mathrm{E}_P(\mathbf{Y}) = \mathbf{0}$ as $\boldsymbol{\beta}_1 \in N(\mathbf{X})$, so we also have $\mathrm{P} \in \mathcal{P}_0$, taking $\boldsymbol{\beta}_2 = \mathbf{0}$ and $\psi_2 = \mathbf{c}'\boldsymbol{\beta}_2 = 0$. Then $\psi_2 \neq \psi_1$, but $\mathcal{P}_{\psi_1} \cap \mathcal{P}_{\psi_2} \neq \emptyset$, as desired. Since the implication (1.23) is false, ψ is not identifiable. □

1.6.2 Contrasts

Linear parametric functions like (1.21) and (1.22) share the property that the coefficients add up to zero. This is characteristic of an expression that compares (or *contrasts*) certain mean responses with others, and indeed that is how such expressions get their name:

Definition 1.30 Let T be the set of treatment combinations in a factorial experiment, ordered in some fixed way, and let $\boldsymbol{\mu}$ be the vector of cell means. A linear parametric function $\mathbf{c}'\boldsymbol{\mu} = \sum_{t\in T} c_t\mu_t$ is a *contrast in cell means*, or simply a *contrast*, if $\sum_{t\in T} c_t = 0$. The coefficient vector $\mathbf{c}$ will be called a *contrast vector*.

Proposition 1.31 *Let T be the set of treatment combinations in a factorial experiment, and let U be the set of contrast vectors. Then U is a vector space, and* $\dim(U) = |T| - 1$.

Proof The vectors in U have length $|T|$. It is easy to see that U is closed under addition and scalar multiplication, and we leave it as an exercise to construct a basis of U consisting of $|T| - 1$ elements.

Alternatively, note that $\mathbf{c} \in U$ iff $\mathbf{c} \perp \mathbf{1}$, that is,

$$U = \mathbf{1}^{\perp}.$$

That U is a subspace is given by Proposition A.60, and its dimension by Corollary A.71. □

It follows from this proposition that the span of any set of contrast vectors will consist of contrast vectors. We will make use of this remark many times.

Contrasts are a key building block in the theory of factorial experiments. While one can form contrasts in any set of parameters, we shall use the term almost exclusively for contrasts in cell means.

1.7 Linear Constraints and Hypotheses

Linear constraints are conditions placed on the parameter vector $\boldsymbol{\beta}$ in a linear model. Constraints arise in two ways: as hypotheses to be tested, and as global assumptions about the model. In either case, we speak of a *constrained model*, or sometimes a *reduced model*. If the constraint is a null hypothesis H_0, the constrained model is also called the *null model*.

For example, an important constraint in a factorial model is the property called "additivity" (see below). While we often test for additivity, it is not uncommon to *assume* an additive model, either for theoretical reasons or because the paucity of data does not allow investigating a more complex model. Another common use of constraints is to remove problems of nonidentifiability, as we will discuss below and in Sect. 2.5.

The simplest type of linear constraint is a statement of the form

$$\mathbf{c}'\boldsymbol{\beta} = 0. \tag{1.24}$$

This includes hypotheses such as

$$\beta_2 = 0$$

in the regression model of Example 1.23, taking $\mathbf{c} = (0, 0, 1)'$, and

$$\mu_1 - \mu_2 = 0$$

in a factorial model such as that in Example 1.24 (here $\mathbf{c} = (1, -1, 0)'$).

Linear constraints can involve more than one equation. For example, the hypothesis

$$\begin{cases} \beta_1 = 0 \\ \beta_2 = 0 \end{cases}$$

in Example 1.23 is the claim that the independent variables x_1 and x_2 have no effect. The hypothesis $\mu_1 = \mu_2 = \mu_3$ in Example 1.24, which we may express as

$$\begin{cases} \mu_1 - \mu_2 = 0 \\ \mu_2 - \mu_3 = 0, \end{cases}$$

similarly asserts that there is no treatment effect. A somewhat more involved example is the following, which introduces ideas that will be explained more fully in Chap. 2.

Example 1.32 We return to the 2×3 experiment described in Sect. 1.5:

		B		
		1	2	3
A	1	μ_{11}	μ_{12}	μ_{13}
	2	μ_{21}	μ_{22}	μ_{23}

As before, we order the cells of the experiment lexicographically and let the resulting vector of cell means be $\boldsymbol{\mu}$.

In Sect. 2.2.1 we will define the hypothesis of "no *A* effect" to be the statement

$$\mu_{1\cdot} - \mu_{2\cdot} = 0,$$

the equality of the row totals $\mu_{1\cdot}$ and $\mu_{2\cdot}$. (The "dot" notation for sums and averages is discussed in the Preface.) This equation is of the form

$$\mathbf{c}'\boldsymbol{\mu} = 0 \tag{1.25}$$

with $\mathbf{c} = (1, 1, 1, -1, -1, -1)'$. Note that a logically equivalent statement is

$$\bar{\mu}_{1\cdot} - \bar{\mu}_{2\cdot} = 0,$$

the equality of the row averages, which is (1.25) with $\mathbf{c} = (1/3)(1, 1, 1, -1, -1, -1)'$. In fact, there is an infinity of equivalent equations, replacing the scalar 1/3 by any other nonzero real number.

The hypothesis of "no *B* effect" will be described by the equality of column totals:

$$\mu_{\cdot 1} = \mu_{\cdot 2} = \mu_{\cdot 3},$$

which we may rewrite as the pair of equations

$$\begin{cases} \mu_{\cdot 1} - \mu_{\cdot 2} = 0 \\ \mu_{\cdot 2} - \mu_{\cdot 3} = 0. \end{cases}$$

The two equalities are of the form (1.25) with $\mathbf{c}_1 = (1, -1, 0, 1, -1, 0)'$ and $\mathbf{c}_2 = (0, 1, -1, 0, 1, -1)'$. There are many other pairs of equations logically equivalent to these, the most obvious resulting from substituting $\mu_{\cdot 1} - \mu_{\cdot 3} = 0$ for either of the above pair.

Finally, we will say that there is *no interaction* between A and B, or that the effects of A and B are *additive*, if the mean responses at each level of B shift by the same constant when we change the level of A. In our example this means that the row differences in each column are equal:

$$\mu_{21} - \mu_{11} = \mu_{22} - \mu_{12} = \mu_{23} - \mu_{13}.$$

This pair of equations can be written in the form (1.25). For example, subtracting the left member from the middle and from the right gives

$$\begin{cases} \mu_{22} - \mu_{12} - \mu_{21} + \mu_{11} = 0, \\ \mu_{23} - \mu_{13} - \mu_{21} + \mu_{11} = 0, \end{cases} \tag{1.26}$$

which are of the form (1.25) with $\mathbf{c} = (1, -1, 0, -1, 1, 0)'$ and $(1, 0, -1, -1, 0, 1)'$.

With these examples as a guide, consider a linear model $\mathbf{Y} = \mathbf{X}\boldsymbol{\beta}$, where $\boldsymbol{\beta} \in \mathbb{R}^p$. A *linear constraint* about $\boldsymbol{\beta}$ is a system of equations

$$\begin{cases} \mathbf{c}_1'\boldsymbol{\beta} = 0 \\ \quad\vdots \\ \mathbf{c}_d'\boldsymbol{\beta} = 0. \end{cases} \tag{1.27}$$

The expressions on the left-hand side may or may not be contrasts. A *linear hypothesis* is a linear constraint that is subject to a statistical test.

A linear constraint can be written in several different ways:

Lemma 1.33 *Let $U \subset \mathbb{R}^p$ be spanned by $\mathbf{c}_1, \ldots, \mathbf{c}_d$, and let these be the columns of a matrix $\mathbf{C}$. Let $W = U^\perp$, the orthocomplement of U, let $\mathbf{w}_1, \ldots, \mathbf{w}_k$ span W, and let these be the columns of a matrix $\mathbf{W}$. The following are equivalent:*

a. $\boldsymbol{\beta}$ satisfies (1.27).
b. $\boldsymbol{\beta}$ satisfies

$$\mathbf{C}'\boldsymbol{\beta} = \mathbf{0}. \tag{1.28}$$

c. $\boldsymbol{\beta}$ satisfies

$$\boldsymbol{\beta} \perp U. \tag{1.29}$$

d. $\boldsymbol{\beta}$ *satisfies*

$$\boldsymbol{\beta} \in W. \tag{1.30}$$

e. There exists a vector $\boldsymbol{\beta}_0$ *such that*

$$\boldsymbol{\beta} = \mathbf{W}\boldsymbol{\beta}_0. \tag{1.31}$$

Sketch of Proof (b) $\Leftrightarrow$ (a): Obvious.

(a) $\Leftrightarrow$ (c): The system (1.27) asserts that $\boldsymbol{\beta} \perp \mathbf{c}_1, \ldots, \mathbf{c}_d$, which is equivalent to saying that $\boldsymbol{\beta} \perp U$, their span (Theorem A.57(c)).

(c) $\Leftrightarrow$ (d): Obvious.

(d) $\Rightarrow$ (e): Since the vectors $\mathbf{w}_1, \ldots, \mathbf{w}_k$ span W,

$$\boldsymbol{\beta} = b_1\mathbf{w}_1 + \cdots + b_k\mathbf{w}_k = \mathbf{W}\boldsymbol{\beta}_0$$

where $\boldsymbol{\beta}_0 = (b_1, \ldots, b_k)$.

(e) $\Rightarrow$ (d): Let $W = R(\mathbf{W})$, the columnspace of $\mathbf{W}$. □

The expressions (1.29) and (1.30) provide two descriptions of a linear constraint that do not depend on choices of bases, and are unique for the given constraint. On the other hand, the expressions (1.27), (1.28) and (1.31) are not unique (since there are infinitely many ways of choosing spanning sets), but are often computationally useful ways of writing a constraint. While some choices may be better than others, either for computation or for interpretation, the choice should not affect the inferential procedures we use or the inferences we draw.

We illustrate forms (1.30) and (1.31) with a couple of examples.

Example 1.34 We saw above that the assumption of additivity in a 2×3 experiment is represented by the equations (1.26). With $\boldsymbol{\mu} = (\mu_{11}, \mu_{12}, \mu_{13}, \mu_{21}, \mu_{22}, \mu_{23})'$, this asserts that $\boldsymbol{\mu} \perp (1, -1, 0, -1, 1, 0)'$ and $(1, 0, -1, -1, 0, 1)'$, or equivalently that $\boldsymbol{\mu} \perp U$, where U is the span of these two vectors. On the other hand, rewriting these equations in the form

$$\mu_{22} = \mu_{21} + \mu_{12} - \mu_{11}$$
$$\mu_{23} = \mu_{21} + \mu_{13} - \mu_{11},$$

we see that

$$\boldsymbol{\mu} = \begin{pmatrix} \mu_{11} \\ \mu_{12} \\ \mu_{13} \\ \mu_{21} \\ \mu_{22} \\ \mu_{23} \end{pmatrix} = \begin{pmatrix} 1 & 0 & 0 & 0 \\ 0 & 1 & 0 & 0 \\ 0 & 0 & 1 & 0 \\ 0 & 0 & 0 & 1 \\ -1 & 1 & 0 & 1 \\ -1 & 0 & 1 & 1 \end{pmatrix} \begin{pmatrix} \mu_{11} \\ \mu_{12} \\ \mu_{13} \\ \mu_{21} \end{pmatrix} = \mathbf{W}\boldsymbol{\mu}_0,$$

say, which is in the form (1.31). Thus $\boldsymbol{\mu} \in W =$ the columnspace of the matrix $\mathbf{W}$, which puts the constraint in the form (1.30). Alternatively, $W = U^{\perp}$.

Example 1.35 Consider the hypothesis $H_0\colon \beta_2 = 2\beta_1$ applied to Examples 1.23 and 1.27. Writing H_0 as $-2\beta_1 + \beta_2 = 0$, we see that it is of the form $\boldsymbol{\beta} \perp U$ where $U = \langle (0, -2, 1)' \rangle$. On the other hand, using H_0 we see that

$$\boldsymbol{\beta} = \begin{pmatrix} \beta_0 \\ \beta_1 \\ \beta_2 \end{pmatrix} = \begin{pmatrix} 1 & 0 \\ 0 & 1 \\ 0 & 2 \end{pmatrix} \begin{pmatrix} \beta_0 \\ \beta_1 \end{pmatrix} = \mathbf{W}\boldsymbol{\beta}_0,$$

which expresses H_0 in the form (1.31). Then H_0 is also of the form (1.30) with W the columnspace of the matrix $\mathbf{W}$.

As one might expect, a constrained model is also a linear model. More precisely:

Theorem 1.36 *If* $\mathrm{E}(\mathbf{Y}) = \mathbf{X}\boldsymbol{\beta}$ *and if* $\boldsymbol{\beta}$ *is subject to a linear constraint* $\boldsymbol{\beta} \in W$, *then the constrained model is also a linear model*

$$\mathrm{E}(\mathbf{Y}) = \mathbf{X}_0\boldsymbol{\beta}_0, \tag{1.32}$$

where $\mathbf{X}_0 = \mathbf{XW}$, *and* $\mathbf{W}$ *and* $\boldsymbol{\beta}_0$ *are as in (1.31). If* $W \cap N(\mathbf{X}) = (0)$, *then we may choose* $\mathbf{X}_0$ *to have full rank.*

Proof If we write the linear constraint in the form (1.31), then $\mathrm{E}(\mathbf{Y}) = \mathbf{XW}\boldsymbol{\beta}_0 = \mathbf{X}_0\boldsymbol{\beta}_0$.

Recall that we view $\mathbf{X}$ as a linear transformation between the parameter space $\mathbb{R}^p$ and observation space $\mathbb{R}^N$. We may write $\mathbf{X}(W)$ for the image of the set $W \subset \mathbb{R}^p$ under the map $\mathbf{X}$.

The vectors $\mathbf{Xw}_1, \ldots, \mathbf{Xw}_k$ are the columns of $\mathbf{X}_0$. These vectors thus span both $\mathbf{X}(W)$ and $R(\mathbf{X}_0)$, so $\mathbf{X}(W) = R(\mathbf{X}_0)$. If $W \cap N(\mathbf{X}) = (0)$, and if the vectors $\mathbf{w}_i$ are linearly independent, then so are the vectors $\mathbf{Xw}_i$, so that $\mathbf{X}_0$ has full rank. □

The significance of this theorem will be apparent when we discuss estimation and testing. Note that the choice of $\mathbf{X}_0$ and $\boldsymbol{\beta}_0$ is not unique, nor is the choice of $\mathbf{W}$ in (1.31). When written in the form (1.32) the constrained model is often called a *reduced model.*

As mentioned above, we sometimes impose a constraint on a linear model in order to remove nonidentifiability of the parameter $\boldsymbol{\beta}$. We do this by replacing a non-full-rank model with one having full rank, whereby the new parameter is identifiable:

Theorem 1.37 *Suppose* $\mathrm{E}(\mathbf{Y}) = \mathbf{X}\boldsymbol{\beta}$ *where* $\mathbf{X}$ *is* $N \times p$ *and* $\mathrm{rank}(\mathbf{X}) = r < p$. *Then there is a constraint of the form* $\boldsymbol{\beta} \in W$, *where* $\dim W = r$, *such that in the constrained model we have* $\mathrm{E}(\mathbf{Y}) = \mathbf{X}_0\boldsymbol{\beta}_0$ *where* $\mathrm{rank}\,\mathbf{X}_0 = r$.

Proof We will find a constraint in the form (1.31), that is, $\boldsymbol{\beta} = \mathbf{W}\boldsymbol{\beta}_0$.

Fix $\boldsymbol{\nu} = \mathrm{E}(\mathbf{Y})$. Since $\boldsymbol{\nu} = \mathbf{X}\boldsymbol{\beta}$, we have $\boldsymbol{\beta} \in \boldsymbol{\beta}^* + N(\mathbf{X})$ where $\mathbf{X}\boldsymbol{\beta}^* = \boldsymbol{\nu}$, and we may choose $\boldsymbol{\beta}^* \perp N(\mathbf{X})$ (Corollary A.66). But then $\boldsymbol{\beta}^* \in R(\mathbf{X}')$ (Theorem A.79). Pick a basis of $R(\mathbf{X}')$, say $\mathbf{w}_1, \ldots, \mathbf{w}_r$ of $\mathbf{X}'$. There are unique constants $\gamma_1, \ldots, \gamma_r$ such that $\boldsymbol{\beta} = \gamma_1\mathbf{w}_1 + \cdots + \gamma_r\mathbf{w}_r = \mathbf{W}\boldsymbol{\beta}_0$ where $\mathbf{W} = (\mathbf{w}_1 \cdots \mathbf{w}_r)$ and $\boldsymbol{\beta}_0 = (\gamma_1, \ldots, \gamma_r)'$. Now the linear transformation defined by $\mathbf{X}$ is one-to-one on $N(\mathbf{X})^\perp$, so the vectors $\mathbf{X}\mathbf{w}_i$ are also linearly independent. But these are the columns of the $n \times r$ matrix $\mathbf{X}_0 = \mathbf{X}\mathbf{W}$, so that $\operatorname{rank} \mathbf{X}_0 = r$. □

Theorem 1.37 makes an assertion *in principle*. While the proof is constructive, it does not necessarily describe how one might construct a full rank model from a non-full rank one in practice. We will discuss this further in the case of factorial designs in Sect. 2.5.

Remark 1.38 We have taken the point of view that hypotheses are formulated in the parameter space $\mathbb{R}^p$ in which $\boldsymbol{\beta}$ resides. One can also view linear hypotheses as statements of the form $\mathrm{E}(\mathbf{Y}) \in V$ for a subspace V of $R(\mathbf{X})$, as Darroch and Silvey [39] and Seber [128] do. One reason for thinking of linear hypotheses that way is that in applications other than linear models $\mathrm{E}(\mathbf{Y})$ is often the parameter vector of primary interest.

These two points of view are equivalent, since $\boldsymbol{\beta} \in W$ implies that $\mathrm{E}(\mathbf{Y}) \in \mathbf{X}(W)$, and, conversely, $\mathrm{E}(\mathbf{Y}) \in V$ implies that $\boldsymbol{\beta} \in \mathbf{X}^{-1}(V)$. However, formulating hypotheses in observation space $\mathbb{R}^N$ forces us to add a constraint to every hypothesis whenever there are repeated observations: namely, the equality of certain components of $\mathrm{E}(\mathbf{Y})$. Compare, for example, [128, page 46]; the added constraint is labeled G.

In separating parameter space $\mathbb{R}^p$ from observation space $\mathbb{R}^N$, we make explicit the role of $\mathbf{X}$ connecting them.

1.8 Exercises

Section 1.1

1.1 One often defines a random vector $\mathbf{Y}$ to be a map from a probability space $(\Omega, \mathcal{A}, \mathrm{P})$ to $\mathbb{R}^N$ (where $\mathbf{Y}$ is $N \times 1$) such that $\mathbf{Y}^{-1}(B)$ belongs to the σ-algebra $\mathcal{A}$ for each Borel set B of $\mathbb{R}$. Show that this definition is equivalent to the one we gave in Sect. 1.1.

1.2 Prove Theorem 1.1. (Write the event $f(\mathbf{X}) \in A$) in the form $\mathbf{X} \in A'$. You can ignore measurability issues, which are taken care of automatically.)

1.3 Prove Eq. (1.5) and Theorem 1.4(a–c).

1.4 Prove Theorem 1.4(d).

1.5 Prove Proposition 1.5. (Use the properties of trace (page 325) along with property (1.4) and the observation that $\mathbf{Y}'\mathbf{A}\mathbf{Y} = \operatorname{tr}(\mathbf{Y}'\mathbf{A}\mathbf{Y})$.)

1.6 Prove Theorem 1.6(b).

1.7 Prove Theorem 1.6(c). (Show that **Y** has the moment-generating function given in part (b) of the theorem.)

1.8 Prove Lemma 1.14.

Section 1.2

1.9. Show that Definition 1.15 is a special case of Definition 1.16.

Section 1.6

1.10. Give a basis of the subspace U in Proposition 1.31.

Section 1.7

1.11. In a 2×2 experiment, consider the hypothesis that μ_{01}, μ_{10}, and μ_{11} all equal μ_{00}, where μ_{ij} is the expected responses to treatment ij. Express this hypothesis in the five different ways described by Lemma 1.33.

Chapter 2
Effects in a Factorial Experiment

Abstract Building on the ideas developed in Chap. 1, we describe the main hypotheses for a factorial (ANOVA) experiment having three or fewer factors, and the lattices formed by these hypotheses (see Fig. 2.1) and by their corresponding subspaces. The goal is to clarify the statistical meaning of the hypotheses in terms of the cell means of the experiment. We contrast this with the factor-effects approach, and spend some time showing its relationship with the cell means model, which is the one we will use almost exclusively throughout the book. The main exception is the modeling of random effects, where the standard approach starts with the factor-effects model, as we discuss in Sect. 2.5.

2.1 One-Factor Designs

A one-factor experiment consists of a set of s treatments, sometimes representing groups or populations. The ith treatment mean may be denoted μ_i, and the n_i observations in that treatment by Y_{ij}, so that

$$E(Y_{ij}) = \mu_i, \; i = 1, \ldots, s, \; j = 1, \ldots n_i. \tag{2.1}$$

The hypothesis of *no treatment effect* is

$$H_0\colon \mu_1 = \cdots = \mu_s. \tag{2.2}$$

There are many equivalent ways to write H_0—for example,

$$\begin{aligned} \mu_1 - \mu_2 &= 0 \\ 2\mu_1 - \mu_2 - \mu_3 &= 0 \\ 3\mu_1 - \mu_2 - \mu_3 - \mu_4 &= 0 \\ &\vdots \\ (s-1)\mu_1 - \mu_2 - \cdots - \mu_s &= 0. \end{aligned}$$

J. H. Beder, *Linear Models and Design*,
https://doi.org/10.1007/978-3-031-08176-7_2

In fact, letting $\boldsymbol{\mu} = (\mu_1, \ldots, \mu_s)'$, it is not hard to see that we have the following result, whose proof is left as an exercise:

Proposition 2.1 *H_0 holds iff every contrast $\mathbf{c}'\boldsymbol{\mu}$ equals 0, or equivalently iff $\boldsymbol{\mu} \perp U$ where U is the subspace of contrast vectors in $\mathbb{R}^s$. If $\mathbf{c}_1, \ldots, \mathbf{c}_{s-1}$ is a basis of U, then H_0 is equivalent to the statement $\mathbf{c}_i'\boldsymbol{\mu} = 0, i = 1, \ldots, s-1$.*

Proposition 1.31 guaranteed that $\dim U = s - 1$. Proposition 2.1 tells us that H_0 may be represented by any set of $s - 1$ linearly independent contrast equations.

2.2 Two-Factor Designs

In an $a \times b$ factorial design, the ab treatment combinations and their means can be displayed as follows:

$$
\begin{array}{cc|c|c|c|c|}
 & & \multicolumn{4}{c}{B} \\
 & & 1 & 2 & \cdots & b \\
\cline{3-6}
 & 1 & \mu_{11} & \mu_{12} & \cdots & \mu_{1b} \\
\cline{3-6}
 & 2 & \mu_{21} & \mu_{22} & \cdots & \mu_{2b} \\
\cline{3-6}
\text{A} & \vdots & \vdots & \vdots & \ddots & \vdots \\
\cline{3-6}
 & a & \mu_{a1} & \mu_{a2} & \cdots & \mu_{ab} \\
\cline{3-6}
\end{array}
\qquad (2.3)
$$

We fix the order of the cells lexicographically[1], which is to say row 1 followed by row 2, etc., and let $\boldsymbol{\mu}$ be the vector of cell means in this order.

2.2.1 *Three Elementary Hypotheses*

Three hypotheses are easy to describe from first principles:

H_0: Only A Present If this hypothesis holds, then the cell means of array (2.3) should look like this:

$$
\begin{array}{c|c|c|c|c|}
 & 1 & 2 & \cdots & b \\
\cline{2-5}
1 & \mu_1 & \mu_1 & \cdots & \mu_1 \\
\cline{2-5}
2 & \mu_2 & \mu_2 & \cdots & \mu_2 \\
\cline{2-5}
\vdots & \vdots & \vdots & \ddots & \vdots \\
\cline{2-5}
a & \mu_a & \mu_a & \cdots & \mu_a \\
\cline{2-5}
\end{array}
\qquad (2.4)
$$

[1] The choice of lexicographic order is arbitrary. In Sect. 5.1 we will see how to express things without having to fix an order. Lexicographic order is defined in general in Example A.1 in the Appendix.

In other words, this hypothesis consists of the equations

$$\begin{aligned} \mu_{11} &= \cdots = \mu_{1b} \\ \mu_{21} &= \cdots = \mu_{2b} \\ &\vdots \\ \mu_{a1} &= \cdots = \mu_{ab}. \end{aligned} \tag{2.5}$$

Each of these $a(b-1)$ equalities is of the form $\mathbf{c}'\boldsymbol{\mu} = 0$ where the left-hand side is a contrast. For example, $\mu_{11} = \mu_{12}$ is of the form $\mathbf{c}'\boldsymbol{\mu} = 0$ with $\mathbf{c}' = (1, -1, 0, \ldots, 0)$. Thus H_0 is specified by $a(b-1)$ contrast equations, and we leave it as an exercise to show that these equations—or their coefficient vectors $\mathbf{c}$ – are independent. For the moment, we denote by $U_{A\,\text{only}}$ the subspace of $\mathbb{R}^{ab}$ spanned by these vectors. Then $U_{A\,\text{only}}$ consists of contrast vectors, and $\dim(U_{A\,\text{only}}) = a(b-1)$. Following the discussion in Sect. 1.7, we see that (2.5) holds iff $\boldsymbol{\mu} \perp U_{A\,\text{only}}$.

H_0**: Only** B **Present** If this hypothesis holds, then the cell means should look like this:

	1	2	$\cdots$	b
1	μ_1	μ_2	$\cdots$	μ_b
2	μ_1	μ_2	$\cdots$	μ_b
$\vdots$	$\vdots$	$\vdots$	$\ddots$	$\vdots$
a	μ_1	μ_2	$\cdots$	μ_b

(2.6)

This is specified by imposing $(a-1)b$ independent contrast equations

$$\begin{aligned} \mu_{11} &= \cdots = \mu_{a1} \\ \mu_{12} &= \cdots = \mu_{a2} \\ &\vdots \\ \mu_{1b} &= \cdots = \mu_{ab}. \end{aligned} \tag{2.7}$$

Again, each equality may be written in the form $\mathbf{c}'\boldsymbol{\mu} = 0$ for some contrast vector $\mathbf{c}$. For now, we denote by $U_{B\,\text{only}}$ the subspace of $\mathbb{R}^{ab}$ spanned by these contrast vectors. Then $U_{B\,\text{only}}$ consists of contrast vectors, and $\dim(U_{B\,\text{only}}) = (a-1)b$. Following the discussion in Sect. 1.7, we see that (2.7) holds iff $\boldsymbol{\mu} \perp U_{B\,\text{only}}$.

H_0: **Additivity No Interaction Between** A **and** B

Definition 2.2 We say that factors A and B are *additive* if a change in the level of A produces an equal change in expected response at every level of B. When the factors are additive, we say that they have *no interaction*,

That is, the cell means in row i' are obtained simply by adding a single constant to the values in row i in the array (2.3). (Of course, the value of the constant may be different for different choices of rows.) Since the change from row to row is additive, we say that a model with no interaction is an *additive* model and that H_0 is the hypothesis of additivity.

It is obvious that additivity holds between *any* pair of rows iff it holds between row 1 and row i, $i = 2, \ldots, a$. Thus additivity holds iff the following $(a-1)(b-1)$ equations hold:

$$\mu_{ij} - \mu_{1j} = \mu_{i1} - \mu_{11}, \quad i = 2 \ldots a,\ j = 2, \ldots, b,$$

or in contrast form,

$$\mu_{ij} - \mu_{1j} - \mu_{i1} + \mu_{11} = 0, \quad i = 2 \ldots a,\ j = 2, \ldots, b. \tag{2.8}$$

The coefficients of the ijth equation in (2.8) can be displayed as follows:

	1	⋯	j	⋯
1	1		−1	
⋮				
i	−1		1	
⋮				

(2.9)

where empty cells are filled with zeros. (Caution: this array contains coefficients c, not cell means μ.)

Since equations (2.8) are symmetric in i and j, we see that there is additivity iff a change in the level of B produces the same change at every level of A.

These equations are of the form $\mathbf{c}'\boldsymbol{\mu} = 0$, the left-hand side being a contrast. Let us write $\mathbf{c}_{ij}$ for the coefficient vectors in (2.8). We leave it as an exercise to show that these equations—or the coefficient vectors $\mathbf{c}_{ij}$—are linearly independent. Let

$$U_{12} = \langle \mathbf{c}_{ij}, i = 2, \ldots a,\ j = 2, \ldots, b \rangle \tag{2.10}$$

be the subspace of $\mathbb{R}^{ab}$ spanned by these vectors. Then U_{12} consists of contrast vectors, and there is additivity iff $\boldsymbol{\mu} \perp U_{12}$. We also see that

$$\dim(U_{12}) = (a-1)(b-1).$$

Note that *"interaction" is defined simply as the absence of additivity*. We will come back to this point shortly.

2.2.2 The Main Effects Hypotheses

We wish to define the hypotheses

no A effect and no B effect

in the form

$$\boldsymbol{\mu} \perp U_1 \qquad \text{and} \qquad \boldsymbol{\mu} \perp U_2$$

for appropriate subspaces $U_i \subset \mathbb{R}^p$. How should these be defined? That is, what sets of equations should represent the absence of the main effect of A or of B?

It seems reasonable to say that

$$\text{no } A \text{ effect and no interaction} \Longleftrightarrow \text{only } B \text{ present},$$

and similarly with respect to the B effect. This should mean that U_1 is defined so that

$$\boldsymbol{\mu} \perp U_1 \text{ and } \boldsymbol{\mu} \perp U_{12} \Longleftrightarrow \boldsymbol{\mu} \perp U_{B\,\text{only}},$$

which means that

$$U_1^{\perp} \cap U_{12}^{\perp} = U_{B\,\text{only}}^{\perp}.$$

From the De Morgan laws (Corollary A.72) we see that we must have

$$U_1 + U_{12} = U_{B\,\text{only}},$$

and we will require in addition that $U_1 \perp U_{12}$ so that the equations defining the effect of A are separated from those defining additivity. This means that we define U_1, and similarly U_2, so that

$$\begin{aligned} U_1 &= U_{B\,\text{only}} \ominus U_{12} = \{\mathbf{c} \in U_{B\,\text{only}} \colon \mathbf{c} \perp U_{12}\}, \\ U_2 &= U_{A\,\text{only}} \ominus U_{12}. \end{aligned} \tag{2.11}$$

Thus, by Corollary A.71, $U_{A\,\text{only}} = U_2 \oplus U_{12}$ and $U_{B\,\text{only}} = U_1 \oplus U_{12}$. Moreover, we have

$$\begin{aligned} \dim(U_1) &= \dim(U_{B\,\text{only}}) - \dim(U_{12}) \\ &= (a-1)b - (a-1)(b-1) = a-1 \end{aligned}$$

and likewise

$$\dim(U_2) = b - 1.$$

Remark 2.3 This is the first use we have made of orthogonality to separate out effects, but it is certainly not the last. Indeed, orthogonality is a mathematical expression of separation, and underlies the analysis of variance, as we shall see in Chap. 4.

We *define* the hypothesis "no A effect" to be the statement $\boldsymbol{\mu} \perp U_1$, and "no B effect" to be $\boldsymbol{\mu} \perp U_2$. Proposition 2.6 below expresses these conditions in equation form. To see exactly what these equations are, we first need to know what contrast vectors belong to U_1 and to U_2.

Proposition 2.4 *We have the following:*

a. $\mathbf{c} \in U_1$ *iff* $\mathbf{c}$ *is a contrast vector and its components* c_{ij} *are independent of* j.
b. $\mathbf{c} \in U_2$ *iff* $\mathbf{c}$ *is a contrast vector and its components* c_{ij} *are independent of* i.

Moreover, $U_1 \perp U_2$.

To be clear, let $\mathbf{c} \in U_1$; according to (a) its components may be displayed as follows:

$$\begin{array}{c|c|c|c|c|} & 1 & 2 & \cdots & b \\ \hline 1 & c_1 & c_1 & \cdots & c_1 \\ \hline 2 & c_2 & c_2 & \cdots & c_2 \\ \hline \vdots & \vdots & \vdots & \ddots & \vdots \\ \hline a & c_a & c_a & \cdots & c_a \\ \hline \end{array} \tag{2.12}$$

where

$$\sum_{i=1}^{a} c_i = 0. \tag{2.13}$$

Written out row-by-row, we would have

$$\mathbf{c} = [\underbrace{c_1, \ldots, c_1}_{b}, \underbrace{c_2, \ldots, c_2}_{b}, \ldots, \underbrace{c_a, \ldots, c_a}_{b}]'$$

for $\mathbf{c} \in U_1$. The characterization of U_2 is analogous. We will say that the vectors $\mathbf{c}$ in U_1 are *constant on rows*, and that those in U_2 are *constant on columns*. The corresponding expressions $\mathbf{c}'\boldsymbol{\mu}$ are thus *contrasts in the rows* or *in the columns*, respectively.

Proof of Proposition 2.4 To prove the first part, let

$$U = \{\mathbf{c} \text{ is a contrast vector and the components} c_{ij} \text{of} \mathbf{c} \text{ are independent of} j\}.$$

We will show that $U \subset U_1$, and then use dimensions to show that we have equality. To show the former, definition (2.11) requires that we establish two things:

$U \subset U_{B\,\text{only}}$: But by Theorem A.70(c) it suffices to show that $\boldsymbol{\mu} \perp U$ implies $\boldsymbol{\mu} \perp U_{B\,\text{only}}$. However, $\boldsymbol{\mu} \perp U$ implies that $\boldsymbol{\mu}$ has the form given in array (2.6), and it is easy to see that if $\mathbf{c}$ has the form (2.12) then $\mathbf{c} \perp \boldsymbol{\mu}$.

$U \perp U_{12}$: But contrast vectors of form (2.12) and (2.9) are perpendicular, as is easily seen by taking the dot product.

Thus $U \subset U_1$. To show equality, we observe from (2.12) that U is closed under addition and scalar multiplication, so that it is not just a set but a vector space, and that $\dim(U) = a - 1$ due to (2.13). But we saw above that $\dim(U_1) = a - 1$, so $U = U_1$, as claimed.

The proof of (b) is the same, *mutatis mutandis*. Finally, from (2.12) and the corresponding array for U_2 it is easy to see that $U_1 \perp U_2$. □

Remark 2.5 It may seem odd to prove $U \subset U_{B\,\text{only}}$ by showing that $U^{\perp} \supset (U_{B\,\text{only}})^{\perp}$. We leave it as an exercise to show directly that $U \subset U_{B\,\text{only}}$.

By construction, U_{12} is perpendicular to both U_1 and U_2. Following [22], we say that a contrast $\mathbf{c}'\boldsymbol{\mu}$ *belongs to the main effect of* A, or simply *belongs to* A, if $\mathbf{c} \in U_1$, that it *belongs to (the main effect of)* B if $\mathbf{c} \in U_2$, and that it *belongs to interaction* if $\mathbf{c} \in U_{12}$.

A contrast $\mathbf{c}'\boldsymbol{\mu}$ belongs to A if $\mathbf{c}$ is given by (2.12), and thus the contrast obviously condenses to an expression

$$\mathbf{c}'\boldsymbol{\mu} = c_1\mu_{1\cdot} + \cdots + c_a\mu_{a\cdot},$$

that is, it is a *contrast in the row totals* of the cell means. Thus the hypothesis of "no A effect" is the statement that all such contrasts are zero. Similarly, the contrast belongs to B if

$$\mathbf{c}'\boldsymbol{\mu} = c_1\mu_{\cdot 1} + \cdots + c_a\mu_{\cdot b},$$

in other words, if it is a *contrast in the column totals*, and there is "no B effect" means that all such contrasts are zero. An equivalent statement is this:

Proposition 2.6 *In an $a \times b$ design with factors A and B,*

- *the hypothesis of "no A effect" is equivalent to*

$$\mu_{1\cdot} = \cdots = \mu_{a\cdot}.$$

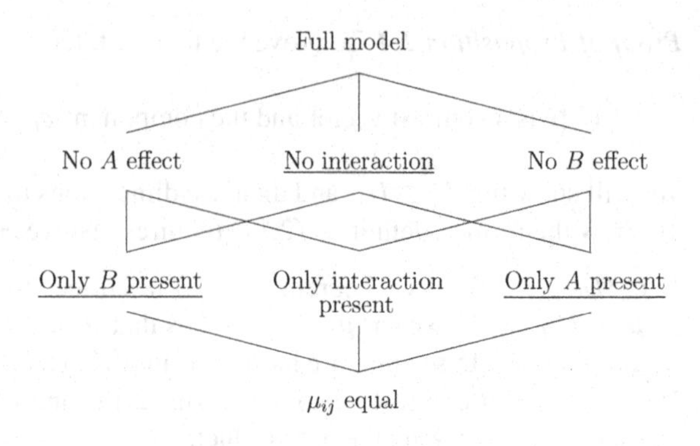

Fig. 2.1 The lattice of hypotheses of an $a \times b$ design. The "elementary" hypotheses of Sect. 2.2.1 are underlined

- *the hypothesis of "no B effect" is equivalent to*

$$\mu_{\cdot 1} = \cdots = \mu_{\cdot b}\,.$$

Thus these hypotheses refer to equality of "marginal sums". Of course, one may substitute equality of "marginal averages" in each case. Proposition 2.6 expresses the commonly held view that the main effect of a factor is a measure of the average change in expected response that occurs when the level of the factor is changed, where the "average" is taken over all other factors in the experiment.[2] The proof of the proposition is left as an exercise.

It may be helpful to place the five hypotheses we have discussed so far in a diagram like Fig. 2.1. The "full model" assumes no constraints on the cell means μ_{ij}, while the hypotheses may be written

$$\begin{aligned} &\text{No } A \text{ effect}: && \boldsymbol{\mu} \perp U_1, \\ &\text{No } B \text{ effect}: && \boldsymbol{\mu} \perp U_2, \\ &\text{Nointeraction}: && \boldsymbol{\mu} \perp U_{12}, \\ &\text{Only } A \text{ present}: && \boldsymbol{\mu} \perp U_2 \oplus U_{12}, \end{aligned}$$

and so on. These hypotheses form a *lattice*. We will revisit this diagram in Sect. 4.6.

We also note that we have in effect decomposed the parameter space $\mathbb{R}^p$ orthogonally. We summarize what we have learned:

Theorem 2.7 *With U_1, U_2 and U_{12} defined by (2.11) and (2.10) and $p = ab$, we have* $\dim(U_1) = a-1$, $\dim(U_2) = b-1$, $\dim(U_{12}) = (a-1)(b-1)$, *and moreover*

$$\mathbb{R}^p = \langle\, \mathbf{1}\,\rangle \oplus U_1 \oplus U_2 \oplus U_{12} \tag{2.14}$$

(orthogonal sum), where $\langle\, \mathbf{1}\,\rangle$ is the space spanned by the vector $\mathbf{1}$.

[2] This is essentially taken from [14].

This underlies the analysis of variance, as we shall see, and is generalized in Sect. 5.3.

2.2.3 *Effects in a Two-Factor Design*

From Proposition 2.4 we may simply take the following as our definitions of U_1, U_2 and U_{12}:

- U_1 consists of contrast vectors $\mathbf{c}$ whose components c_{ij} depend only on i;
- U_2 consists of contrast vectors $\mathbf{c}$ whose components c_{ij} depend only on j;
- U_{12} consists of contrast vectors $\mathbf{c}$ orthogonal to both U_1 and U_2.

Our definitions imply a general procedure: First find U_1 and U_2, then find U_{12} by orthogonality. We illustrate this with a small example.

Example 2.8 The simplest multifactor design is the 2×2. With an eye toward later developments, we will index the levels of each factor by 0 and 1 rather than by 1 and 2. (Often the levels mean something like "off" and "on", so the use of 0 and 1 is not out of place.) If we order the cells lexicographically, then one choice of contrast vectors is this:

cell	A	B	AB
00	1	1	1
01	1	−1	−1
10	−1	1	−1
11	−1	−1	1

As an element of U_1, the column A must have the form $(c, c, -c, -c)'$, and we have picked $(1, 1, -1, -1)'$ as a basis for U_1. Column B is chosen similarly. Column AB must be orthogonal to A and to B, and its elements must sum to 0. This imposes three equations on the four components, the solution being all scalar multiples of $(1, -1, -1, 1)'$.

Of course, the column AB could also be determined directly as in (2.9), applied to a 2×2 array of cells.

Remark 2.9 It is certainly possible to have a set of cell means which are non-additive but for which one or both main effects are absent. For example, one can have $\boldsymbol{\mu} \perp U_1$ but $\not\perp U_{12}$. (We leave it as an exercise to construct a simple 2×2 example.) One may ask whether this makes sense—can A and B interact if one or both of them has no effect?

Data sets do arise which statistically give this impression when the appropriate hypotheses are tested. The problem may only be apparent, and may be simply a matter of semantics. While the word "interaction" conjures many kinds of relationships, we are using the word in a very specific sense to mean "non-additivity". This suggests that the latter term is preferable to "interaction" in that it doesn't carry colloquial implications. Similarly, we have chosen to describe the main effect of a factor in a very specific way. It is quite conceivable that there is an effect of A, say, that is not captured by our specific description of "main effect" but whose only manifestation is non-additivity in the presence of B. Perhaps alternate terminology should also be developed for what we now call main effects.

The description of the main-effects hypotheses given in Proposition 2.6, or in the definitions of the contrasts for main effects given at the beginning of this subsection, are not new. We have justified them by showing that they are forced on us once we accept (a) additivity as the definition of "no interaction", (b) the definitions of "only A present" and "only B present", and (c) the use of orthogonal differencing to separate effects. There are other ways of justifying these contrasts, although one may ask whether they are more direct. We leave this question as an exercise.

2.3 Multifactor Designs

Consider an $a \times b \times c$ design, that is, a design with three factors, which we will label A, B and C. A treatment combination is now an ordered triple (i, j, k) and its expected response is μ_{ijk}, where i, j and k denote the levels of A, B and C, respectively. The set T of treatment combinations can be viewed as a 3-dimensional array, and "rows" and "columns" must be replaced by other sets:

- there are a "slices" determined by the a levels of factor A; similarly, there are b slices determined by factor B and c determined by factor C;
- there are ab "tubes" determined by the combined levels of A and B; similarly, there are ac tubes determined by the levels of A and C, and bc tubes determined by the levels of B and C.

We will use the generic term "blocks" for these sets, which are pictured in Fig. 2.2. (We will meet them again in Sect. 5.3.)

We may now define these sets of contrast vectors, where as before we order cells lexicographically:

$$
\begin{aligned}
U_1 &= \{\text{contrast vectors } \mathbf{c} \text{ that are constant on the blocks determined by } A\}, \\
U_2 &= \{\text{contrast vectors } \mathbf{c} \text{ that are constant on the blocks determined by } B\}, \\
U_3 &= \{\text{contrast vectors } \mathbf{c} \text{ that are constant on the blocks determined by } C\},
\end{aligned} \tag{2.15}
$$

$$
\begin{aligned}
U_{12} = \{&\text{contrast vectors } \mathbf{c} \text{ that are constant on the blocks determined by} A \text{ and } B \\
&\text{and are} \perp U_1 \text{ and } U_2\}, \\
U_{13} = \{&\text{contrast vectors } \mathbf{c} \text{ that are constant on the blocks determined by} A \text{ and } C \\
&\text{and are} \perp U_1 \text{ and } U_3\},
\end{aligned}
$$

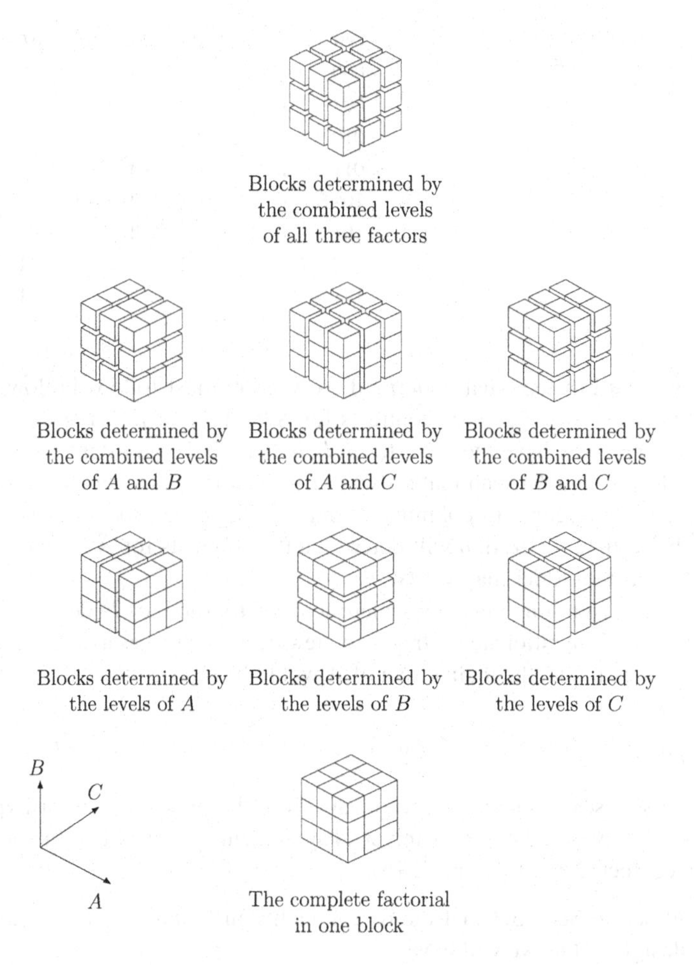

Fig. 2.2 Basic blockings (partitions) of an $a \times b \times c$ design (for purposes of illustration, $a = b = c = 3$)

$$U_{23} = \{\text{contrast vectors } \mathbf{c} \text{ that are constant on the blocks determined by} B \text{ and } C$$
$$\text{and are} \perp U_2 \text{ and } U_3\},$$
$$U_{123} = \{\text{contrast vectors } \mathbf{c} \text{ that are} \perp \text{all the above}\}.$$

If $\mathbf{c} \in U_1$, then the contrast $\mathbf{c}'\boldsymbol{\mu}$ belongs to the main effect of A, and similarly for U_2 and U_3. If $\mathbf{c} \in U_{12}$, then the contrast $\mathbf{c}'\boldsymbol{\mu}$ belongs to the interaction between A and B, and so on. If $\mathbf{c} \in U_{123}$, then the contrast $\mathbf{c}'\boldsymbol{\mu}$ belongs to the three-factor (or second-order) interaction of A, B and C.

Example 2.10 (The $2 \times 2 \times 2$ *design)* As in Example 2.8, we may index the levels of each factor by 0 and 1. Each main effect will be represented by one vector,

Table 2.1 Contrast vectors in a 2^3 design, as constructed in Example 2.10

cell	A	B	C	AB	AC	BC	ABC
000	1	1	1	1	1	1	1
001	1	1	−1	1	−1	−1	−1
010	1	−1	1	−1	1	−1	−1
011	1	−1	−1	−1	−1	1	1
100	−1	1	1	−1	−1	1	−1
101	−1	1	−1	−1	1	−1	1
110	−1	−1	1	1	−1	−1	1
111	−1	−1	−1	1	1	1	−1

and it is not hard to see what patterns these vectors must follow. Following that, orthogonalization would give us contrasts for AB, AC and BC. For example, the column for AB must have the form $(a, a, b, b, c, c, d, d)'$ (constant on the blocks determined by A and B) such that $a + b + c + d = 0$ (it is a contrast vector) and such that it is orthogonal to columns A and B. The same process gives AC and BC. Further orthogonalization will determine the contrasts for ABC. A full set is in Table 2.1, as the reader may verify.

There is a convention to insert a scalar factor of 1/4 (and for 2^k designs, $1/2^{k-1}$) in these vectors. The rationale for this is to view each contrast as a difference of two averages. For example, the main effect of A would be represented by

$$\frac{1}{4}(\mu_{000} + \mu_{001} + \mu_{010} + \mu_{011}) - \frac{1}{4}(\mu_{100} + \mu_{101} + \mu_{110} + \mu_{111}).$$

As we will see, scalar factors are irrelevant from the point of view of hypothesis testing, and in any case there is no universal agreement on what scalar factors should be used (see Sect. 2.5.3, Example 2.15).

We will see in Sect. 5.3 that the orthogonality in Example 2.10 is true for all factorial designs. Thus we will have

$$\mathbb{R}^p = \langle \mathbf{1} \rangle \oplus U_1 \oplus U_2 \oplus U_3 \oplus U_{12} \oplus U_{13} \oplus U_{23} \oplus U_{123}, \tag{2.16}$$

where $p = abc$.

A factorial design with more than three factors has a set of contrast vectors U_I for each $I \subset \{1, \ldots, k\}$. These are defined inductively beginning with main effects and continuing to progressively higher orders of interaction by orthogonalization. We will describe this construction more explicitly in Sect. 5.3. The reader may already sense that the general construction would benefit from introducing some combinatorial language and more convenient notation, and we will take this up in Sect. 5.2.

Even in the case of a three-factor design, it's clear that the orthogonalization process such as that used in Examples 2.8 and 2.10 would become quite onerous. We will give a simpler computational method in Sect. 5.4.

The reflective reader may have noticed that the notion of an "effect" has been defined by what it isn't! For example, we define the main effect of factor A by saying when it is absent, namely when certain relations (contrasts) hold between cell means. This is written succinctly in the form $\boldsymbol{\mu} \perp U_1$, where U_1 contains the coefficient vectors of these relations. Similarly, the $B \times C$ interaction is absent if $\boldsymbol{\mu} \perp U_{23}$, and so on. Thus we may identify an *effect* with a set U of contrast vectors: the effect is absent when $\boldsymbol{\mu} \perp U$. Note that we are including interactions as "effects".

Of course, any set of contrast vectors could be said to define an effect. Moreover, the relation $\boldsymbol{\mu} \perp U$ shows that there is no loss of generality in assuming that U is a *subspace* of contrast vectors, since a set of vectors may be replaced by its span. We will therefore adopt the following terminology:

Definition 2.11 In a factorial model $\mathrm{E}(\mathbf{Y}) = \mathbf{X}\boldsymbol{\mu}$, where $\boldsymbol{\mu}$ is $p \times 1$, an *effect* is a subspace $U \subset \mathbb{R}^p$ consisting of contrast vectors. The effect is *absent* if $\boldsymbol{\mu} \perp U$.

2.4 Quantitative Factors

A factorial experiment may include factors whose levels are *quantitative*—for example, temperature, chemical concentration, etc.—rather than simply categorical. In such a case, the mean response μ may be modeled as a polynomial in the corresponding independent variables. While this suggests a regression approach, it is common instead to continue to use a factorial model, and to seek an orthogonal basis of each main effect that separates the effect into a linear component, a quadratic component, and so on.

Consider first the case of a one-factor experiment with s quantitative treatment levels, say $r_1 < \cdots < r_s$, and let $\boldsymbol{\mu} = (\mu_1, \ldots, \mu_s)'$ be the vector of mean responses. Initially,

$$\mu_r = \beta_0 + \beta_1 r + \cdots + \beta_{s-1} r^{s-1},$$

so that

$$\boldsymbol{\mu} = \begin{pmatrix} \mu_1 \\ \vdots \\ \mu_s \end{pmatrix} = \begin{pmatrix} \beta_0 + \beta_1 r_1 + \beta_1 r_1^2 + \cdots + \beta_{s-1} r_1^{s-1} \\ \vdots \\ \beta_0 + \beta_1 r_s + \beta_1 r_s^2 + \cdots + \beta_{s-1} r_s^{s-1} \end{pmatrix}$$

$$= \begin{pmatrix} 1 & r_1 & r_1^2 & \cdots & r_1^{s-1} \\ \vdots & \vdots & \vdots & & \vdots \\ 1 & r_s & r_s^2 & \cdots & r_s^{s-1} \end{pmatrix} \begin{pmatrix} \beta_0 \\ \beta_1 \\ \vdots \\ \beta_{s-1} \end{pmatrix} = \mathbf{R}\boldsymbol{\beta},$$

say. The matrix $\mathbf{R}$ is a square *Vandermonde matrix*, and it is well known (see, e.g., [85]) that $\det \mathbf{R} = \prod_{i<j}(r_j - r_i)$. Since we are assuming that the numbers r_i are distinct, this determinant is nonzero and so $\mathbf{R}$ is nonsingular. Thus we have reparametrized the model, replacing $\boldsymbol{\mu}$ with $\boldsymbol{\beta}$. In particular, the polynomial

representing μ_r cannot have degree higher than $s-1$, as otherwise $\boldsymbol{\beta}$ would not be identifiable.

Let $\mathbf{r}_0 = \mathbf{1}$, $\mathbf{r}_1, \ldots, \mathbf{r}_{s-1}$ be the columns of $\mathbf{R}$. By the above, they are linearly independent, and so span $\mathbb{R}^s$. Applying the *Gram-Schmidt process* to them yields a set of s orthogonal vectors $\mathbf{1}, \mathbf{c}_1, \ldots, \mathbf{c}_{s-1}$. We make several observations:

a. The vectors $\mathbf{c}_1, \ldots, \mathbf{c}_{s-1}$ must be contrast vectors as they are orthogonal to $\mathbf{1}$.
b. Their span, $U = \langle \mathbf{c}_1, \ldots, \mathbf{c}_{s-1} \rangle = \mathbf{1}^\perp$, defines the hypothesis H_0: $\mu_1 = \cdots = \mu_s$, as this is equivalent to $\boldsymbol{\mu} \perp U$ (Proposition 2.1).
c. For each $1 \le d \le s-1$ we have

$$\langle \mathbf{1}, \mathbf{c}_1, \ldots, \mathbf{c}_d \rangle = \langle \mathbf{1}, \mathbf{r}_1, \ldots, \mathbf{r}_d \rangle, \tag{2.17}$$

by construction. This is clear from the Gram-Schmidt equations (A.15).

Equation (2.17) tells us that to every $\boldsymbol{\beta}$ there is a $\boldsymbol{\gamma}$ such that

$$\beta_0\mathbf{1} + \beta_1\mathbf{r}_1 + \cdots + \beta_d\mathbf{r}_d = \gamma_0\mathbf{1} + \gamma_1\mathbf{c}_1 + \cdots + \gamma_d\mathbf{c}_d$$

for each $1 \le d \le s-1$. This means that *we can equally use either* $\mathbf{r}_1, \ldots, \mathbf{r}_d$ *or* $\mathbf{c}_1, \ldots, \mathbf{c}_d$ *to represent the components of* $\boldsymbol{\mu}$ *as a polynomial of degree* d. Because of this, the contrasts $\mathbf{c}_i'\boldsymbol{\mu}$ are known as *polynomial effects*. In particular, the contrast $\mathbf{c}_1'\boldsymbol{\mu}$ is said to represent the *linear effect of treatment*, $\mathbf{c}_2'\boldsymbol{\mu}$ represents the *quadratic effect of treatment*, and so on. The reason for this is that if, for example, $\boldsymbol{\mu} \perp \mathbf{c}_k$ for $k > 2$, then $\boldsymbol{\mu} = a_0\mathbf{1} + a_1\mathbf{c}_1 + a_2\mathbf{c}_2$, so that μ_r is a quadratic function of r.

Gram-Schmidt orthogonalization[3] produces vectors $\mathbf{c}_i$ satisfying (2.17), but such vectors may be modified by multiplication by scalars, as this does not change property (2.17) or orthogonality. In application it is typical to simplify each vector by multiplying by a convenient scalar, especially if there are equivalent vectors with integer components. This is generally possible only in special cases, in particular when the values $r_1, \ldots, r_s$ are equispaced, in which case they can be recoded to be $1, \ldots, s$.

Example 2.12 If $s = 4$ and the numbers $r_1, \ldots, r_4$ are equally spaced, then up to scalar multiples the polynomial contrast vectors are $\mathbf{c}_1 = (-3, -1, 1, 3)'$, $\mathbf{c}_2 = (1, -1, -1, 1)'$, and $\mathbf{c}_3 = (-1, 3, -3, 1)'$ (Problem 2.9). Tables of such contrast vectors are given in many books on experimental design and regression; see, for example, [151, Appendix G] and [51, Section 22.2]. These vectors are often referred to as *orthogonal polynomials*, for reasons having to do with regression—see Sect. 4.6.2 below.

For non-equispaced values r_i one must do the calculations directly. See Exercises 2.10 and 2.11.

[3] We do not need *orthonormalization*, which produces unit vectors.

Remark 2.13 There are many computer packages and online websites that will perform Gram-Schmidt orthogonalization. Alternatively, we have noted (page 315) that while formulas (A.15) can be used inductively, one can also compute $\mathbf{c}_k = \mathbf{r}_k - \hat{\mathbf{r}}_k$ where $\hat{\mathbf{r}}_k$ is the orthogonal projection of $\mathbf{r}_k$ on $\mathbf{r}_1, \ldots, \mathbf{r}_{k-1}$. Statisticians can take some satisfaction in using regression software for this, since least squares fitting is orthogonal projection. (Least squares fitting will be discussed in Sect. 3.1.) This could be done as follows:

1. Compute

$$\mathbf{c}_1 = \mathbf{r}_1 - \frac{\mathbf{r}_1 \cdot \mathbf{1}}{\mathbf{1} \cdot \mathbf{1}} \mathbf{1} = \mathbf{r}_1 - \bar{r}_1 \mathbf{1},$$

   where $\bar{r}_1$ is the average of the components of $\mathbf{r}_1$.
2. For $k \geq 2$, regress $\mathbf{r}_k$ on $\mathbf{r}_1, \ldots, \mathbf{r}_{k-1}$, and store the residual vector $\mathbf{c}_k = \mathbf{r}_k - \hat{\mathbf{r}}_k$.

The residual vectors are precisely the desired orthogonal contrast vectors. If desired, one may multiply or divide each by a convenient constant to make the entries easy to work with (for example, to make them small integers in the equispaced case).

With a multifactor design, a similar process may be used for any main effect, but the components must be repeated so that the contrast vectors belong to the given effect. In an $a \times b$ design, for example, these vectors need to be constant on rows in order to produce $a - 1$ contrasts belonging to the main effect of A. Thus the linear contrast vector for A in a 4×2 design would be $(-3, -3, -1, -1, 1, 1, 3, 3)'$. Furthermore, when there are two quantitative factors, one can compute interaction contrasts for effects that are called linear-by-linear, linear-by-quadratic, and so on. The method for doing this is given in Sect. 5.4. Exercise 5.8 requires carrying this out in a $3 \times 3 \times 2$ experiment.

2.5 The Factor-Effects Parametrization

Many readers will be familiar with models of the form

$$\mathrm{E}(Y_{ij}) = \mu + \tau_i$$

and

$$\mathrm{E}(Y_{ijk}) = \mu + \alpha_i + \beta_j + \gamma_{ij}$$

for factorial designs with one or two factors. In this section we describe such models with an emphasis on the meaning of the parameters and the formulation of hypotheses, emphasizing the problems of identifiability and other ambiguities. Issues of estimation and testing will be taken up in Chaps. 3 and 4.

2.5.1 The One-Factor Model

The one-factor model (2.1) is often written

$$E(Y_{ij}) = \mu + \tau_i, \ i = 1, \ldots, s, \ j = 1, \ldots, n_i, \tag{2.18}$$

where μ represents an overall expected response and τ_i is the additional response due to treatment i. The hypothesis of "no treatment effect" is the statement

$$H_0 \tau_i = 0, \ i = 1, \ldots, s. \tag{2.19}$$

Letting $\mu_i = E(Y_{ij})$, we have

$$\mu_i = \mu + \tau_i, \tag{2.20}$$

from which we see that H_0 is equivalent to the hypothesis (2.2) that we originally understood to mean "no treatment effect".

If we let $\boldsymbol{\beta} = (\mu, \tau_1, \ldots, \tau_s)'$ and let $\mathbf{Y}$ be the vector of observations (ordered consistent with $\boldsymbol{\mu}$), then we may write this model in the usual form

$$E(\mathbf{Y}) = \mathbf{X}\boldsymbol{\beta}. \tag{2.21}$$

For $s = 3$ treatments and $n_i = 2$ observations per treatment, the model takes the form

$$E\begin{pmatrix} Y_{11} \\ Y_{12} \\ Y_{21} \\ Y_{22} \\ Y_{31} \\ Y_{32} \end{pmatrix} = \begin{pmatrix} 1\,1\,0\,0 \\ 1\,1\,0\,0 \\ 1\,0\,1\,0 \\ 1\,0\,1\,0 \\ 1\,0\,0\,1 \\ 1\,0\,0\,1 \end{pmatrix} \begin{pmatrix} \mu \\ \tau_1 \\ \tau_2 \\ \tau_3 \end{pmatrix}. \tag{2.22}$$

Consider the relation (2.20). For any given value of μ_i there are infinitely many possible values of μ and τ_i that satisfy this relation. The parameters μ and τ_i are *not identifiable*. That is, while μ_i has a definite (if unknown) value, the quantities μ and τ_i don't. We also say that the model (2.18) is *overparametrized*, as it uses $s + 1$ parameters to describe a model that needs only s.

Moreover, it is not hard to see that when we write the model in the form (2.21) the design matrix $\mathbf{X}$ is $N \times (s + 1)$ but has rank s. For example, columns 2 through $s + 1$ are clearly linearly independent (in fact, orthogonal) while column 1 equals their sum. This is simply a reflection of overparametrization. In fact, if $n_i = 1$ for all i, then $\mathbf{X}$ is simply the matrix of the equations in (2.20) when written in the form $\boldsymbol{\mu} = \mathbf{X}\boldsymbol{\beta}$, and since $\mathbf{X}$ does not have full rank the solution $\boldsymbol{\beta}$ is not unique. In

Chaps. 3 and 4 we will examine the implications of not being a full rank model in estimation and in hypothesis testing.

The problem of non-identifiability goes beyond these practical difficulties, to the *meaning* of the model parameters. For example, the quantity $\mu + \tau_i$ has a clear meaning (it is $\mathrm{E}(Y_{ij})$), but μ and τ_i by themselves do not. The hypothesis (2.19) is meaningful, but the hypothesis $H_0 \tau_2 = 0$ is not.

In order to cope with this problem, it is typical to impose linear constraints on the parameters, the most common of which are these:

- the "zero-sum constraint" [151]

$$\sum_i \tau_i = 0.$$

  Summing both sides of (2.20) and applying this constraint, we see that we have defined

$$\mu = \bar{\mu}., \quad \tau_i = \mu_i - \bar{\mu}. \, ,$$

  where $\bar{\mu}.$ is the average of the treatment means μ_i. Clearly τ is now interpreted as the excess of the ith treatment over this average. The zero-sum constraint is probably the most common of all.
- the constraint

$$\tau_1 = 0. \tag{2.23}$$

  With this assumption, we have $\mu = \mu_1$ and $\tau_i = \mu_i - \mu_1$ for $i \geq 2$. This views treatment 1 as a baseline or control, and treatment effects τ_i as measuring the difference from the control, because of which (2.23) is sometimes called a "baseline constraint" [151]. (Of course, any treatment could be considered the baseline.)
- the constraint

$$\sum_i \frac{n_i}{N} \tau_i = 0,$$

  where n_i is the number of observations taken on treatment i and $N = \sum_i n_i$. Applying this constraint to (2.20), we find that μ is a *weighted* average of the means μ_i (with weights n_i/N) and τ_i is the difference between μ_i and μ. An illustration of this is given in [83, pages 703–4]. Obviously this constraint reduces to the zero-sum constraint when the sample sizes n_i are equal.

These constraints are special cases of

$$\sum_i w_i \tau_i = 0, \tag{2.24}$$

where w_i are *weights* satisfying $w_i \geq 0$ and $\sum_i w_i = 1$. It is easy to see that this constraint implies that $\mu = \sum_i w_i \mu_i$, the weighted average of the treatment means, and τ_i is the excess of the mean response μ_i above this average. In other words, each parameter now has a definite meaning, albeit dependent on the choice of weights w_i.

To see that such constraints turn this into a full-rank model, we make use of the zero-sum constraint (2.24) to rewrite the model, noting in particular that there are now only s independent parameters. For example,

$$\tau_s = -\sum_{i=1}^{s-1} \tau_i,$$

so that the model (2.22) may be written

$$E(\mathbf{Y}) = \begin{pmatrix} 1 & 1 & 0 \\ 1 & 1 & 0 \\ 1 & 0 & 1 \\ 1 & 0 & 1 \\ 1 & -1 & -1 \\ 1 & -1 & -1 \end{pmatrix} \begin{pmatrix} \mu \\ \tau_1 \\ \tau_2 \end{pmatrix}.$$

One easily checks that the columns of the design matrix are linearly independent, so that the matrix has full rank. It is instructive to compare this model with its cell-means version (1.9), which is obviously of full rank.

2.5.2 *Models with Two Factors*

Similarly, a two-factor design with factors A and B is sometimes modeled by

$$E(Y_{ijk}) = \mu + \alpha_i + \beta_j + \gamma_{ij}, \; i = 1, \ldots, a, \; j = 1, \ldots, b, \tag{2.25}$$

where Y_{ijk} is the kth response to treatment combination ij. Here μ again represents an overall expected response, α_i the additional expected response to the ith level of A, β_j the analogous quantity for B, and γ_{ij} an interaction term for the ith level of A and the jth level of B. One expects the main hypotheses to look like this:

$$\begin{aligned} H_0 &: \text{No } A \text{ effect: } \alpha_i = 0, \; i = 1, \ldots, a; \\ H_0 &: \text{No } B \text{ effect: } \beta_j = 0, \; j = 1, \ldots, b. \\ H_0 &: \text{No interaction: } \gamma_{ij} = 0, \; \text{all } i, j. \end{aligned} \tag{2.26}$$

Indeed, under the third hypothesis the model (2.25) reduces to

$$\mathrm{E}(Y_{ijk}) = \mu + \alpha_i + \beta_j, \ i = 1, \ldots, a, \ j = 1, \ldots, b,$$

which is clearly additive in the sense of Definition 2.2. However, as it stands there is no way to link the first two hypotheses to the main effects hypotheses of Proposition 2.6. Here identifiability is an essential obstruction, one that didn't arise with the one-factor model. Without further conditions, the individual terms α_i and β_j (and, for that matter, γ_{ij}) have no precise meaning.

The ab cell means μ_{ij} are expressed in (2.25) in terms of $1 + a + b + ab$ parameters, that is,

$$\mu_{ij} = \mu + \alpha_i + \beta_j + \gamma_{ij}, \tag{2.27}$$

and so we need to impose $a + b + 1$ constraints. A general set of constraints is this:

$$\begin{aligned} &\sum_i u_i \alpha_i = 0, \quad \sum_j v_j \beta_j = 0, \\ &\qquad \sum_i u_i \gamma_{ij} = 0 \quad \text{for each } j, \quad \sum_j v_j \gamma_{ij} = 0 \quad \text{for each } i. \end{aligned} \tag{2.28}$$

(The careful reader will note that (2.28) contains $a + b + 2$ equations. We leave it as an exercise to show that there are $a + b + 1$ *independent* equations.) Here the weights u_i and v_j are nonnegative and $\sum_i u_i = 1 = \sum_j v_j$. As in the one-factor model there are three common choices of weight:

- $u_1 = \cdots = u_a = 1/a$, $v_1 = \cdots = v_b = 1/b$. This choice gives "zero sum" constraints. We will call these *uniform weights*.
- $u_1 = 1$, $v_1 = 1$, all other weights = zero. This choice gives "baseline" constraints (or "corner point" constraints, since the (1, 1) corner cell is the baseline). As in the one-factor case, any other cell can be used as the baseline.
- $u_i = n_{i\cdot}/N$, $v_j = n_{\cdot j}/N$ where $N = \sum_i \sum_j n_{ij}$. We will discuss the use of this choice in a special case in Sect. 4.6.1.

Scheffé [121, page 91] offers an example of weights chosen to reflect a stratified sampling scheme. He and others develop equations (2.28) not as a set of constraints but as the result of defining a natural set of parameters μ, α_i, β_j, and γ_{ij}. He declares that if the parameters just satisfy the model (2.25) by itself, this "is not sufficient for them to be the general mean, main effects, and interactions, unless the side conditions [(2.28)] are satisfied ...". This opinion is not universally held (see, for example, [123, page 147]).

Because models such as this express the effects of interest directly through their parameters, we will call them *factor-effects models*, a name that appears to have been introduced in [100][4]. Other terms are *effects models* [81, page 183] and *canonical models* [73, page 120]. These terms are typically used when a system of constraints is imposed, but we may occasionally abuse the terminology (*pace* Scheffé) to describe models like (2.18) and (2.25) even without constraints.

Applying the general constraints (2.28) to the model (2.27) and defining weighted row and column averages by

$$A_i = \sum_j v_j \mu_{ij}, \quad B_j = \sum_i u_i \mu_{ij}, \tag{2.29}$$

the reader can verify that the parameters of (2.25) may be expressed directly in terms of the cell means as follows:

$$\begin{aligned} \mu &= \sum_i \sum_j u_i v_j \mu_{ij}, \\ \alpha_i &= A_i - \mu, \quad \beta_j = B_j - \mu, \\ \gamma_{ij} &= \mu_{ij} - A_i - B_j + \mu \end{aligned} \tag{2.30}$$

Thus μ represents an overall weighted average of the expected responses, α_i the excess of the ith row average over the grand average, and β_j the excess of the jth column average over μ.

Example 2.14 Consider the 2×3 factorial experiment with cell means as indicated below. Rows indicate the levels of factor A and columns those of factor B.

μ_{11}	μ_{12}	μ_{13}
μ_{21}	μ_{22}	μ_{23}

Using the zero-sum constraints, we find that

$$\begin{aligned} \mu &= (1/6)\mu_{..}, \\ \alpha_1 &= (1/6)(\mu_{1.} - \mu_{2.}), \\ \beta_1 &= (1/6)(2\mu_{.1} - \mu_{.2} - \mu_{.3}), \\ \beta_2 &= (1/6)(-\mu_{.1} + 2\mu_{.2} - \mu_{.3}), \\ \gamma_{11} &= (1/6)(2\mu_{11} - \mu_{12} - \mu_{13} - 2\mu_{21} + \mu_{22} + \mu_{23}), \\ \gamma_{12} &= (1/6)(-\mu_{11} + 2\mu_{12} - \mu_{13} + \mu_{21} - 2\mu_{22} + \mu_{23}), \end{aligned} \tag{2.31}$$

[4] See especially [100, pages 552 and 693]. This is an earlier edition of [83]

where, as usual, $\mu_{i\cdot} = \sum_j \mu_{ij}$, $\mu_{\cdot j} = \sum_i \mu_{ij}$, and $\mu_{\cdot\cdot} = \sum_i \sum_j \mu_{ij}$. The other parameters are gotten from these by applying the zero-sum constraints; for example, $\alpha_2 = -\alpha_1$.

Let us instead use the baseline constraints with the (2, 3) cell as the baseline, so that $u_2 = v_3 = 1$ and all other weights equal 0. Using primes to distinguish the solutions from those using the zero-sum constraints, we have

$$\begin{aligned}
\mu' &= \mu_{23}, \\
\alpha_1' &= \mu_{13} - \mu_{23}, \\
\beta_1' &= \mu_{21} - \mu_{23}, \\
\beta_2' &= \mu_{22} - \mu_{23}, \\
\gamma_{11}' &= \mu_{11} - \mu_{13} - \mu_{21} + \mu_{23}, \\
\gamma_{12}' &= \mu_{12} - \mu_{13} - \mu_{22} + \mu_{23},
\end{aligned} \tag{2.32}$$

the other parameters equaling zero. □

We notice that in either set of weights the parameters (except for μ and μ') are expressed as contrasts in cell means. This is actually true for any set of weights (Theorem 2.18 below). It is obvious that corresponding expressions (say for α and α') represent rather different comparisons between cell means, due entirely to the system of side conditions that have been imposed. We discuss this problem further in Sect. 2.5.4.

2.5.3 *Models with Three or More Factors*

For designs with three or more effects, the limitations of the alphabet necessitate a more flexible notation to accommodate a large number of terms. One common scheme, which would replace γ in the two-factor model (2.25) by the expression $(\alpha\beta)$ (including parentheses), writes a three-factor model in the form

$$\mathrm{E}(Y_{ijk\ell}) = \mu + \alpha_i + \beta_j + \gamma_k + (\alpha\beta)_{ij} + (\alpha\gamma)_{ik} + (\beta\gamma)_{jk} + (\alpha\beta\gamma)_{ijk},$$
$$i = 1, \ldots, a,\ j = 1, \ldots, b,\ k = 1, \ldots, c.$$

An alternative, somewhat more flexible scheme writes

$$\begin{aligned}
\mathrm{E}(Y_{ijk\ell}) &= \mu + \alpha_i^A + \alpha_j^B + \alpha_k^C + \alpha_{ij}^{AB} + \alpha_{ik}^{AC} + \alpha_{jk}^{BC} + \alpha_{ijk}^{ABC}, \\
i &= 1, \ldots, a,\ j = 1, \ldots, b,\ k = 1, \ldots, c.
\end{aligned} \tag{2.33}$$

The same problems of identifiability confront us with such models. To write down the usual constraints we must introduce another set of weights for each additional factor. Thus for an $a \times b \times c$ model we need a set of weights $w_k, k = 1, \ldots, c$ in addition to u_i and v_j as above. We may express the large number of constraints succinctly by denoting *weighted* averages by

$$\bar{\alpha}_{\cdot}^{A} = \sum_i u_i \alpha_i^A, \quad \bar{\alpha}_{i\cdot}^{AB} = \sum_j v_j \alpha_{ij}^{AB}, \quad \bar{\alpha}_{ij\cdot}^{ABC} = \sum_i w_k \alpha_{ijk}^{ABC},$$

and so on. For the model (2.33) the constraints now take the form

$$\begin{aligned}
&\bar{\alpha}_{\cdot}^{A} = \bar{\alpha}_{\cdot}^{B} = \bar{\alpha}_{\cdot}^{C} = 0,\\
&\bar{\alpha}_{i\cdot}^{AB} = \bar{\alpha}_{\cdot j}^{AB} = \bar{\alpha}_{i\cdot}^{AC} = \bar{\alpha}_{\cdot k}^{AC} = \bar{\alpha}_{j\cdot}^{BC} = \bar{\alpha}_{\cdot k}^{BC} = 0 \quad \text{for each } i, j, k, \text{ respectively},\\
&\bar{\alpha}_{ij\cdot}^{ABC} = \bar{\alpha}_{i\cdot k}^{ABC} = \bar{\alpha}_{\cdot jk}^{ABC} = 0 \quad \text{for each pair among } i, j, k, \text{ respectively.}
\end{aligned}$$

This leads to the following expressions:

$$\begin{aligned}
&\mu = \bar{\mu}_{\cdots}, \quad \alpha_i^A = \bar{\mu}_{i\cdot\cdot} - \bar{\mu}_{\cdots}, \quad \alpha_j^B = \bar{\mu}_{\cdot j\cdot} - \bar{\mu}_{\cdots}, \quad \alpha_k^C = \bar{\mu}_{\cdot\cdot k} - \bar{\mu}_{\cdots},\\
&\alpha_{ij}^{AB} = \bar{\mu}_{ij\cdot} - \bar{\mu}_{i\cdot\cdot} - \bar{\mu}_{\cdot j\cdot} + \bar{\mu}_{\cdots}, \quad \alpha_{ik}^{AC} = \bar{\mu}_{i\cdot k} - \bar{\mu}_{i\cdot\cdot} - \bar{\mu}_{\cdot\cdot k} + \bar{\mu}_{\cdots}, \qquad (2.34)\\
&\alpha_{jk}^{BC} = \bar{\mu}_{\cdot jk} - \bar{\mu}_{\cdot j\cdot} - \bar{\mu}_{\cdot\cdot k} + \bar{\mu}_{\cdots},\\
&\alpha_{ijk}^{ABC} = \mu_{ijk} - \bar{\mu}_{ij\cdot} - \bar{\mu}_{i\cdot k} - \bar{\mu}_{\cdot jk} + \bar{\mu}_{i\cdot\cdot} + \bar{\mu}_{\cdot j\cdot} + \bar{\mu}_{\cdot\cdot k} - \bar{\mu}_{\cdots}.
\end{aligned}$$

It is not hard to see that these expressions (except that for μ) are contrasts in cell means. We illustrate with a special example.

Example 2.15 Consider the model (2.33) for the $2 \times 2 \times 2$ factorial experiment with the equal weights (zero-sum) constraints. To be consistent with previous notation, let us assume that the indices i, j and k equal 0 or 1. One can show (Exercise 2.15) that when $i = j = k = 0$, the contrasts given by (2.34) are those of Table 2.1 multiplied by 1/8. Scheffé [121, page 121] notes the departure from the usual convention of $1/2^{k-1}$ that we indicated in Example 2.10.

To put this another way, let $\mathbf{X}$ be the 8×8 matrix consisting of the seven columns of Table 2.1 preceded by a column of ones:

$$\mathbf{X} = \begin{bmatrix}
1 & 1 & 1 & 1 & 1 & 1 & 1 & 1\\
1 & 1 & 1 & -1 & 1 & -1 & -1 & -1\\
1 & 1 & -1 & 1 & -1 & 1 & -1 & -1\\
1 & 1 & -1 & -1 & -1 & -1 & 1 & 1\\
1 & -1 & 1 & 1 & -1 & -1 & 1 & -1\\
1 & -1 & 1 & -1 & -1 & 1 & -1 & 1\\
1 & -1 & -1 & 1 & 1 & -1 & -1 & 1\\
1 & -1 & -1 & -1 & 1 & 1 & 1 & -1
\end{bmatrix}.$$

We note that the columns of $\mathbf{X}$ are mutually orthogonal and that in fact

$$\mathbf{X}'\mathbf{X} = 8\mathbf{I}. \tag{2.35}$$

Let $\boldsymbol{\mu}$ be the vector of cell means, ordered as in that table, and let

$$\boldsymbol{\beta} = (\mu, \alpha_0^A, \alpha_0^B, \ldots, \alpha_{000}^{ABC})', \tag{2.36}$$

consisting of the eight factor-effects parameters in (2.34) with $i = j = k = 0$. By what we have just observed,

$$\boldsymbol{\beta} = (1/8)\mathbf{X}'\boldsymbol{\mu}.$$

But then

$$\mathbf{X}\boldsymbol{\beta} = (1/8)\mathbf{X}\mathbf{X}'\boldsymbol{\mu} = \boldsymbol{\mu}, \tag{2.37}$$

and so if $\mathbf{Y}$ is a vector of observations, one per cell, then $\mathbf{Y}$ satisfies the linear model

$$\mathrm{E}(\mathbf{Y}) = \mathbf{X}\boldsymbol{\beta}. \tag{2.38}$$

Remark 2.16 An $n \times n$ matrix $\mathbf{H}$ of ± 1s satisfying $\mathbf{H}'\mathbf{H} = n\mathbf{I}$ is called a *Hadamard matrix* of order n. Equation (2.35) shows that the matrix $\mathbf{X}$ is a Hadamard matrix of order 8. In (2.37) we have made use of the fact that for such a matrix $\mathbf{H}$ we also have $\mathbf{H}\mathbf{H}' = n\mathbf{I}$, as is easily verified.

2.5.4 *The Different Systems of Weights*

As we noted after Example 2.14, different sets of weights (or of side conditions) cause the factor effects parameters to represent rather different comparisons between cell means. These are all comparisons of interest, but it is not clear for example whether α_i or α_i', if either, has greater claim to measuring "the effect of the ith level of A". Moreover, if we accept the idea that (2.26) represents the primary hypotheses of interest, then the hypotheses themselves depend on this choice. Sensitive to this problem, Scheffé gives the following result:

Theorem 2.17 ([121, page 93, Theorem 1]) *If the interactions $\{\gamma_{ij}\}$ are all zero for some system of weights $\{u_i\}$ and $\{v_j\}$, then they are all zero for every system of weights. In that case every contrast in the main effects $\{\alpha_i\}$ or $\{\beta_j\}$ has a value that does not depend on the system of weights $\{u_i\}$ and $\{v_j\}$, and the same is true for contrasts in the means $\{A_i\}$ and $\{B_j\}$ for the levels of A and B, respectively.*

The first part of this theorem may be rephrased to say that if additivity (non-interaction) holds in one system of weights, then it holds in all systems. It follows in fact that the *truth* of the hypothesis of additivity is invariant to the choice of weights: if it is true (false) in one system, then it is true (false) in all systems. This is reflected in our example: it is immediate that the expressions for γ'_{11} and γ'_{12} both belong to interaction as originally defined (the coefficient vectors are in U_{12}), and the reader may verify that the same is true of γ_{11} and γ_{12}.

When additivity holds, the theorem does *not* assert that the main effect parameters themselves are invariant to the choice of weights, but merely that *contrasts in them* are invariant (for example, the expression $\alpha_1 - \alpha_2$ would not depend on the choice of weights). Assuming additivity would be enough to let us assert that the truth of each main effect hypothesis is independent of this choice, and so the theorem is helpful *if one takes the position that one should only test the hypotheses concerning main effects when additivity holds.* We note that Scheffé does not share this philosophy [121, page 116]. We will have more to say about this position in Chap. 4.

Of course, we have already established definitions of the main effects hypotheses as well as that for interaction in Sect. 2.2, and so we may ask which choice of weights corresponds to these hypotheses. An examination of Example 2.14 shows that the contrasts for α_i belong to the main effect of A in the sense of Sect. 2.2, and those for β_j belong to B—that is, they are contrasts in row or column totals, respectively—but this is not true of α'_i and β'_j. This is not accidental, according to the following theorem, which also characterizes the choice of uniform weights in terms of orthogonality.

Theorem 2.18 *Consider the model (2.25) with constraints (2.28).*

a. The parameters α_i, β_j, and γ_{ij} are all contrasts in the cell means μ_{ij}.
b. The contrasts for γ_{ij} belong to `interaction` *no matter what system of weights is used.*
c. The contrasts for $\alpha_1, \ldots, \alpha_a$ belong to the main effect of A iff the weights $v_1, \ldots, v_b$ are equal, and similarly for β_j, B and u_i.
d. The contrast vectors for α_i, β_j, and γ_{ij} are mutually orthogonal if and only if $u_1 = \cdots = u_a$ and $v_1 = \cdots = v_b$.

In order to prove this, we need to represent each factor-effects parameter as a linear function of cell means. The coefficients of these functions can be read off of equations (2.30), as the reader can easily check. Let δ be the Kronecker delta ($\delta_{mn} = 1$ if $m = n$, and = 0 otherwise).

Lemma 2.19 *Write each factor-effect parameter as a linear combination of cell means. Then*

- *the ijth coefficient for a particular $\alpha_{i'}$ is*

$$(\delta_{ii'} - u_i)v_j\,, \tag{2.39}$$

- *the ijth coefficient for a particular $\beta_{j'}$ is*

$$u_i(\delta_{jj'} - v_j)\,.$$

- *the ijth coefficient for a particular $\gamma_{i'j'}$ is*

$$(\delta_{ii'} - u_i)(\delta_{jj'} - v_j)\,.$$

Proof of Theorem 2.18

(a) It is easy to see in each case that summing the coefficients over i and j gives zero.

(b) Let $\gamma_{i'j'} = \mathbf{e}'\boldsymbol{\mu}$. To show that $\mathbf{e} \in U_{12}$, we must show that $\mathbf{e} \perp U_1$ and U_2. Let $\mathbf{c}$ be an $ab \times 1$ vector whose ijth component c_{ij} is independent of j. (This is a bit more general than being an element of U_1.) Then there are constants c_i such that $c_{ij} \equiv c_i$ for all i and j, and

$$\begin{aligned}\mathbf{e} \cdot \mathbf{c} &= \sum_i \sum_j (\delta_{ii'} - u_i)(\delta_{jj'} - v_j)c_i \\ &= \sum_i c_i(\delta_{ii'} - u_i) \sum_j (\delta_{jj'} - v_j) \\ &= \sum_i c_i(\delta_{ii'} - u_i)(1 - 1) = 0,\end{aligned}$$

so that $\mathbf{e} \perp U_1$. Similarly, $\mathbf{e} \perp U_2$, and since $\mathbf{e}$ is a contrast vector, it must belong to U_{12}, as claimed.

(c) The coefficient vector $\mathbf{c}$ for $\alpha_{i'}$ belongs to U_1 if and only if its components (2.39) do not depend on j, that is, if and only if

$$(\delta_{ii'} - u_i)v_j = (\delta_{ii'} - u_i)v_{j'} \tag{2.40}$$

for all i, j and j'. Suppose this holds for every i'. Pick an index i' such that $u_{i'} \neq 1$, so that v is not the Kronecker delta at i'. Then $\delta_{ii'} - u_i \neq 0$ for some i, and with that choice of i we see that (2.40) holds iff $v_j = v_{j'}$ for all j and j'—that is, iff the weights v_j are equal, as claimed. The proof concerning $\beta_1, \ldots, \beta_b$ is similar.

(d) Let $\mathbf{c}_i$, $\mathbf{d}_j$, and $\mathbf{e}_{ij}$ be the coefficient vectors for α_i, β_j, and γ_{ij}, respectively. Now

$$\begin{aligned}\mathbf{c}_{i'} \cdot \mathbf{d}_{j'} &= \sum_i \sum_j (\delta_{ii'} - u_i)v_j\, u_i(\delta_{jj'} - v_j) \\ &= \sum_i (\delta_{ii'} - u_i)u_i \sum_j v_j(\delta_{jj'} - v_j),\end{aligned}$$

which equals 0 if and only if

$$\sum_i (\delta_{ii'} - u_i)u_i = 0 \quad \text{or} \quad \sum_j v_j(\delta_{jj'} - v_j) = 0. \tag{2.41}$$

Assume that (2.41)—that is, $\mathbf{c}_{i'} \perp \mathbf{d}_{j'}$ – holds for all i' and j'. If there is a j' such that $\sum_j v_j(\delta_{jj'} - v_j) \neq 0$ then we have $\sum_i (\delta_{ii'} - u_i)u_i = u_{i'} - \sum_i u_i^2 = 0$ for all i', so that $u_1 = \cdots = u_a$. If not, then $v_1 = \cdots = v_b$.

Assume that the weights u_i are equal. (The proof when v_j are equal is similar.) Now

$$\begin{aligned}\mathbf{e}_{i'j'} \cdot \mathbf{c}_{k'} &= \sum_i \sum_j (\delta_{ii'} - u_i)(\delta_{jj'} - v_j)\,(\delta_{ik'} - u_i)v_j \\ &= \sum_i (\delta_{ii'} - u_i)(\delta_{ik'} - u_i) \sum_j (\delta_{jj'} - v_j)v_j,\end{aligned}$$

which equals zero if and only if

$$\sum_i (\delta_{ii'} - u_i)(\delta_{ik'} - u_i) = 0 \quad \text{or} \quad \sum_j (\delta_{jj'} - v_j)v_j = 0. \tag{2.42}$$

But

$$\begin{aligned}\sum_i (\delta_{ii'} - u_i)(\delta_{ik'} - u_i) &= \sum_i \delta_{ii'}\delta_{ik'} - u_i \sum_i \delta_{ii'} - u_i \sum_i \delta_{ik'} + \sum_i u_i^2 \\ &= \delta_{i'k'} - \frac{1}{a} - \frac{1}{a} + \frac{a}{a^2} \\ &= \delta_{i'k'} - \frac{1}{a},\end{aligned}$$

which is never zero. Thus (2.42) holds (that is, $\mathbf{e}_{i'j'} \perp \mathbf{c}_{k'}$) for all i', j', and k' if and only if $\sum_j (\delta_{jj'} - v_j)v_j = 0$ for all j', which implies that $v_1 = \cdots = v_b$. □

Regarding part (b) we note that since there are $(a-1)(b-1)$ independent parameters γ_{ij}, and since $\dim U_{ij} = (a-1)(b-1)$, the contrast vectors corresponding to the parameters γ_{ij} actually span U_{12}. When equal weights are used, similar statements hold for the parameters α_i and β_j with respect to U_1 and U_2, respectively.

Interestingly, there is another inner product with respect to which the contrasts for the factor-effects parameters have the same orthogonality as in Theorem 2.18(d) if a different set of weights is used to define them; see Theorem 4.46.

Theorem 2.18 has a natural extension to experiments with three or more factors. Scheffé does not give a generalization of Theorem 2.17 to such designs.

2.6 The Cell-Means Philosophy

Models such as

$$E(Y_{ijk}) = \mu_{ij}$$

are generally known as *cell-means models*, since they are parametrized in terms of the cell means μ_{ij}. They became the focus of attention in the 1960s and '70s as alternatives to factor-effects models although they actually pre-date such models, as Urquhart, Weeks, and Henderson [142] point out. Indeed, the definition of main effects and interactions that we have used were described by Bose [22] in 1947, surely not the first such statement. Scheffé [121, Section 4.1] begins with cell means and builds the factor-effects parameters from them. The side conditions are then natural outgrowths of the model rather than ad hoc assumptions.

The renewed attention to cell means on the part of Hocking and Speed [73, 74, 134] and others occurred because of perceived inadequacies with models such as:

- the presence of inestimable quantities and untestable hypotheses in non-full-rank models. Cell-means models are always full-rank.
- the difficulty in determining the hypothesis actually being tested (the so-called *effective hypothesis*), particularly when there are empty cells (i.e., cells with no data). These questions are typically resolved by referring to cell means.

We may add to this

- the non-identifiability of the terms in non-full-rank models, and the ambiguity that remains due to different choices of constraints, as discussed above.

This ambiguity persists in practice. For example, SAS software uses the zero-sum constraints in formulating and testing hypotheses but uses baseline constraints for estimating effects (see, for example, pages 60 and 64 of [87]). Thus, using the same data one may fail to reject the hypothesis that $\alpha_i = 0$ for all i and yet find that the estimates for some of the α_i are significantly different from zero, or vice versa.

Even when full-rank, factor-effects models have a problem of

- interpretability. While cell means have an obvious meaning, the interpretation of factor-effects parameters is less direct.

The cell means are, of course, the expected values of observations. It is true that the factor-effects parameters are expected values of certain linear combinations of observations,[5] but these linear combinations do not have natural interpretations. Of course, one can simply say that the parameter μ is a "general mean", or that the quantity A_i in (2.29) is the mean for the ith level of A, but one may ask what these

[5] We deal with *estimability* in Chap. 3.

signify: what does it mean to compute an average of a set of expected values? One answer is to view a factor-effects model as a hierarchical model in which the weights function as prior distributions on rows, columns, or cells. This comes close to the example suggested by Scheffé [121, page 91]. The factor-effects parameters are then viewed as conditional or unconditional expected values (see Exercise 2.17).

A final issue might be called

- flexibility. Factor-effects models are designed to facilitate the formulation of basic hypotheses concerning main effects and interactions. They are not convenient for other hypotheses, such as arise in post hoc analysis.

Since the cell-means approach avoids these problems, one may ask why factor-effects models remain so widely used. Undoubtedly it is because of their intuitive appeal: the *absence* of a particular effect is expressed by the *absence* of the corresponding parameters. In the cell-means formulation, by contrast, the *absence* of an effect is expressed by the *presence* of certain relations between cell means.

Searle [123, Sections 7.5 and 8.1f] has a good discussion on the advantages of the cell-means approach.

2.7 Random Effects: Components of Variance

The one-factor model (2.18) is often written in the *signal + noise* form

$$Y_{ij} = \mu + \tau_i + e_{ij}, \tag{2.43}$$

where the "noise" terms e_{ij} are independent zero-mean random variables. In certain applications we also take the quantities τ_i to be zero-mean random variables with the same variance, generally assumed independent (and independent of e_{ij}). This is the simplest case of a *random effects model.* The term τ_i is the *random effect.* We often assume that τ_i and e_{ij} are normally distributed, in which case the observations Y_{ij} are as well.

Example 2.20 According to Scheffé[6] [119], perhaps the earliest instance of this model occurred in 1861, when mathematician and Astronomer Royal Sir George Biddell Airy used it to describe measurement error in astronomical observations, where τ_i is the error peculiar to conditions on the ith night, while e_{ij} are the additional errors of each measurement each night.

Example 2.21 One of the most influential applications of this model occurs in biology, where Y_{ij} is the phenotype (observed trait) of the jth offspring of the

[6] Scheffé credits Churchill Eisenhart for information about the early role of astronomers in using such models.

ith father (sire), τ_i are sire effects, and e_{ij} are random effects due to environment, genetic variation among mothers, and other sources. The sire effects are viewed as random because the fathers are viewed merely as a random sample of all possible sires.

Because of the assumption of independence, we see that

$$\sigma_Y^2 = \sigma_\tau^2 + \sigma_e^2, \tag{2.44}$$

and it is a consequence of equations such as (2.44) that models with random effects are known as *variance components models*. A second consequence is that the observations Y are no longer independent, as they are typically assumed to be in fixed-effects models. For example, in the model (2.43) we easily verify that

$$\text{Cov}(Y_{ij}, Y_{ij'}) = \sigma_\tau^2$$

for $j \neq j'$. In the animal model, this means that the phenotypes of half-sibs (sharing the same father) are correlated, as might be expected. We thus have

$$\begin{aligned} \text{Cov}(Y_{ij}, Y_{i'j'}) &= \sigma_\tau^2 + \sigma_e^2, \quad && i = i', j = j', \\ &= \sigma_\tau^2, && i = i', j \neq j', \\ &= 0, && i \neq i'. \end{aligned} \tag{2.45}$$

The mean and covariance structure of model (2.43) may be summarized as follows. Assume that there are n_i observations for treatment i, where $i = 1, \ldots, a$, and let us put the observations in a single vector $\mathbf{Y} = (Y_{11}, \ldots, Y_{1n_1}, \ldots, Y_{a1}, \ldots, Y_{an_a})'$. Then $\mathbf{Y}$ has mean vector

$$\boldsymbol{\mu} = \mu \mathbf{1}$$

and, according to (2.45), a block-diagonal covariance matrix

$$\boldsymbol{\Sigma} = \begin{bmatrix} \boldsymbol{\Sigma}_1 & \mathbf{0} & \cdots & \mathbf{0} \\ \mathbf{0} & \boldsymbol{\Sigma}_2 & \ddots & \vdots \\ \vdots & \ddots & \ddots & \mathbf{0} \\ \mathbf{0} & \cdots & \mathbf{0} & \boldsymbol{\Sigma}_a \end{bmatrix}$$

where $\boldsymbol{\Sigma}_i$ is an $n_i \times n_i$ matrix of the form $\sigma_\tau^2 \mathbf{J} + \sigma_e^2 \mathbf{I}$, $\mathbf{I}$ is an identity matrix, $\mathbf{J}$ is a matrix of ones, $\mathbf{0}$ is a matrix of zeros, and $\mathbf{I}$, $\mathbf{J}$ and $\mathbf{0}$ are of appropriate (and varying) sizes. If the sample sizes n_i are equal with common value n, say, then the matrices on the diagonal are all equal to $\sigma_\tau^2 \mathbf{J}_n + \sigma_e^2 \mathbf{I}_n$, where the subscripts on $\mathbf{I}$ and $\mathbf{J}$ denote the dimensions, and $\mathbf{\Sigma}$ itself can be written as a *Kronecker product*

$$\mathbf{\Sigma} = \mathbf{I}_a \otimes (\sigma_\tau^2 \mathbf{J}_n + \sigma_e^2 \mathbf{I}_n).$$

This form is convenient for some computations.

Consider two-factor model

$$Y_{ijk} = \mu + \alpha_i + \beta_j + \gamma_{ij} + e_{ijk} \tag{2.46}$$

where e_{ijk} are assumed to be independent with zero mean and finite variance σ_e^2. A fixed-effects model would impose side conditions on α_1, β_j and γ_{ij}, as in Sect. 2.5.2. A random-effects model assumes that the variables α, β, γ and e are random and independent with mean 0 and with finite variances $\sigma_\alpha^2, \sigma_\beta^2, \sigma_\gamma^2$ and σ_e^2, respectively.

A *third* possibility is a *mixed model* in which, say, factor A is random and B is fixed. This means that the terms α_i and γ_{ij} are random with zero mean, while β_j are fixed and random terms are independent. In this case we must impose a side condition such as

$$\sum_j \beta_j = 0. \tag{2.47}$$

With this, we see that the mean of Y satisfies the one-factor model

$$\mathrm{E}(Y_{ijk}) = \mu + \beta_j \quad \text{for all } i, k$$

while the covariances are

$$\begin{aligned} \mathrm{Cov}(Y_{ijk}, Y_{i'j'k'}) &= \sigma_\alpha^2 + \sigma_\gamma^2 + \sigma_e^2, & i = i', j = j', k = k', \\ &= \sigma_\alpha^2 + \sigma_\gamma^2, & i = i', j = j', k \neq k', \\ &= \sigma_\alpha^2, & i = i', j \neq j', \\ &= 0 & i \neq i'. \end{aligned}$$

The term *variance components model* includes both random-effects and mixed models, and so has become standard.

The matrix expression of the mean vector and (especially) the covariance matrix of the observation vector $\mathbf{Y}$ for models with two or more factors is much more complicated than for one-factor models. For balanced experiments, though, the Kronecker product greatly simplifies this expression. For example, for the mixed model above let $\mathbf{Y}$ be the vector of observations Y_{ijk} are ordered lexicographically, k within j within i, and suppose that there are n observations per ij-cell. Putting

$$\boldsymbol{\nu} = [\mu + \beta_1, \ldots, \mu + \beta_b]', \ \mathbf{B} = \sigma_\alpha^2 \mathbf{J}_n, \ \text{and } \mathbf{D} = \sigma_e^2 \mathbf{I}_n + \sigma_\gamma^2 \mathbf{J}_n,$$

we see (Exercise 2.18) that $\mathbf{Y}$ has mean vector

$$\boldsymbol{\mu} = \mathbf{1}_a \otimes \boldsymbol{\nu} \otimes \mathbf{1}_n \tag{2.48}$$

and covariance matrix

$$\boldsymbol{\Sigma} = \mathbf{I}_a \otimes (\mathbf{J}_b \otimes \mathbf{B} + \mathbf{I}_b \otimes \mathbf{D}), \tag{2.49}$$

where as usual A has a levels and B has b levels.

Remark 2.22 In mixed models, any interaction term is assumed to be random if it involves a random factor. Thus in the model (2.46) where we assume that α is random and β fixed, γ must also be random. Because the interaction also includes a fixed effect, the literature sometimes suggests a side condition on γ corresponding to the fixed effect, in this instance

$$\sum_j \gamma_{ij} = 0 \text{ for each } i. \tag{2.50}$$

Since γ_{ij} are random variables, the constraints (2.50) are assumed to hold with probability 1, and for each i the variables γ_{ij} are correlated. There is no general agreement on whether to assume (2.50). See Section 4.3c(iv) of [125] for a discussion.

Scheffé develops one approach to such constraints in [121, Section 8.1]. As he states in [120], his initial motivation is his objection to the usual assumption of independence of the parameters in the mixed model. He starts instead with a two-factor model

$$Y_{ijk} = m_{ij} + e_{ijk}$$

where the quantities m and e are both random and independent but where m_{ij} satisfy several assumptions that he believes are reasonable. From these he *defines* quantities α_i, β_j and γ_{ij} satisfying (2.46), and then deduces their covariance structure, somewhat different from the usual one. This is similar to the way he creates the factor-effects parameters from cell means in a fixed-effects model [121, Section 4.1], and in fact he refers to m_{ij} as "cell means". As it turns out, his parameters γ do satisfy (2.50) (with the roles of i and j reversed as he assumes B to be the random effect).

The hypothesis that a random effect is absent is that the corresponding variance component is zero. Thus in the one-factor model (2.43) the hypothesis of no effect is

$$H_0\colon \sigma_\tau^2 = 0.$$

In the two-factor model (2.46) with factors A and B, if both factors are random then the hypotheses to be tested are

$$H_0\colon \sigma_\alpha^2 = 0 \quad \text{(No } A \text{ effect)}$$
$$H_0\colon \sigma_\beta^2 = 0 \quad \text{(No } B \text{ effect)}$$
$$H_0\colon \sigma_\gamma^2 = 0 \quad \text{(No interaction)}$$

These are of course very different from the hypotheses we test in the fixed-effects model. In a mixed model where factor B is random, the hypotheses about the B effect and about interaction are as above, while the hypothesis of no A effect is the usual one[7] for a one-factor experiment.

We will give a brief overview of estimation and testing in variance components models in Section 4.9. The text by Searle, Casella and McCulloch [125] is a standard reference on the subject.

Remark 2.23 A history of variance components models is given in [119, Section 2], and more recently in [125, Chapter 2]. An exposition and discussion from the cell-means point of view is given in [73]. We will touch on this briefly at the end of Sect. 4.9.

Fisher's seminal 1918 paper on population genetics notes equation (2.44) [55, page 405, with different notation], and indeed his goal is to break apart total variance into constituent parts.[8] This paper introduced the terms *variance* and *analysis of variance*.

2.8 Exercises

Section 2.1

2.1 Prove Proposition 2.1.

Section 2.2

2.2 (i) Show that the equations in display (2.5) are linearly independent.
(ii) Show that the equations in display (2.8) are linearly independent.

2.3 In the proof of Proposition 2.4, give an alternate, direct proof that $U \subset U_{B\,\text{only}}$. That is, describe the contrasts of $U_{B\,\text{only}}$ and show that it contains all contrasts of the form (2.12). (See Remark 2.5.)

2.4 Prove Proposition 2.6.

2.6 Display a basis of each of U_1, U_2 and U_{12} in a 2×3 experiment.

---

[7] Assuming the zero-sum side condition (2.47).

[8] Fisher does not explicitly write down a model such as (2.43) in [55].

2.6 Construct a 2×2 example having cell means showing non-additivity and a main effect of B but such that there is no main effect of A. (See Remark 2.9.)

2.7 In Remark 2.9 we raised the question of giving an alternate rationale for the description of the two main-effects hypotheses that we derived in Proposition 2.6. Can you provide such a rationale?

Section 2.3

2.8 Use the definitions of U_{12} and U_{123} in (2.15) to determine the contrast vectors for AB and for ABC.

Section 2.4

2.9 Verify the contrast vectors in Example 2.12.

2.10 Exercise 7 of [81, Chapter 6], gives the results of a three-factor soil science experiment in which the two quantitative factors are water content of the soil and salinity of the water, each at three levels. A statistical package has been used to calculate the linear and quadratic contrast vectors. The water content has been set at 0, 5 and 15 percent, and the package computed the following contrasts:

Linear:	−0.617	−0.154	0.772
Quadratic:	0.535	−0.802	−0.267

These numbers are rounded, and are not easy to interpret. Show that the vectors $(-4, -1, 5)$ and $(2, -3, 1)$ are exact linear and quadratic contrasts.

2.11 Table 3.51 of [151] gives data for a 3-factor "muzzle velocity" experiment in which one factor, the Discharge Hole Area, is measured at levels 0.016, 0.030, 0.048, and 0.062 inches. Find the contrast vectors for the linear, quadratic and cubic effects of this factor, expressed in small integers. (Answer: the cubic effect vector is $(9, -23, 23, -9)'$.)

Section 2.5

2.12 Show that (2.28) contains $a+b+1$ independent equations. In particular, show that the $a+b$ equations constraining the parameters γ_{ij} contain $a+b-1$ independent equations.

2.13 Derive equations (2.30).

2.14 In Example 2.14:

(i) Show that γ_{11} and γ_{12} belong to interaction in the sense that their coefficient vectors belong to U_{12}.

(ii) Show that if additivity is assumed, then $\alpha_1' - \alpha_2' = \alpha_1 - \alpha_2$, as predicted by Theorem 2.17.

2.15 In the $2 \times 2 \times 2$ design, indexing levels by 0 and 1, show that when $i = j = k = 0$, the contrasts given by (2.34) are those of Table 2.1 multiplied by 1/8, as asserted in Example 2.15.

2.16 Show that if $\mathbf{H}$ is a Hadamard matrix of order n, then $\mathbf{HH}' = n\mathbf{I}$.

Section 2.6

2.17 Assume a population has been stratified by level of factor A ("rows") and of B ("columns"). Suppose the A-strata occur in proportions $u_1, \ldots, u_a$, and B-strata, $v_1, \ldots, v_b$, so that $\sum_i u_i = \sum_j v_j = 1$. Assume that a cell is chosen at random such that the probability of cell ij is $u_i v_j$. Let Y be an observation from the population with conditional mean $\mu_{ij} = \mathrm{E}(Y|\text{cell } ij)$. Show how to interpret the parameters A_i and B_j (Eq. (2.29)) as conditional expected values of Y, and the parameter μ as $\mathrm{E}(Y)$ (unconditional). What do α_i, β_j, and γ_{ij} represent? (Formulas (2.30) may help.)

Section 2.7

2.18 Verify formulas (2.48) and (2.49). (For the latter, it may help to build $\mathbf{\Sigma}$ in steps. The vector of responses in cell (i, j) has covariance matrix $\mathbf{B} + \mathbf{D}$. For fixed i, the covariance matrix of the vector of responses is a block matrix of the form $\mathbf{J}_b \otimes \mathbf{B} + \mathbf{I}_b \otimes \mathbf{D}$.)

Chapter 3
Estimation

Abstract This brief chapter introduces least squares estimation in a linear model, in particular the error sum of squares, and studies the basic distribution theory of the resulting estimators. It introduces t-tests and t-intervals as well, in anticipation of the next chapter. The Moore-Penrose inverse of the regression/design matrix $\mathbf{X}$ also makes its first appearance.

Given a linear model

$$\mathrm{E}(\mathbf{Y}) = \mathbf{X}\boldsymbol{\beta}, \tag{3.1}$$

our primary interest will be in estimating $\boldsymbol{\beta}$ as well as linear parametric functions $\mathbf{c}'\boldsymbol{\beta}$. We will also estimate σ^2 when the model assumes that $\mathbf{Y}$ has covariance matrix $\boldsymbol{\Sigma} = \sigma^2\mathbf{I}$. As before, we assume that $\mathbf{Y}$ is $N \times 1$ and $\boldsymbol{\beta}$ is $p \times 1$. *We will assume throughout that* $N \geq p$.

Suppose that we simply index the observations by the numbers 1 through N. Then each Y_j in model (3.1) satisfies

$$\mathrm{E}(Y_j) = \mathbf{x}^{(j)}\boldsymbol{\beta}, \quad j = 1, \ldots, N, \tag{3.2}$$

where $\mathbf{x}^{(j)}$ is the jth *row* of $\mathbf{X}$. For example, in a polynomial regression model (1.13) of degree $p-1$ there are numbers $x_1, \ldots, x_N$, not necessarily distinct, such that

$$\mathrm{E}(Y_j) = \beta_0 + \beta_1 x_j + \beta_2 x_j^2 + \cdots + \beta_{p-1} x_j^{p-1}, \quad j = 1, \ldots, N. \tag{3.3}$$

In this case we would have $x^{(j)} = (1, x_j, x_j^2, \ldots, x_j^{p-1})$. For a given set of observations, estimating $\boldsymbol{\beta}$ would amount to fitting a polynomial function to the data points (x_j, Y_j). Using the estimates $\hat{\beta}_i$, the quantities

$$\hat{Y}_j = \hat{\beta}_0 + \hat{\beta}_1 x_j + \hat{\beta}_2 x_j^2 + \cdots + \hat{\beta}_{p-1} x_j^{p-1} \tag{3.4}$$

J. H. Beder, *Linear Models and Design*,
https://doi.org/10.1007/978-3-031-08176-7_3

are called *fitted values*. In general, if $\hat{\boldsymbol{\beta}}$ is an estimate of $\boldsymbol{\beta}$, then $\hat{\mathbf{Y}} = \mathbf{X}\hat{\boldsymbol{\beta}}$ is the *vector of fitted values*. This applies to factorial as well as to regression models.

Typically we have $N \gg p$. In the extreme case that $N = p$, and assuming that $\mathbf{X}$ is nonsingular, we could estimate $\boldsymbol{\beta}$ by *equating* each observed value Y_j with its fitted value, that is, replacing E($\mathbf{Y}$) in (3.1) by $\mathbf{Y}$, and simply solve for $\boldsymbol{\beta}$. For the polynomial regression model (3.3) with distinct values x_j, this would amount to passing a curve through the data points (x_j, y_j) where y_j is the observed value of Y_j. Keeping in mind that y_j is simply one value of a random variable, we understand that this would amount to *overfitting* the data by starting with a model with too many terms. And of course, if $N > p$ then this will not even be possible. Thus we need methods of estimation in which the the fitted values are *close to* the observed values y_j in some overall sense. There are many ways to do this, the oldest and still the most common being that of *least squares*.

In what follows, we will not distinguish notationally between the random variable Y_j and a particular observed value y_j, using Y_j for both. Context will tell which is meant. Thus, when we write E(Y_j) we clearly mean the random variable Y_j, while estimation will be performed "pointwise", that is, at each observed value of Y_j.

The case that $N < p$ introduces particular problems, as we indicate in an exercise. While we will not pursue this topic further, we should note that it has become an area of active research in recent years due to the proliferation of data sets with very large numbers of parameters (where, in fact, $p \gg N$). The survey [77], along with accompanying papers, describes situations in which such data arise and various approaches to statistical inference in such cases.

3.1 The Method of Least Squares

We continue to index the observations by 1 through N for the moment. Let us use $\hat{Y}_j$ to represent the fitted value of Y at $\mathbf{x}^{(j)}$, that is,

$$\hat{Y}_j = \mathbf{x}^{(j)}\boldsymbol{\beta}.$$

In asking that $\hat{Y}_j$ be "close to" its corresponding observed value, we are choosing $\boldsymbol{\beta}$ to minimize the quantities

$$|Y_j - \hat{Y}_j|$$

simultaneously. As its name implies, the method of least squares does this by minimizing the quantity

$$\sum_{j=1}^{N}(Y_j - \hat{Y}_j)^2. \tag{3.5}$$

We recognize this expression as representing a squared distance in $\mathbb{R}^N$ in the usual Euclidean metric. That is, letting $\mathbf{Y}$ and $\hat{\mathbf{Y}}$ be the vectors of observed and fitted values, respectively, we must choose $\boldsymbol{\beta}$ to minimize

$$\|\mathbf{Y} - \hat{\mathbf{Y}}\|^2, \tag{3.6}$$

where $\|\mathbf{v}\| = \sum_j v_j^2$. Writing the sum (3.5) in this form is notationally convenient, as we no longer need to index the observations or fitted values by the numbers 1 through N. It is also conceptually essential.

Remark 3.1 Other distance measures could be used, for example, $\|\mathbf{v}\| = \sum_j |v_j|$, the L^1-norm, or more generally $\sum_j(|v_j|^p)^{1/p}$, the L^p norm. There is no question that the Euclidean norm ($p = 2$) is the most commonly used, probably because the resulting mathematical theory is simplest.

The minimization of (3.6) is constrained by the condition that

$$\hat{\mathbf{Y}} = \mathbf{X}\boldsymbol{\beta} \tag{3.7}$$

for some $\boldsymbol{\beta}$. This means that $\hat{\mathbf{Y}} \in V = R(\mathbf{X})$, the columnspace[1] of $\mathbf{X}$. The vector $\mathbf{Y}$ is an element of $\mathbb{R}^N$, V is a subspace of $\mathbb{R}^N$, and $\hat{\mathbf{Y}}$ is the element of V closest to $\mathbf{Y}$. Theorem A.64 guarantees that such a $\hat{\mathbf{Y}}$ exists and is uniquely determined by the condition

$$\mathbf{Y} - \hat{\mathbf{Y}} \perp V. \tag{3.8}$$

That is, we find $\hat{\mathbf{Y}}$ by "dropping a perpendicular" from $\mathbf{Y}$ to V. From (3.7) we may write

$$\hat{\mathbf{Y}} = \beta_1\mathbf{x}_1 + \cdots + \beta_p\mathbf{x}_p$$

where $\mathbf{x}_i$ are the columns of $\mathbf{X}$. Since these vectors span V, the condition (3.8) is equivalent to

$$\mathbf{Y} - \hat{\mathbf{Y}} \perp \mathbf{x}_1, \ldots, \mathbf{x}_p$$

(Theorem A.57(c)). We may write this equivalently as

$$\mathbf{x}_i'(\mathbf{Y} - \hat{\mathbf{Y}}) = 0, \; i = 1, \ldots, p,$$

[1] We use the notation $R(\mathbf{X})$ because it represents the range of $\mathbf{X}$ viewed as a linear transformation; see Section A.4.8.

or

$$\mathbf{x}_i'\mathbf{Y} = \mathbf{x}_i'\hat{\mathbf{Y}},$$

or finally

$$\mathbf{X}'\mathbf{Y} = \mathbf{X}'\hat{\mathbf{Y}}.$$

But (3.7) allows us to rewrite this as

$$\mathbf{X}'\mathbf{Y} = \mathbf{X}'\mathbf{X}\boldsymbol{\beta}. \tag{3.9}$$

Equation (3.9) specifies a system of equations for $\beta_1, \ldots, \beta_p$, known as the *normal equations*. We say somewhat colloquially that *we have regressed Y on $x_1, \ldots, x_p$* (or $\mathbf{Y}$ *on* $\mathbf{x}_1, \ldots, \mathbf{x}_p$).

We summarize what we have shown:

Theorem 3.2 *The vector $\hat{\mathbf{Y}} = \mathbf{X}\hat{\boldsymbol{\beta}}$ minimizes (3.6) over all $\hat{\mathbf{Y}}$ satisfying (3.7) if and only if $\hat{\boldsymbol{\beta}}$ satisfies the normal equations (3.9).*

We note that $\hat{\mathbf{Y}}$ exists and is unique, by the Minimization Theorem. This implies that the normal equations are solvable for $\boldsymbol{\beta}$, no matter what the value of $\mathbf{Y}$. But rank($\mathbf{X}'\mathbf{X}$) = rank($\mathbf{X}$) (Theorem A.99). Thus if $\mathbf{X}$ has full rank (p), then the $p \times p$ matrix $\mathbf{X}'\mathbf{X}$ is invertible, and the *least squares estimator of* $\boldsymbol{\beta}$ is

$$\hat{\boldsymbol{\beta}} = (\mathbf{X}'\mathbf{X})^{-1}\mathbf{X}'\mathbf{Y}. \tag{3.10}$$

Moreover, from (3.7) we have

$$\hat{\mathbf{Y}} = \mathbf{X}(\mathbf{X}'\mathbf{X})^{-1}\mathbf{X}'\mathbf{Y} \tag{3.11}$$

Proposition 3.3 *The matrix*

$$\mathbf{P} = \mathbf{X}(\mathbf{X}'\mathbf{X})^{-1}\mathbf{X}' \tag{3.12}$$

is the matrix of the orthogonal projection P of $\mathbb{R}^N$ on V, the columnspace of $\mathbf{X}$.

Remark 3.4 Proposition 3.3 can be stated in a slightly different way that is often useful: Given any subspace $V \subset \mathbb{R}^N$, the orthogonal projection of $\mathbb{R}^N$ on V is given by the matrix (3.12), where $\mathbf{X}$ is any matrix whose columns are a basis of V. Note that the projection map is unique, so $\mathbf{P}$ is the same no matter what basis is used.

The matrix $\mathbf{P}$ is sometimes called the "hat matrix", as $\mathbf{PY} = \hat{\mathbf{Y}}$ ("Y-hat").

If rank($\mathbf{X}$) $< p$, then $\mathbf{X}'\mathbf{X}$ will not be invertible. In fact, in this case there will be infinitely many solutions $\hat{\boldsymbol{\beta}}$ to (3.9), although they all express the same element $\hat{\mathbf{Y}}$

in (3.7). For each value of $\mathbf{Y}$ the set of solutions can be given as $\hat{\boldsymbol{\beta}}_0 + N(\mathbf{X}'\mathbf{X})$, where $\hat{\boldsymbol{\beta}}_0$ is a particular solution and $N(\mathbf{X}'\mathbf{X})$ is the nullspace of the linear transformation given by $\mathbf{X'X}$, that is, the set of solutions of the homogeneous equation $\mathbf{X}'\mathbf{X}\boldsymbol{\beta} = \mathbf{0}$ (Theorem A.39). (By Corollary A.80 the solution set is $\hat{\boldsymbol{\beta}}_0 + N(\mathbf{X})$.) There is no canonical choice for the particular solution. This should not surprise us, as $\boldsymbol{\beta}$ itself is not identifiable when $\mathbf{X}$ is not of full rank. We are trying to estimate a quantity that doesn't have a well-defined value.

There are quite a few methods of defining a matrix $\mathbf{G}$ that gives a particular solution $\hat{\boldsymbol{\beta}} = \mathbf{G}\mathbf{X}'\mathbf{Y}$. Such matrices are called *generalized inverses* of $\mathbf{X}'\mathbf{X}$.

Definition 3.5 ([113, page 153]) Given an $m \times n$ matrix $\mathbf{A}$, a *generalized inverse* of $\mathbf{A}$ is an $n \times m$ matrix $\mathbf{G}$ such that for all $\mathbf{z} \in R(\mathbf{A})$ we have

$$\mathbf{Ax} = \mathbf{z} \quad \text{iff} \quad \mathbf{x} = \mathbf{Gz}. \tag{3.13}$$

Note that the condition $\mathbf{z} \in R(\mathbf{A})$ is precisely the condition that the equation $\mathbf{Ax} = \mathbf{z}$ has a solution. One can show [113, Lemma 1] that $\mathbf{G}$ is generalized inverse of $\mathbf{A}$ if and only if

$$\mathbf{AGA} = \mathbf{A}, \tag{3.14}$$

a condition that is often taken as a definition of a generalized inverse. A theorem of Bjerhammer [18, Theorem 1.2] asserts that if (3.14) holds then we also have

$$\mathbf{GAG} = \mathbf{G} \tag{3.15}$$

if and only if $\text{rank}(\mathbf{G}) = \text{rank}(\mathbf{A})$. A generalized inverse satisfying (3.15) is said to be *reflexive*.[2]

In general, a matrix $\mathbf{A}$ may have many generalized inverses. The *Moore-Penrose inverse* of $\mathbf{A}$, for example, gives us the solution $\mathbf{x}$ of $\mathbf{Ax} = \mathbf{z}$ of smallest norm (guaranteed to exist by Corollary A.66). Two classical sources on the theory of generalized inverses are [18] and [115]; the latter includes a lot of applications to statistics. Both give methods of construction.

When $\mathbf{X}$ does not have full rank, the question of whether any generalized solutions $\hat{\boldsymbol{\beta}}$ to the normal equations should be called "estimators of $\boldsymbol{\beta}$" seems unresolved in the literature. Scheffé [121, page 9] and Christensen [37, Corollary 2.2.2] do, although they are careful to use the indefinite article (e.g., "*a* least squares estimate"). Searle [123, page 169] is rather emphatic in *not* using the term "estimator" in this case, referring only to "a solution" of the normal equations.

The vector $\hat{\mathbf{Y}}$ of fitted values does not suffer from such complications. We know that it exists and is uniquely determined by $\mathbf{Y}$, and is given by projecting

[2] Ben-Israel and Greville [18] define generalized inverses more broadly, so that $\mathbf{G}$ may be a matrix satisfying (3.15) but not (3.14).

$\mathbf{Y}$ orthogonally on $R(\mathbf{X})$. Let $\mathbf{P}$ be the matrix of this orthogonal projection, so that $\hat{\mathbf{Y}} = \mathbf{PY}$. In the full-rank case, $\mathbf{P}$ is the "hat matrix" (3.12). In the non-full-rank case, we may take $\mathbf{P} = \mathbf{XGX}'$ where $\mathbf{G}$ is a generalized inverse of $\mathbf{X}'\mathbf{X}$. This requires computing a generalized inverse. Alternatively, we may simply choose a submatrix $\mathbf{X}_0$ of $\mathbf{X}$ consisting of $r = \text{rank}(\mathbf{X})$ linearly independent columns. Then $\mathbf{X}_0$ has full rank, and $\mathbf{P}$ is the hat matrix based on $\mathbf{X}_0$.

A significant practical difficulty occurs when $\mathbf{X}$ has full rank but the columns are *nearly* linearly dependent. This is generally avoidable in factorial models but can easily occur in multiple regression models, a phenomenon called *multicollinearity* that we described in Sect. 1.4. In such a case it is difficult to solve the normal equations accurately (the problem is said to be *ill-conditioned*). Unless one or more independent variables can be removed from the model on theoretical grounds, estimation is generally carried out in a modified form via techniques such as *ridge regression*[3]. Christensen [37, Chapter 14] discusses multicollinearity (referred to there as "collinearity") and reviews several approaches to deal with it.

...

Least squares is a distribution-free method of estimation. The only assumption we have made about $\mathbf{Y}$ is the form of its expected value. In the next section we will study the properties of least squares estimators as we add various distributional assumptions.

3.2 Properties of Least Squares Estimators

In this section we will deal not only with the least squares estimator $\hat{\boldsymbol{\beta}}$ but also with estimators of linear parametric functions $\mathbf{c}'\boldsymbol{\beta}$.

When $\mathbf{X}$ has full rank, $\hat{\boldsymbol{\beta}}$ is given by (3.10), and so from the results given in Sect. 1.1 we immediately have the following facts. Their proof is left as an exercise.

Theorem 3.6 *Suppose* $\mathbf{Y}$ *satisfies the linear model* $\text{E}(\mathbf{Y}) = \mathbf{X}\boldsymbol{\beta}$, *where* $\mathbf{X}$ *has full rank.*

a. *The least squares estimator* $\hat{\boldsymbol{\beta}}$ *is unbiased for* $\boldsymbol{\beta}$.
b. *If* $\text{Var}(\mathbf{Y}) = \sigma^2\mathbf{I}$ *then* $\text{Var}(\hat{\boldsymbol{\beta}}) = \sigma^2(\mathbf{X}'\mathbf{X})^{-1}$.
c. *If* $\mathbf{Y}$ *is normally distributed, then so is* $\hat{\boldsymbol{\beta}}$.
d. *If* $\text{Var}(\mathbf{Y}) = \sigma^2\mathbf{I}$ *and* $\mathbf{Y}$ *is normally distributed, then* $\hat{\boldsymbol{\beta}}$ *is the MLE of* $\boldsymbol{\beta}$.

Proof The first two parts of the theorem come directly from Theorem 1.4, the latter two from Theorem 1.6.

(a) $\text{E}(\hat{\boldsymbol{\beta}}) = \text{E}((\mathbf{X}'\mathbf{X})^{-1}\mathbf{X}'\mathbf{Y}) = (\mathbf{X}'\mathbf{X})^{-1}\mathbf{X}'\mathbf{X}\boldsymbol{\beta} = \boldsymbol{\beta}$.
(b) $\text{Var}(\hat{\boldsymbol{\beta}}) = (\mathbf{X}'\mathbf{X})^{-1}\mathbf{X}'\sigma^2\mathbf{I}\mathbf{X}(\mathbf{X}'\mathbf{X})^{-1} = \sigma^2(\mathbf{X}'\mathbf{X})^{-1}\mathbf{X}'\mathbf{X}(\mathbf{X}'\mathbf{X})^{-1} = \sigma^2(\mathbf{X}'\mathbf{X})^{-1}$.
(c) This follows immediately from Theorem 1.6(a).

[3] Or *Tikhonov regularization*.

(d) The exponent of the likelihood function of $\boldsymbol{\beta}$ is $-1/2$ times

$$(\mathbf{y}-\mathbf{X}\boldsymbol{\beta})'(\sigma^2\mathbf{I})^{-1}(\mathbf{y}-\mathbf{X}\boldsymbol{\beta}) = \sigma^{-2}\|\mathbf{y}-\mathbf{X}\boldsymbol{\beta}\|^2.$$

Thus the likelihood is maximized iff this expression is minimized.

□

Special care is needed in framing these results when $\mathbf{X}$ does not have full rank. A version of Theorem 3.6 is given as an exercise. No such issues surround the vector $\hat{\mathbf{Y}}$ of fitted values:

Theorem 3.7 *Suppose* $\mathbf{Y}$ *satisfies the linear model* $\mathrm{E}(\mathbf{Y}) = \mathbf{X}\boldsymbol{\beta}$, *and let* $\hat{\mathbf{Y}} = \mathbf{P}\mathbf{Y}$ *be the vector of fitted values, where* $\mathbf{P}$ *is the matrix of the orthogonal projection of* $\mathbb{R}^n$ *on* $R(\mathbf{X})$.

a. $\mathrm{E}(\hat{\mathbf{Y}}) = \mathbf{X}\boldsymbol{\beta}$.
b. If $\mathrm{Var}(\mathbf{Y}) = \sigma^2\mathbf{I}$ *then* $\mathrm{Var}(\hat{\mathbf{Y}}) = \sigma^2\mathbf{P}$.
c. If $\mathbf{Y}$ *is normally distributed, then so is* $\hat{\mathbf{Y}}$.

Note that this theorem holds independent of whether or not $\mathbf{X}$ has full rank. The proof of the theorem is left as an exercise.

The vector

$$\mathbf{e} = \mathbf{Y} - \hat{\mathbf{Y}} \tag{3.16}$$

is known as the *vector of residuals*. The residuals are the basis for many diagnostics that are used to check the validity of a particular analysis, such as the assumptions of normality and homoscedasticity (equal variance). Such tests are covered in many textbooks on regression and analysis of variance, and will not be discussed here. Underlying these tests are the following properties.

Theorem 3.8 *Let* $\mathbf{Y}$ *and* $\mathbf{P}$ *be as in Theorem 3.7.*

a. $\mathrm{E}(\mathbf{e}) = \mathbf{0}$.
b. If $\mathrm{Var}(\mathbf{Y}) = \sigma^2\mathbf{I}$ *then* $\mathrm{Var}(\mathbf{e}) = \sigma^2(\mathbf{I}-\mathbf{P})$.
c. $\mathrm{Cov}(\hat{\mathbf{Y}}, \mathbf{e}) = \mathbf{0}$.
d. If $\mathbf{X}$ *has full rank then* $\mathrm{Cov}(\hat{\boldsymbol{\beta}}, \mathbf{e}) = \mathbf{0}$.
e. If $\mathbf{Y}$ *is normally distributed, then so is* $\mathbf{e}$.

For many common models, the residuals (the components of $\mathbf{e}$) sum to zero. This and the proof of Theorem 3.8 are left as exercises.

3.2.1 Estimability

We have seen in Sect. 1.6.1 that a linear parametric function $\mathbf{c}'\boldsymbol{\beta}$ is identifiable if and only if $\mathbf{c} \in R(\mathbf{X}')$, that is, iff $\mathbf{c} = \mathbf{X}'\mathbf{a}$ for some $\mathbf{a} \in \mathbb{R}^N$. In particular, all such functions are identifiable if $\mathbf{X}$ has full rank. We now see how to estimate them.

Definition 3.9 Suppose $\mathbf{Y}$ satisfies a linear model $\mathrm{E}(\mathbf{Y}) = \mathbf{X}\boldsymbol{\beta}$. A real-valued estimator is said to be *linear* if it is of the form $\mathbf{a}'\mathbf{Y}$. An identifiable function $\mathbf{c}'\boldsymbol{\beta}$ is said to be *estimable* if it has a linear unbiased estimator (abbreviated LUE). An LUE of $\mathbf{c}'\boldsymbol{\beta}$ is *best (BLUE)* if it has minimum variance among all LUEs of $\mathbf{c}'\boldsymbol{\beta}$.

Lemma 3.10 *In a linear model* $\mathrm{E}(\mathbf{Y}) = \mathbf{X}\boldsymbol{\beta}$, *all identifiable functions* $\mathbf{c}'\boldsymbol{\beta}$ *are estimable. In particular, if* $\mathbf{a}$ *is any solution of* $\mathbf{X}'\mathbf{a} = \mathbf{c}$, *then* $\mathbf{a}'\mathbf{Y}$ *is an LUE of* $\mathbf{c}'\boldsymbol{\beta}$.

Proof If $\mathbf{c}'\boldsymbol{\beta}$ is identifiable, the solution $\mathbf{a}$ exists (Proposition 1.29). We then have $\mathrm{E}(\mathbf{a}'\mathbf{Y}) = \mathbf{a}'\mathbf{X}\boldsymbol{\beta} = \mathbf{c}'\boldsymbol{\beta}$. □

Note that LUEs are not unique, since solutions to $\mathbf{X}'\mathbf{a} = \mathbf{c}$ are not. Thus we may ask for the optimal one.

Theorem 3.11 (Gauss-Markov) *Suppose* $\mathbf{Y}$ *satisfies a linear model* $\mathrm{E}(\mathbf{Y}) = \mathbf{X}\boldsymbol{\beta}$ *and that* $\mathrm{Var}(\mathbf{Y}) = \sigma^2\mathbf{I}$. *If* $\mathbf{c}'\boldsymbol{\beta}$ *is identifiable then it has a unique BLUE* $\mathbf{a}'\mathbf{Y}$. *The vector* $\mathbf{a}$ *is the unique shortest solution of* $\mathbf{X}'\mathbf{a} = \mathbf{c}$, *and is also the unique solution orthogonal to* $N(\mathbf{X}')$.

Proof The solutions $\mathbf{a}$ of $\mathbf{X}'\mathbf{a} = \mathbf{c}$ are a set of the form $\mathbf{a} + N(\mathbf{X}')$, where $\mathbf{a}$ is a particular solution (Theorem A.39(c)). Now $\mathrm{Var}(\mathbf{a}'\mathbf{Y}) = \mathbf{a}'\sigma^2\mathbf{I}\,\mathbf{a} = \sigma^2\|\mathbf{a}\|^2$, so we are seeking the solution of minimum length. But this vector exists and is unique, according to Corollary A.66. □

Corollary 3.12 *If* $\mathbf{X}$ *has full rank, then the BLUE of* $\mathbf{c}'\boldsymbol{\beta}$ *is* $\mathbf{c}'\hat{\boldsymbol{\beta}}$ *where* $\hat{\boldsymbol{\beta}}$ *is the least-squares estimator of* $\boldsymbol{\beta}$. *We have* $\mathrm{Var}(\mathbf{c}'\hat{\boldsymbol{\beta}}) = \sigma^2\mathbf{c}'(\mathbf{X}'\mathbf{X})^{-1}\mathbf{c}$.

Proof If $\mathbf{X}$ has full rank, then $\mathbf{c}'\hat{\boldsymbol{\beta}} = \mathbf{c}'(\mathbf{X}'\mathbf{X})^{-1}\mathbf{X}'\mathbf{Y} = \mathbf{a}'\mathbf{Y}$ where

$$\mathbf{a} = \mathbf{X}(\mathbf{X}'\mathbf{X})^{-1}\mathbf{c}. \tag{3.17}$$

We need just show that $\mathbf{a} \perp N(\mathbf{X}')$. But by Theorem A.79 this holds iff $\mathbf{a} \in R(\mathbf{X})$, which is obviously true from the expression (3.17).

The variance of the estimator comes from Theorem 1.4(b), applied to $\hat{\boldsymbol{\beta}}$ (rather than to $\mathbf{Y}$). □

A version of Corollary 3.12 holds for identifiable functions $\mathbf{c}'\boldsymbol{\beta}$ even if $\mathbf{X}$ does not have full rank. This is left as an exercise. It is natural to refer to $\mathbf{c}'\hat{\boldsymbol{\beta}}$ as a *least squares estimator* of $\mathbf{c}'\boldsymbol{\beta}$, although it is $\boldsymbol{\beta}$ and not $\mathbf{c}'\boldsymbol{\beta}$ that is estimated via least squares.

If we make the additional assumption that $\mathbf{Y}$ is normally distribution, then Theorem 3.6 tells us that $\hat{\boldsymbol{\beta}} \sim N(\boldsymbol{\beta}, \sigma^2(\mathbf{X}'\mathbf{X})^{-1})$, from which we immediately have the following:

Proposition 3.13 *If* $\mathbf{Y} \sim N(\mathbf{X}\boldsymbol{\beta}, \sigma^2\mathbf{I})$ *and if* $\hat{\boldsymbol{\beta}}$ *is the least squares estimator of* $\boldsymbol{\beta}$*, then* $\mathbf{c}'\hat{\boldsymbol{\beta}} \sim N(\mathbf{c}'\boldsymbol{\beta}, \sigma^2\mathbf{c}'(\mathbf{X}'\mathbf{X})^{-1}\mathbf{c})$.

Remark 3.14 Typically Lemma 3.10 is phrased to say that $\mathbf{c}'\boldsymbol{\beta}$ is estimable if and only if $\mathbf{c} \in R(\mathbf{X}')$. In the present exposition, we have used the latter condition to characterize identifiability, not estimability . Once $\mathbf{c}'\boldsymbol{\beta}$ is identifiable, we can find a linear estimator of it. The missing "only if" statement is really a principle: if $\mathbf{c}'\boldsymbol{\beta}$ is not identifiable, then it can't be estimated – by any function of the data, linear or not. Rao [113, page 156] simply uses the term "estimable" for identifiable.

The term *estimable* in the sense of Definition 3.9 is generally credited to Bose [21]. Plackett [105] reviews the history of the Gauss-Markov Theorem, in particular the roles of Gauss and Markov.

3.2.2 The Moore-Penrose Inverse of X

We may for a moment take a closer look at the matrix $\mathbf{X}(\mathbf{X}'\mathbf{X})^{-1}$ in equation (3.17). For given $\mathbf{c} \in \mathbb{R}^p$ it gives the unique shortest solution of $\mathbf{X}'\mathbf{a} = \mathbf{c}$, and is therefore the Moore-Penrose inverse of $\mathbf{X}'$. We may call this $\mathbf{T}'$, so that

$$\mathbf{T} = (\mathbf{X}'\mathbf{X})^{-1}\mathbf{X}'. \tag{3.18}$$

Note that the estimator $\hat{\boldsymbol{\beta}}$ has the form $\hat{\boldsymbol{\beta}} = \mathbf{TY}$.

Since we are assuming that $\mathbf{X}$ has full rank, we see that if $\mathbf{Xv} = \mathbf{z}$ is consistent—that is, if $\mathbf{z} \in R(\mathbf{X})$—then there is a unique solution $\mathbf{v} \in \mathbb{R}^p$, given by $\mathbf{v} = \mathbf{Tz}$, as is easily verified. Thus $\mathbf{T}$ is the Moore-Penrose inverse of $\mathbf{X}$. We summarize these and other useful properties of $\mathbf{T}$ in the following.

Lemma 3.15 *Let* $\mathbf{T}$ *be defined by (3.18), where* $\mathbf{X}$ $(N \times p)$ *has rank* p*. Then*

a. $\mathbf{TX} = \mathbf{X}'\mathbf{T}' = \mathbf{I}$, *where* $\mathbf{I}$ *is the* $p \times p$ *identity matrix.*
b. $\mathbf{XT} = \mathbf{T}'\mathbf{X}' = \mathbf{P}$, *the "hat matrix" representing the orthogonal projection of* $\mathbb{R}^N$ *on* $R(\mathbf{X})$.
c. $\mathbf{T}'$ *maps* $\mathbb{R}^p$ *into* $\mathbb{R}^N$ *in a one-to-one manner.* $\mathbf{T}$ *maps* $\mathbb{R}^N$ *onto* $\mathbb{R}^p$*, and is one-to-one on* $R(\mathbf{X})$.
d. *If* $\mathbf{u}, \mathbf{w} \in \mathbb{R}^p$ *and* $\mathbf{u} \perp \mathbf{w}$ *then* $\mathbf{T}'\mathbf{u} \perp \mathbf{Xw}$.

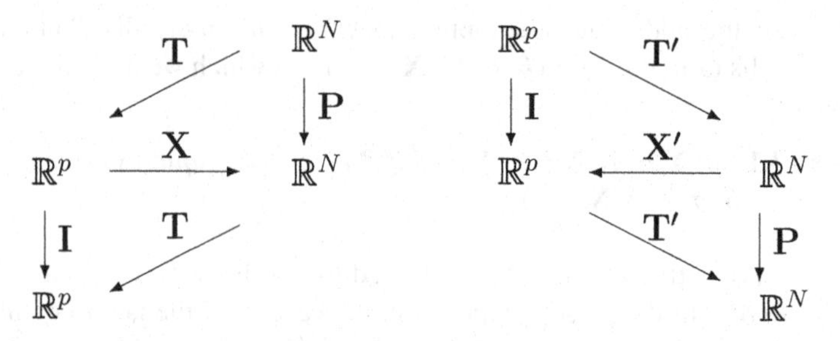

Fig. 3.1 The relationships between $\mathbf{X}$ and $\mathbf{T} = (\mathbf{X}'\mathbf{X})^{-1}\mathbf{X}'$, and between their transposes, as described in Lemma 3.15. $\mathbf{P} = \mathbf{XT}$ = the "hat matrix" = the orthogonal projection on $R(\mathbf{X})$ ($\mathbf{P}$ results when the arrow for $\mathbf{X}$ *follows* that for $\mathbf{T}$). $\mathbf{I}$ is the identity matrix

Relations described in this lemma are depicted in Fig. 3.1. Part (a) says that $\mathbf{T}$ is a *left-inverse* of $\mathbf{X}$ and that $\mathbf{T}'$ is a *right-inverse* of $\mathbf{X}'$.

Proof Matrix multiplication gives (a) and (b), the latter using (3.12).

(c) $\mathbf{T}'$ defines a one-to-one map since both $\mathbf{X}$ and $(\mathbf{X}'\mathbf{X})^{-1}$ are full-rank. The fact that $R(\mathbf{T}') = \mathbb{R}^p$ follows, for example, from Theorem A.79(d) and the one-to-oneness of $\mathbf{T}'$. Finally, since the maps $\mathbf{X}$ and $\mathbf{TX}$ ($= \mathbf{I}$) are one-to-one, $\mathbf{T}$ must be one-to-one on $R(\mathbf{X})$.

(d) Since $\mathbf{TX} = \mathbf{I}$, we have $(\mathbf{T}'\mathbf{u}) \cdot (\mathbf{Xw}) = \mathbf{u}'\mathbf{TXw} = \mathbf{u}'\mathbf{w} = 0$. □

3.3 Estimating σ^2: Sum of Squares, Mean Square

We now add to the linear model

$$\mathrm{E}(\mathbf{Y}) = \mathbf{X}\boldsymbol{\beta} \tag{3.19}$$

the assumption that

$$\mathrm{Var}(\mathbf{Y}) = \sigma^2\mathbf{I}, \tag{3.20}$$

and ask for an estimator of σ^2.

As before, we let $\hat{\mathbf{Y}}$ be the vector of fitted values using least squares, and let

$$SSE = \|\mathbf{Y} - \hat{\mathbf{Y}}\|^2$$

be the *sum of squares for error*. (It is a sum of squares since $\|\mathbf{v}\|^2 = \sum_i v_i^2$.) We interpret this quantity as follows:

> SSE measures the amount of variation in the data not accounted for by the model.

Note that $SSE = \|\mathbf{e}\|^2$, where $\mathbf{e}$ is the vector of residuals. Since in many models the residuals sum to zero, as we've remarked, this variation "balances out."

We note that $\mathbf{Y} - \hat{\mathbf{Y}} = (\mathbf{I} - \mathbf{P})\mathbf{Y}$ where $\mathbf{P}$ is the matrix of the orthogonal projection of $\mathbb{R}^N$ on $R(\mathbf{X})$, where N is the length $\mathbf{Y}$. Since $\mathbf{I} - \mathbf{P}$ is an orthogonal projection (Corollary A.91), we need to study the distribution of $\|\mathbf{QY}\|^2$ for orthogonal projection matrices $\mathbf{Q}$. Recall that such matrices are characterized by being symmetric and idempotent (Theorem A.107), so that

$$\|\mathbf{QY}\|^2 = \mathbf{Y}'\mathbf{Q}'\mathbf{QY} = \mathbf{Y}'\mathbf{QY},$$

a *quadratic form* in $\mathbf{Y}$ (see Remark 3.18 below).

Theorem 3.16 *Let $\mathbf{Y}$ be an $N \times 1$ satisfying a linear model* $\mathrm{E}(\mathbf{Y}) = \mathbf{X}\boldsymbol{\beta}$, *and let $\mathbf{Q}$ be an orthogonal projection matrix of rank $r > 0$. Let $\delta = \boldsymbol{\beta}'\mathbf{X}'\mathbf{QX}\boldsymbol{\beta}$.*

a. If $\mathrm{Var}(\mathbf{Y}) = \sigma^2\mathbf{I}$, *then*

$$\mathrm{E}(\|\mathbf{QY}\|^2) = r\sigma^2 + \delta. \tag{3.21}$$

b. If in addition $\mathbf{Y}$ is normally distributed, then

$$\frac{\|\mathbf{QY}\|^2}{\sigma^2} \sim \chi^2(r, \delta/\sigma^2). \tag{3.22}$$

Proof Let $\mathbf{O}$ be an orthogonal matrix such that $\mathbf{O}'\mathbf{QO} = \mathbf{D}$ where $\mathbf{D}$ is the diagonal matrix $\mathrm{diag}(\underbrace{1, \ldots, 1}_{r}, \underbrace{0, \ldots, 0}_{N-r})$ (Corollary A.113), and put $\mathbf{Z} = \mathbf{O}'\mathbf{QY}$. Then $\mathbf{QY} = \mathbf{OZ}$, so

$$\|\mathbf{QY}\|^2 = \|\mathbf{OZ}\|^2 = \|\mathbf{Z}\|^2 = \sum_{i=1}^{N} Z_i^2, \tag{3.23}$$

where $\mathbf{Z} = (Z_1, \ldots, Z_N)'$.

Let $\mu_i = \mathrm{E}(Z_i)$ and $\boldsymbol{\mu} = (\mu_1, \ldots, \mu_N)'$. Then

$$\boldsymbol{\mu} = \mathbf{O}'\mathbf{Q}\mathbf{X}\boldsymbol{\beta}$$

and

$$\mathrm{Var}(\mathbf{Z}) = \mathbf{O}'\mathbf{Q}(\sigma^2\mathbf{I})\mathbf{Q}'\mathbf{O} = \sigma^2\mathbf{O}'\mathbf{Q}\mathbf{O} = \sigma^2\mathbf{D}.$$

Note that $Z_{r+1}, \ldots, Z_N$ have zero variance and thus equal their means with probability 1. Thus

$$\mathrm{E}(Z_i^2) = \mathrm{Var}(Z_i) + \mu_i^2 = \begin{cases} \sigma^2 + \mu_i^2, & i \leq r; \\ \mu_i^2, & i > r. \end{cases},$$

so

$$\mathrm{E}(\|\mathbf{Z}\|^2) = \sum_{i=1}^{N} \mathrm{E}(Z_i^2) = r\sigma^2 + \sum_{i=1}^{N} \mu_i^2 = r\sigma^2 + \|\boldsymbol{\mu}\|^2.$$

Since

$$\|\boldsymbol{\mu}\|^2 = \|\mathbf{O}'\mathbf{Q}\mathbf{X}\boldsymbol{\beta}\|^2 = \boldsymbol{\beta}'\mathbf{X}'\mathbf{Q}'\mathbf{O}\mathbf{O}'\mathbf{Q}\mathbf{X}\boldsymbol{\beta} = \boldsymbol{\beta}'\mathbf{X}'\mathbf{Q}\mathbf{X}\boldsymbol{\beta} = \delta,$$

we have (3.21).

Before proving (3.22), we observe that $\mu_i = 0$ for $i > r$. To prove this, we note that $\mathbf{O}'\mathbf{Q} = \mathbf{D}\mathbf{O}'$ (multiply $\mathbf{O}'\mathbf{Q}\mathbf{O} = \mathbf{D}$ on the right by $\mathbf{O}'$), so

$$\boldsymbol{\mu} = \mathbf{D}\mathbf{O}'\mathbf{X}\boldsymbol{\beta}.$$

But the entries of the last $N - r$ rows of $\mathbf{D}$ are all zero, so the same is true of $\boldsymbol{\mu}$, as claimed. Now since $\mathbf{Y}$ is normally distributed, so is $\mathbf{Z}$; specifically, $\mathbf{Z} \sim N(\boldsymbol{\mu}, \sigma^2\mathbf{D})$, so that

$$\begin{aligned} Z_i &\sim N(\mu_i, \sigma^2), \quad i \leq r, \\ &= 0 \quad \text{with probability 1}, \quad i > r \end{aligned}$$

and $Z_1, \ldots, Z_r$ are independent. Thus $Z_i/\sigma \sim N(\mu_i/\sigma^2, 1)$ for $i \leq r$, so by Theorem 1.9 we have

$$\|\mathbf{Z}\|^2/\sigma^2 = \sum_{i=1}^{r} (Z_i/\sigma)^2 \quad \text{with probability 1}$$

$$\sim \chi^2(r, \sum_{i=1}^{r} \mu_i^2/\sigma^2)$$

$$= \chi^2(r, \|\boldsymbol{\mu}\|^2/\sigma^2) = \chi^2(r, \delta/\sigma^2),$$

which is (3.22). □

From this we easily get our desired result:

Corollary 3.17 *Assume that* $\mathrm{E}(\mathbf{Y}) = \mathbf{X}\boldsymbol{\beta}$, *with* $r = \mathrm{rank}(\mathbf{X})$. *Let* $\hat{\mathbf{Y}}$ *be the vector of fitted values, and let* $SSE = \|\mathbf{Y} - \hat{\mathbf{Y}}\|^2$. *If* $\mathrm{Var}(\mathbf{Y}) = \sigma^2\mathbf{I}$, *the quantity* $SSE/(N-r)$ *is unbiased for* σ^2. *If in addition* **Y** *is normally distributed, then* $SSE/\sigma^2 \sim \chi^2(N-r)$.

Proof Let **P** be the matrix of the orthogonal projection of $\mathbb{R}^N$ on $R(\mathbf{X})$, where **Y** is $N \times 1$. We apply Theorem 3.16 with $\mathbf{Q} = \mathbf{I} - \mathbf{P}$. Our result follows as $\mathbf{QX} = \mathbf{0}$, so that $\delta = 0$. □

The integer $N - r$ is known as the *degrees of freedom for error*, and the quantity

$$MSE = SSE/(N - r)$$

is known variously as the *mean squared error* or the *mean square for error*. Corollary 3.17 says that under the usual variance assumption (3.20) the MSE is unbiased for σ^2, and that $(N-r)MSE/\sigma^2 \sim \chi^2(N-r)$ if **Y** is normally distributed. The MSE is often denoted s^2, which one must be careful to distinguish from the ordinary sample variance. Like the sample variance, the MSE is defined by dividing a measure of sample variability by the number of "independent" pieces of data. In the present case that number is the rank of $\mathbf{I}-\mathbf{P}$. This is in keeping with the comment made in Sect. 1.1 that "degrees of freedom" generally represents the dimension of a vector space. Other mean squares will be introduced in succeeding sections, each defined by the formula SS/df.

Remark 3.18 We have noted that $\|\mathbf{QY}\|^2 = \mathbf{Y}'\mathbf{QY}$ when **Q** is symmetric and idempotent. An expression of the form $\mathbf{Y}'\mathbf{AY} = \sum_i \sum_j a_{ij} Y_i Y_j$ is called a *quadratic form* in **Y** . The results of Theorem 3.16 and the corollary are usually expressed in terms of such forms. For example, the linear substitution $\mathbf{Z} = \mathbf{O}'\mathbf{QY}$ *diagonalized* the form $\mathbf{Y}'\mathbf{QY}$, as we see in (3.23).

There is a converse to Theorem 3.16(b) asserting that if $\mathbf{Y}'\mathbf{AY}$ has a noncentral chi-square distribution, then **A** is symmetric and idempotent; see [128, page 7].

Example 3.19 Consider a one-way factorial model with p treatments, n_i observations on the ith treatment, and put $N = \sum_i n_i$. Let Y_{ij} be the jth observation on the ith treatment and $\mu_i = \mathrm{E}(Y_{ij})$, and let

$$\boldsymbol{\mu} = (\mu_1, \ldots, \mu_p)' \quad \text{and} \quad \mathbf{Y} = (Y_{11}, \cdots, Y_{1n_1}, \cdots, Y_{p1}, \cdots, Y_{pn_p})'.$$

Then $E(\mathbf{Y}) = \mathbf{X}\boldsymbol{\mu}$ where the $N \times p$ design matrix is

$$\mathbf{X} = \begin{pmatrix} \mathbf{1}_{n_1} & & \\ & \ddots & \\ & & \mathbf{1}_{n_p} \end{pmatrix},$$

where $\mathbf{1}_n$ is the $n \times 1$ vector of ones. Here $\text{rank}(\mathbf{X}) = p$ and we have

$$\mathbf{X}'\mathbf{X} = \begin{pmatrix} n_1 & & \\ & \ddots & \\ & & n_p \end{pmatrix} \quad \text{and} \quad \mathbf{X}'\mathbf{Y} = \begin{pmatrix} Y_{1\cdot} \\ \vdots \\ Y_{p\cdot} \end{pmatrix}.$$

From $\hat{\boldsymbol{\mu}} = (\mathbf{X}'\mathbf{X})^{-1}\mathbf{X}'\mathbf{Y}$ and $\hat{\mathbf{Y}} = \mathbf{X}\hat{\boldsymbol{\mu}}$ we have

$$\hat{\boldsymbol{\mu}} = (\bar{Y}_{1\cdot}, \ldots, \bar{Y}_{p\cdot})' \quad \text{and} \quad \hat{\mathbf{Y}} = (\underbrace{\bar{Y}_1, \ldots, \bar{Y}_1}_{n_1}, \ldots, \underbrace{\bar{Y}_p, \ldots, \bar{Y}_p}_{n_p})',$$

so that

$$SSE = \|\mathbf{Y} - \hat{\mathbf{Y}}\|^2 = \sum_{i=1}^{p}\sum_{j=1}^{n_i}(Y_{ij} - \bar{Y}_{i\cdot})^2.$$

There are $N - p$ df for error, and $MSE = SSE/(N - p)$.

Example 3.20 We apply a similar procedure to the simple linear regression model in which $E(Y_i) = \beta_0 + \beta_1 x_i$, $i = 1, \ldots, N$. Here we put $\mathbf{Y} = (Y_1, \ldots, Y_N)'$, $\mathbf{x} = (x_1, \ldots, x_N)'$, $\boldsymbol{\beta} = (\beta_0, \beta_1)'$, and $\mathbf{X} = (\mathbf{1}\ \mathbf{x})$ (an $N \times 2$ matrix), so that $E(\mathbf{Y}) = \mathbf{X}\boldsymbol{\beta}$. Let $S_{xx} = \sum_i (x_i - \bar{x})^2$. We leave it as an exercise to show:

a. $\det \mathbf{X}'\mathbf{X} = N S_{xx}$.

b. $\hat{\boldsymbol{\beta}} = \dfrac{1}{S_{xx}} \begin{pmatrix} \sum_i x_i^2 \bar{Y} - \bar{x} \sum_i x_i Y_i \\ \sum_i x_i Y_i - N\bar{x}\bar{Y} \end{pmatrix}$.

c. $\hat{\beta}_0 = \bar{Y} - \hat{\beta}_1 \bar{x}$. That is, the point $(\bar{x}, \bar{Y})$ lies on the *estimated regression line* $y = \hat{\beta}_0 + \hat{\beta}_1 x$.

d. There are $N - 2$ degrees of freedom for error.

We have $\hat{\mathbf{Y}} = \hat{\beta}_0\mathbf{1} + \hat{\beta}_1\mathbf{x}$, and $SSE = \|\mathbf{Y} - \hat{\mathbf{Y}}\|^2 = \sum_{i=1}^{N}(Y_i - \hat{\beta}_0 - \hat{\beta}_1 x_i)^2$. There are various ways of writing SSE (or MSE), none of them terribly simple—see, for example, [65, page 178].

3.4 t-Tests, t-Intervals

In this section we briefly leave the topic of estimation to deal with hypothesis tests and confidence intervals. These are taken up more fully in Chap. 4.

Corollary 3.12 to the Gauss-Markov Theorem found the BLUE of $\mathbf{c}'\boldsymbol{\beta}$ to be $\mathbf{c}'\hat{\boldsymbol{\beta}}$ where $\hat{\boldsymbol{\beta}}$ is the least squares estimator of $\boldsymbol{\beta}$. Proposition 3.13 asserted that $\mathbf{c}'\hat{\boldsymbol{\beta}} \sim N(\mathbf{c}'\boldsymbol{\beta}, \sigma^2\mathbf{c}'(\mathbf{X}'\mathbf{X})^{-1}\mathbf{c})$. In practice, σ^2 is unknown, and according to Corollary 3.17 it is natural to replace it by the mean square error.

Theorem 3.21 *Let* $\mathbf{Y} \sim N(\mathbf{X}\boldsymbol{\beta}, \sigma^2\mathbf{I})$, *where* $\mathbf{Y}$ *is* $N \times 1$ *and* $\mathbf{X}$ *has full rank* p. *Let* $\hat{\boldsymbol{\beta}}$ *be the least squares estimator of* $\boldsymbol{\beta}$. *Then*

$$\frac{\mathbf{c}'\hat{\boldsymbol{\beta}} - \mathbf{c}'\boldsymbol{\beta}}{\sqrt{MSE\,\mathbf{c}'(\mathbf{X}'\mathbf{X})^{-1}\mathbf{c}}} \sim t(N-p). \tag{3.24}$$

The proof is a standard application of Definition 1.11, and is left as an exercise. Theorem 3.21 gives us the standard *t-test* of hypotheses of the form $H_0 : \mathbf{c}'\boldsymbol{\beta} = a$. We use the test statistic

$$T = \frac{\mathbf{c}'\hat{\boldsymbol{\beta}} - a}{\sqrt{MSE\,\mathbf{c}'(\mathbf{X}'\mathbf{X})^{-1}\mathbf{c}}}, \tag{3.25}$$

rejecting H_0 at level α if

$T > t_{N-p,\alpha}$ if the alternative hypothesis is H_1: $\mathbf{c}'\boldsymbol{\beta} > a$;
$T < -t_{N-p,\alpha}$ if the alternative hypothesis is H_1: $\mathbf{c}'\boldsymbol{\beta} < a$;
$|T| > t_{N-p,\alpha/2}$ if the alternative hypothesis is H_1: $\mathbf{c}'\boldsymbol{\beta} \neq a$.

We note that a one-sided alternative has a one-tailed test, and the two-sided alternative, a two-tailed test.

We may form a level $1-\alpha$ *confidence interval* for $\mathbf{c}'\boldsymbol{\beta}$ by inverting the test, that is, by finding all values of a in (3.25) that would *not* be rejected by a given test (see Sect. 1.2.3). For the two-tailed test, the interval would consist of those a for which

$$\left|\frac{\mathbf{c}'\hat{\boldsymbol{\beta}} - a}{\sqrt{MSE\,\mathbf{c}'(\mathbf{X}'\mathbf{X})^{-1}\mathbf{c}}}\right| \le t_{N-p,\alpha/2}.$$

giving the usual *t-interval*

$$\mathbf{c}'\hat{\boldsymbol{\beta}} - t_{N-p,\alpha/2}\sqrt{MSE\,\mathbf{c}'(\mathbf{X}'\mathbf{X})^{-1}\mathbf{c}} \le \mathbf{c}'\boldsymbol{\beta} \le \mathbf{c}'\hat{\boldsymbol{\beta}} + t_{N-p,\alpha/2}\sqrt{MSE\,\mathbf{c}'(\mathbf{X}'\mathbf{X})^{-1}\mathbf{c}}. \tag{3.26}$$

If we invert one of the one-tailed tests, we get an interval with ∞ or $-\infty$ as an endpoint, in which case the finite endpoint is called a *confidence bound*..

Note in particular that if we choose $\mathbf{c} = [0, \ldots, 1, \ldots, 0]'$, with 1 as the ith coordinate and 0's elsewhere, then (3.26) is a confidence interval for β_i.

Example 3.22 Consider the simple linear regression model in Example 3.20. Suppose we wish to find a confidence interval for the expected response at a particular x—not necessarily one of the x_i at which we originally collected data. The expected response is $\mathrm{E}(Y) = \beta_0 + \beta_1 x = \mathbf{c}'\boldsymbol{\beta}$ where

$$\mathbf{c}' = [1, x].$$

With $\mathbf{X}$ as in Example 3.20, one can show (Exercise 3.11) that

$$\mathbf{c}'(\mathbf{X}'\mathbf{X})^{-1}\mathbf{c} = \frac{1}{n} + \frac{(x-\bar{x})^2}{S_{xx}}, \tag{3.27}$$

where $S_{xx} = \sum_i (x_i - \bar{x})^2$, so that the confidence interval will have endpoints

$$\hat{\beta}_0 + \hat{\beta}_1 x \pm t_{N-2,\alpha/2}\sqrt{MSE\left(\frac{1}{N} + \frac{(x-\bar{x})^2}{S_{xx}}\right)}. \tag{3.28}$$

In particular, the narrowest interval will occur for $x = \bar{x}$, the average of the points $x_1, \ldots, x_N$ that were actually sampled.

The two-tailed t-test is a special case of a likelihood ratio test (or *Wald* test) that will be developed in Sects. 4.2 and 4.7.

3.5 Exercises

Section 3.1

3.1 Let $\mathbf{X}$ be $N \times p$, and suppose $N < p$. As before, $R(\mathbf{X})$ is the columnspace of $\mathbf{X}$, or the range of $\mathbf{X}$ as a linear transformation.

(i) Show that for any $\hat{\mathbf{Y}} \in R(\mathbf{X})$, equation (3.7) has infinitely many solutions $\boldsymbol{\beta}$.

(ii) Suppose for simplicity that $\mathbf{X}$ has full rank (namely N). Show that we minimize $\|\mathbf{Y} - \hat{\mathbf{Y}}\|^2$ over all $\hat{\mathbf{Y}} \in R(\mathbf{X})$ by taking $\hat{\mathbf{Y}} = \mathbf{Y}$. (Hint: In this case, what is the relationship between $\mathbb{R}^N$ and $R(\mathbf{X})$?)

(iii) In [123, page 79] it is asserted that there is no estimation problem when $N \le p$, since a value of $\boldsymbol{\beta}$ can be derived so that $\mathbf{Y} = \mathbf{X}\boldsymbol{\beta}$ exactly. What do you think of that assertion?

3.2 Show that $\mathbf{G}$ is a generalized inverse of $\mathbf{A}$ if and only if (3.14) holds. (If: Equation (3.13) holds in particular when $\mathbf{z}$ is a column of $\mathbf{A}$. Only if: Show that $\mathbf{AGAx} = \mathbf{Ax}$ for all $\mathbf{x}$).

Section 3.2

3.3 Prove the following version of Theorem 3.6, applicable when $\mathbf{X}$ does not have full rank.

Theorem 3.23 *Suppose* $\mathbf{Y}$ *satisfies the linear model* $\mathrm{E}(\mathbf{Y}) = \mathbf{X}\boldsymbol{\beta}$. *Let* $\mathbf{G}$ *be a generalized inverse of* $\mathbf{X}'\mathbf{X}$, *and let* $\hat{\boldsymbol{\beta}} = \mathbf{G}\mathbf{X}'\mathbf{Y}$.

(i) $\mathbf{G}\mathbf{X}'\mathbf{X}\boldsymbol{\beta}$ *is identifiable, and* $\mathrm{E}(\hat{\boldsymbol{\beta}}) = \mathbf{G}\mathbf{X}'\mathbf{X}\boldsymbol{\beta}$.
(ii) If $\mathrm{Var}(\mathbf{Y}) = \sigma^2\mathbf{I}$ *and* $\mathbf{G}$ *is reflexive, then* $\mathrm{Var}(\hat{\boldsymbol{\beta}}) = \sigma^2\mathbf{G}$.
(iii) If $\mathbf{Y}$ *is normally distributed, then so is* $\hat{\boldsymbol{\beta}}$.
(iv) If $\mathrm{Var}(\mathbf{Y}) = \sigma^2\mathbf{I}$ *and* $\mathbf{Y}$ *is normally distributed, then* $\hat{\boldsymbol{\beta}}$ *is an MLE of* $\boldsymbol{\beta}$.

3.4 Prove Theorem 3.7. You do not neet to know the form of $\mathbf{P}$, or whether $\mathbf{X}$ has full rank, just that $\mathbf{P}$ is the orthogonal projection on $R(\mathbf{X})$. See Theorem A.107.

3.5 Prove Theorem 3.8. Is part(d) valid if $\mathbf{X}$ does not have full rank?

3.6 In both a regression model with a constant term and a factorial model, show that

(i) $\bar{\hat{Y}} = \bar{Y}$, that is, the average of the fitted values equals the average of the data.
(ii) the residuals sum to zero.

(For both, start by showing that $\mathbf{1} \in R(\mathbf{X})$, the columnspace of the regression/design matrix $\mathbf{X}$.)

3.7 Prove this version of Corollary 3.12:

Corollary 3.24 *Let* $\hat{\beta} = \mathbf{G}\mathbf{X}'\mathbf{Y}$ *where* $\mathbf{G}$ *is a generalized inverse of* $\mathbf{X}'\mathbf{X}$. *If* $\mathbf{c}'\boldsymbol{\beta}$ *is identifiable, then* $\mathbf{c}'\hat{\boldsymbol{\beta}}$ *has a value independent of the choice of* $\mathbf{G}$, *and is the BLUE of* $\mathbf{c}'\boldsymbol{\beta}$. *We have* $\mathrm{Var}(\mathbf{c}'\hat{\boldsymbol{\beta}}) = \sigma^2\mathbf{c}'\mathbf{G}\mathbf{c}$.

(Imitate the proof of Corollary 3.12, which will give the needed uniqueness.)

Section 3.3

3.8 In Example 3.20, compute $\mathbf{X}'\mathbf{X}$ and $\mathbf{X}'\mathbf{Y}$, and use them to verify the results enumerated there.

Section 3.4

3.9 Prove Theorem 3.21. (Divide the numerator and denominator in (3.24) by the standard deviation of $\mathbf{c}'\hat{\boldsymbol{\beta}}$, simplify, and apply Definition 1.11. Be sure to verify the independence of $\hat{\boldsymbol{\beta}}$ and MSE.)

3.10 If you invert the t-test for testing $H_0 : \mathbf{c}'\boldsymbol{\beta} = c$ *vs.* $H_1 : \mathbf{c}'\boldsymbol{\beta} > c$, do you get an upper or lower confidence bound for $\mathbf{c}'\boldsymbol{\beta}$?

3.11 Prove formula (3.27).

Chapter 4
Testing

Abstract This chapter gives an extended exposition of the theory of hypothesis testing and confidence sets in a linear model. Considering both regression and factorial models, we revisit the relevant lattice of subspaces of the parameter space, and study in detail the link between them and subspaces of the observation space, a link afforded by the regression/design matrix **X**. Using this, we examine the relationship between adjusted and sequential sums of squares, exploring the cases where they agree and approaches to take when they don't. After discussing confidence sets and the Scheffé method of simultaneous inference, we conclude with an introduction to hypothesis testing in variance components models.

The most fundamental idea in testing a linear hypothesis H_0 will be this: We fit two models, one the initial or *full* linear model $\mathrm{E}(\mathbf{Y}) = \mathbf{X}\boldsymbol{\beta}$, the other the model restricted by H_0, and compare the two error sums of squares (SSE). Denoting the SSE of the restricted model by SSE_R, we have $SSE_R \geq SSE$, since a restricted minimum obviously cannot be less than an unrestricted one. Based on the interpretation of SSE that we gave on page 71, we will *not* reject H_0 if these two quantities are close, since we give benefit of doubt to H_0. Thus we will reject H_0 if $SSE_R \gg SSE$, that is, if SSE_R/SSE is sufficiently large. The method of fitting will be least squares. The criterion of "sufficiently large" will be given by an F-test, as we shall see.

As mentioned in Sect. 1.7, we may view the $N \times p$ matrix **X** as a linear transformation from the parameter space $\mathbb{R}^p$ to the observation space $\mathbb{R}^N$. Hypotheses are formulated in $\mathbb{R}^p$, while the process of least-squares fitting occurs in $\mathbb{R}^N$. We denote by $\mathbf{X}(W)$ the image of W under the mapping defined by **X**.

J. H. Beder, *Linear Models and Design*,
https://doi.org/10.1007/978-3-031-08176-7_4

4.1 Testing a Linear Hypothesis

We have already described fitting an unrestricted model in Chap. 3. We saw that the principle of least squares amounted to projecting $\mathbf{Y}$ orthogonally on $V = R(\mathbf{X})$, the columnspace of $\mathbf{X}$. We called the projected value $\hat{\mathbf{Y}}$, and defined $SSE = \|\mathbf{Y} - \hat{\mathbf{Y}}\|^2$.

The process of fitting a restricted model is similar. We write the hypothesis in the form H_0: $\boldsymbol{\beta} \in W$, where W is a subspace of $\mathbb{R}^p$, and let $V_0 = \mathbf{X}(W)$, a subspace of V. To fit the restricted model, we find the value $\hat{\mathbf{Y}}_0 \in V_0$ closest to the data $\mathbf{Y}$. That is, $\hat{\mathbf{Y}}_0$ is the orthogonal projection of $\mathbf{Y}$ on V_0, and

$$SSE_R = \|\mathbf{Y} - \hat{\mathbf{Y}}_0\|^2.$$

The situation can be pictured as in Fig. 4.1.

To carry out our test, we would need to know the distribution of the ratio SSE_R/SSE. Assuming normality, and rewriting the restricted model in the form $\mathrm{E}(\mathbf{Y}) = \mathbf{X}_0\boldsymbol{\beta}_0$ with $\mathbf{X}(W) = R(\mathbf{X}_0)$ (Theorem 1.36), we may apply Corollary 3.17 to conclude that SSE_R has a non-central chi-square distribution with $N - r_0$ df, where $r_0 = \mathrm{rank}(\mathbf{X}_0)$, central if H_0 holds. Since SSE also has a chi-square distribution, we might be tempted to make SSE_R/SSE into an F-ratio, inserting degrees of freedom as appropriate. Unfortunately, this ratio would not have an F distribution since SSE_R and SSE are not independent, as we will soon see. (An indication of this, though not a proof, is that $\mathbf{Y} - \hat{\mathbf{Y}}$ and $\mathbf{Y} - \hat{\mathbf{Y}}_0$ are correlated, as the reader may show.)

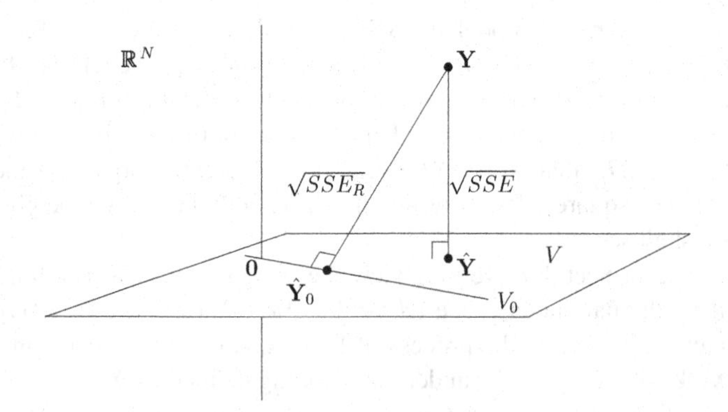

Fig. 4.1 Geometric representation of $\mathbf{Y}$, $\hat{\mathbf{Y}}$, and $\hat{\mathbf{Y}}_0$. $\mathbb{R}^N$ is represented schematically as three-dimensional, the subspace $V = R(\mathbf{X})$ as a plane, and the subspace V_0 as a line lying in the plane. (The line and plane would actually extend indefinitely.) We have dropped two perpendiculars from $\mathbf{Y}$, one to V and the other to V_0. The squared lengths of the perpendiculars are the respective sums of squares

Instead, we consider the triangle formed by $\mathbf{Y}$, $\hat{\mathbf{Y}}$, and $\hat{\mathbf{Y}}_0$ in Fig. 4.1. Since $\hat{\mathbf{Y}}-\hat{\mathbf{Y}}_0$ lies in V, this is clearly a right triangle, and the Pythagorean Theorem gives us

$$\|\mathbf{Y}-\hat{\mathbf{Y}}_0\|^2 = \|\mathbf{Y}-\hat{\mathbf{Y}}\|^2 + \|\hat{\mathbf{Y}}-\hat{\mathbf{Y}}_0\|^2. \tag{4.1}$$

If we let[1]

$$SS(H_0) = \|\hat{\mathbf{Y}}-\hat{\mathbf{Y}}_0\|^2,$$

then (4.1) may be written

$$SSE_R = SSE + SS(H_0), \tag{4.2}$$

so that

$$\frac{SSE_R}{SSE} = 1 + \frac{SS(H_0)}{SSE}.$$

Clearly SSE_R/SSE is large if and only if $SS(H_0)/SSE$ is large, and so we could base our test on the latter ratio. We call $SS(H_0)$ the *sum of squares for testing* H_0, or simply *for* H_0. If we let $\mathbf{P}$ and $\mathbf{P}_0$ define the orthogonal projections of $\mathbb{R}^N$ on V and on V_0, respectively, then $\hat{\mathbf{Y}} = \mathbf{PY}$ and $\hat{\mathbf{Y}}_0 = \mathbf{P}_0\mathbf{Y}$, so that

$$SS(H_0) = \|(\mathbf{P}-\mathbf{P}_0)\mathbf{Y}\|^2. \tag{4.3}$$

Theorem 4.1 *Assume that* $\mathbf{Y} \sim N(\mathbf{X}\boldsymbol{\beta}, \sigma^2\mathbf{I})$, *and let* H_0: $\boldsymbol{\beta} \in W$ *be a linear hypothesis. Put* $V = R(\mathbf{X})$, $V_0 = \mathbf{X}(W)$, $r = \dim(V) = \operatorname{rank}(\mathbf{X})$ *and* $r_0 = \dim(V_0)$. *Let* $\mathbf{P}$ *and* $\mathbf{P}_0$ *be the orthogonal projections of* $\mathbb{R}^N$ *on* V *and on* V_0. *Then:*

a. $SS(H_0)/\sigma^2 \sim \chi^2(r-r_0, \delta/\sigma^2)$ *where* $\delta = \boldsymbol{\beta}'\mathbf{X}'(\mathbf{P}-\mathbf{P}_0)\mathbf{X}\boldsymbol{\beta}$. *If* H_0 *holds, then* $SS(H_0)/\sigma^2 \sim \chi^2(r-r_0)$.
b. $SS(H_0)$ *and* SSE *are independent.*

Proof (a) Let $\mathbf{Q} = \mathbf{P}-\mathbf{P}_0$. Since $\mathbf{Q}$ is the orthogonal projection of $\mathbb{R}^N$ on $V \ominus V_0$ (Corollary A.96), we have $\operatorname{rank}(\mathbf{Q}) = r - r_0$. The distribution of $SS(H_0)$ is then a direct application of Theorem 3.16. Moreover, if $\boldsymbol{\beta}$ is constrained by H_0, then $\mathbf{X}\boldsymbol{\beta} \in \mathbf{X}(W) = V_0$, so $\mathbf{QX}\boldsymbol{\beta} = \mathbf{0}$, and so $\delta = 0$.

(b) It is left as an exercise to show that $\mathbf{Y}-\hat{\mathbf{Y}}$ and $\hat{\mathbf{Y}}-\hat{\mathbf{Y}}_0$ are uncorrelated. Since they are normally distributed, they are independent. But then SSE and $SS(H_0)$ are independent. □

[1] We will soon write SSE_R as SST (total sum of squares). Equation (4.2) is then $SST = SSE + SS(H_0)$. It is the basic equation of the analysis of variance.

This result, together with Corollary 3.17, gives the following:

Corollary 4.2 *Under the assumptions of Theorem 4.1 and with the same notation, let F be given by*

$$F = \frac{SS(H_0)/(r - r_0)}{SSE/(N - r)}. \tag{4.4}$$

Then $F \sim F(r-r_0, N-r, \delta/\sigma^2)$, and when H_0 holds we have $F \sim F(r-r_0, N-r)$. In particular, the test that rejects H_0 at significance level α if $F > F_{r-r_0,N-r,\alpha}$ has constant power[2] *α over all null values of $\boldsymbol{\beta}$.*

This test can be developed as a *likelihood ratio test*; see, e.g., [121, Section 2.5]. Since the power function of the test is constant under H_0, we can define the size of this test unambiguously without introducing a supremum over all null-distributions (as in Definition 1.21).

In Sect. 3.3 we called the denominator in (4.4) the *mean square for error (MSE)*. We now define the numerator,

$$MS(H_0) = SS(H_0)/(r - r_0),$$

to be the *mean square for testing* H_0. The F-statistic in (4.4) can thus be written

$$F = \frac{MS(H_0)}{MSE}.$$

The number $r - r_0$ in Theorem 4.1 is the *degrees of freedom for* H_0, which we will denote by $\mathrm{df}(H_0)$:

$$\mathrm{df}(H_0) = r - r_0.$$

We will give an alternate formula for $\mathrm{df}(H_0)$ in Corollary 4.5 below.

The notations $SS(H_0)$, $MS(H_0)$ and $\mathrm{df}(H_0)$ are not standard. For testing that the slope $\beta_1 = 0$ in a simple linear regression, the first two are often written SSR and MSR, the *sum of squares* and *mean square for regression*. For testing that the means are equal in a one-way factorial model, they are similarly written $SSTr$ and $MSTr$, the *sum of squares* and *mean square for treatments*. The number $\mathrm{df}(H_0)$ is likewise the *degrees of freedom for treatments* or *for regression*.

The quantity SSE_R is commonly written SST and called the *total sum of squares*. The terminology comes from (4.2) which is the basic equation for the

[2] Tests for which the power function is constant on the "boundary" between H_0 and H_1 are said to be *similar on the boundary*, or just *similar*; see [89, p. 110]. Corollary 4.2 says that this F-test is such a test, where we understand the boundary to be all of H_0—that is, all of the subspace $W \subset \mathbb{R}^p$.

analysis of variance (ANOVA). As we have seen, the total sum of squares plays no direct role in testing H_0, and so a corresponding mean square is not computed.

It is customary to display these quantities in an *ANOVA table*. "Source" means "source of variation":

Source	SS	df	MS	F
H_0	$SS(H_0)$	$r - r_0$	$SS(H_0)/(r - r_0)$	$MS(H_0)/MSE$
Error	SSE	$N - r$	$SSE/(N - r)$	
Total	SST	$N - r_0$		

Note that, according to Theorem 1.36, $\mathbf{X}(W) = R(\mathbf{X}_0)$ if the reduced model is written $\mathrm{E}(\mathbf{Y}) = \mathbf{X}_0\boldsymbol{\beta}_0$, and $r_0 = \mathrm{rank}(\mathbf{X}_0)$, the rank of the reduced model. This is convenient in applying Theorem 4.1 to the following examples.

Example 4.3 In Example 3.19 we used the theory developed there to recover the well-known formula for SSE in a one-way factorial experiment, and found the degrees of freedom for error to be $N - p$ when there are p treatments. In this model the parameter vector is $\boldsymbol{\mu} = (\mu_1, \ldots, \mu_p)'$, and the main hypothesis of interest is H_0: $\mu_1 = \cdots = \mu_p$. If we call the common unknown value μ then under H_0 we have $\boldsymbol{\mu}_0 = \mu\mathbf{1}_p$ (where $\mathbf{1}_p$ is the $p \times 1$ vector of ones) and $\mathrm{E}(\mathbf{Y}) = \mu\mathbf{1}_N$, so that $\mathbf{X}_0 = \mathbf{1}_N$. Since $\mathbf{X}_0'\mathbf{X}_0 = [N]$, a 1×1 matrix, the orthogonal projection on $V_0 = \langle \mathbf{1}_N \rangle$ is given by

$$\mathbf{P}_0 = (1/N)\mathbf{1}_N\mathbf{1}_N', \tag{4.5}$$

and so the fitted value under H_0 is

$$\hat{\mathbf{Y}}_0 = \mathbf{P}_0\mathbf{Y} = (\bar{Y}_{..})\mathbf{1}_N,$$

where $\bar{Y}_{..}$ is the grand mean of the observations. Using the expression for $\hat{\mathbf{Y}}$ in Example 3.19, we see that the sum of squares for H_0 is given by the well-known formula

$$SSTr = \|\hat{\mathbf{Y}} - \hat{\mathbf{Y}}_0\|^2 = \sum_i \sum_j (\bar{Y}_{i.} - \bar{Y}_{..})^2 = \sum_i n_i(\bar{Y}_{i.} - \bar{Y}_{..})^2,$$

and since $\mathrm{rank}(\mathbf{X}_0) = 1$ we see that the df for treatments is $r - r_0 = p - 1$.

The ANOVA table looks like this:

Source	SS	df	MS	F
Treatments	$SSTr$	$p - 1$	$SSTr/(p - 1)$	$MSTr/MSE$
Error	SSE	$N - p$	$SSE/(N - p)$	
Total	SST	$N - 1$		

Example 4.4 In Example 3.20 we found an expression for SSE in a simple linear regression in which $\mathrm{E}(Y) = \beta_0 + \beta_1 x$, and found the degrees of freedom for error to be $N - 2$. As we have seen, the regression matrix $\mathbf{X}$ is $N \times 2$ where N is the number of observations, as usual, and evidently has full rank $r = 2$ except in a very trivial case of no practical importance.

The most important hypothesis is $\beta_1 = 0$, which would say that the explanatory variable x has no effect, and that the regression model can be replaced by the simpler model in which $\mathrm{E}(Y_j) = \beta$, the same for all observations Y_j. That is why $SS(H_0)$ is known as the sum of squares due to regression, as noted above. Under H_0 we may write $\mathrm{E}(\mathbf{Y}) = \beta \mathbf{1}_N$, so again $\mathbf{X}_0 = \mathbf{1}_N$, which has rank $r_0 = 1$, and $\hat{\mathbf{Y}}_0 = \bar{Y}.\mathbf{1}$. Thus the total sum of squares is

$$SST = \sum_j (Y_j - \bar{Y}.)^2.$$

A formula for SSE was given in Example 3.20, and the regression sum of squares can be gotten by subtraction. We thus have an ANOVA table of this form:

Source	SS	df	MS	F
Regression	SSR	1	$SSR/1$	MSR/MSE
Error	SSE	$N-2$	$SSE/(N-2)$	
Total	SST	$N-1$		

When $\mathbf{X}$ is full rank it is not hard to give a formula for $\mathrm{df}(H_0)$ that is directly linked to H_0:

Corollary 4.5 *If* $\mathbf{X}$ *has full rank* r, *and if* H_0 *is the statement* $\boldsymbol{\beta} \in W$, *then* $\mathrm{df}(H_0) = r - \dim(W)$. *If* H_0 *is the statement* $\boldsymbol{\beta} \perp U$, *then* $\mathrm{df}(H_0) = \dim U$.

Proof In Theorem 4.1 $r_0 = \dim \mathbf{X}(W)$. Since $\mathbf{X}$ has full rank, it represents a one-to-one linear transformation, so that $\mathbf{X}(W)$ and W are isomorphic, and in particular, $r_0 = \dim W$, so that $\mathrm{df}(H_0) = r - \dim(W)$. But this equals $\dim(U)$, by equation (A.19). □

Put another way, this corollary asserts that $\dim(V \ominus V_0) = \dim(U)$. We will use this shortly to show that $V \ominus V_0$ and U are actually isomorphic under $\mathbf{T}'$ (Proposition 4.11 below).

We have not given a formula for SSR in the regression case, and the simplicity of $SSTr$ in a one-way factorial experiment seems to be simply a bit of luck. In general the process of finding $SS(H_0)$ is at this point a matter of fitting two models and computing $SS(H_0) = \|\hat{\mathbf{Y}} - \hat{\mathbf{Y}}_0\|^2$, the squared distance between the two fitted vectors. One would like a result, similar to Corollary 4.5, that expresses this sum of squares in a manner that more directly involves H_0 itself. This is the conclusion of Theorem 4.8 in the next section.

Finally, the quantities SSE, $SSTr$ and SSR that we have computed are sometimes said to be *corrected* (or *adjusted*) *for the mean*. The "uncorrected" total sum of squares is simply $\|\mathbf{Y}\|^2$, and the other sums of squares are due to a sequential fitting of terms in the model. (We will discuss sequential sums of squares in Sect. 4.5.) Many texts still incorporate the term $\|\mathbf{Y}\|^2$ as a separate line in analysis of variance tables, although it is not clear what purpose it serves. One author writes that "it is effectively the error sum of squares after fitting no model at all" [124, p. 27]. In fact, it does represent the sum of squares SSE_R for a restricted model, although one that is hardly ever of interest. We leave it as an exercise to determine the constraint or hypothesis that leads to this sum of squares. Suffice it to say that we will not make any use of "uncorrected" sums of squares. We caution the reader that we will use the term "adjusted" for sums of squares in a different sense in Sect. 4.4.

4.1.1 Testing in Constrained Models

There are times when we wish to test a linear hypothesis concerning a linear model that includes a constraint. That is, the model is $\mathrm{E}(\mathbf{Y}) = \mathbf{X}\boldsymbol{\beta}$ subject to $\boldsymbol{\beta} \in W_1$, and we wish to test H_0: $\boldsymbol{\beta} \in W_0$. Since under the constraint the hypothesis is really $\boldsymbol{\beta} \in W_0 \cap W_1$, we may assume that $W_0 \subset W_1$. (In the language of Sect. 4.5, we may say that the hypothesis $\boldsymbol{\beta} \in W_0$ is *nested* in the constraint $\boldsymbol{\beta} \in W_1$.) There are two ways we may deal with this:

- In the preceding discussion, we may simply replace $\mathbb{R}^p$ by W_1 and W by W_0, let $V = \mathbf{X}(W_1)$ and $V_0 = \mathbf{X}(W_0)$, and proceed as above.
- According to Theorem 1.36, the constrained model may be written in the form $\mathrm{E}(\mathbf{Y}) = \mathbf{X}_0\boldsymbol{\beta}_0$ with $\boldsymbol{\beta}_0 \in \mathbb{R}^k$. In this case the hypothesis $\boldsymbol{\beta} \in W_0$ can be rewritten as $\boldsymbol{\beta}_0 \in W_0^*$ for an appropriate subspace $W_0^* \subset \mathbb{R}^k$. Moreover, if the parameter $\boldsymbol{\beta}_0 = (b_1, \ldots, b_k)'$ is chosen appropriately, the hypothesis may be written as $\beta_{j+1} = \cdots = \beta_k$ for some j. The reader is referred to the exercises.

It goes without saying that while a linear constraint has the same form as a linear hypothesis, a constraint must be viewed as an assumption, and cannot be tested.

4.1.2 Replication. Lack of Fit and Pure Error

Replication is the drawing of a random sample of two or more measurements of a response variable Y under the same condition. In a regression model $\mathrm{E}(Y) = \beta_0 + \beta_1 x_1 + \cdots + \beta_k x_k$, a condition is a fixed value of $(x_1, \ldots, x_k)$. In a factorial model, a condition is a treatment combination. There may be replication at several conditions or at all of them. If we observe each condition once, we have a *single-replicate design*; if we observe each n times, we have an *equireplicate design*.

Suppose that there are s distinct conditions, and that condition i is observed n_i times, so that there are $N = \sum_i n_i$ observations. Let $Y_{i1}, \ldots, Y_{in_i}$ be a random sample observed at condition i, and suppose we form $\mathbf{Y} = (Y_{11}, \ldots, Y_{sn_s})'$ by stacking the columns $(Y_{i1}, \ldots, Y_{in_i})'$ in order. We may make some simple observations:

a. If the response is described by a linear model

$$\mathrm{E}(\mathbf{Y}) = \mathbf{X}\boldsymbol{\beta}, \tag{4.6}$$

where $\boldsymbol{\beta}$ is $p \times 1$, replication implies that the $N \times p$ design matrix $\mathbf{X}$ has repeated rows. Specifically, there will be s distinct rows, the ith row repeated n_i times.
b. Since $Y_{i1}, \ldots, Y_{in_i}$ is a random sample, these n_i variables have a common expected value, say μ_i. If we let $\boldsymbol{\mu} = (\mu_1, \ldots, \mu_s)'$, then $\mathbf{Y}$ also satisfies a linear model

$$\mathrm{E}(\mathbf{Y}) = \mathbf{Z}\boldsymbol{\mu}, \tag{4.7}$$

where the $N \times s$ matrix $\mathbf{Z}$ has the form given in Eq. (1.19). We note that the rows of $\mathbf{Z}$ have the same repetition pattern as those of $\mathbf{X}$.

If we allow $\boldsymbol{\mu}$ in model (4.7) to be arbitrary, then model (4.6) is in general more constrained. For example, if (4.6) is a regression model, then it assumes that $\mathrm{E}(Y)$ is given by a specific regression equation, while (4.7) makes no assumptions at all. This allows us to create a *test for lack of fit*[3] of the model (4.6). We should emphasize that this model, $\mathrm{E}(\mathbf{Y}) = \mathbf{X}\boldsymbol{\beta}$, is now a hypothesis about the more general model (4.7).

To explore the relationship between the two models above, we might define the *core* of $\mathbf{X}$ to be the $s \times p$ matrix $\mathbf{X}^*$ formed by eliminating duplicate rows from $\mathbf{X}$, so that $\mathbf{X}^*$ has one row of each type from $\mathbf{X}$. Then $\mathbf{Y} = \mathbf{X}\boldsymbol{\beta}$ implies that

$$\boldsymbol{\mu} = \mathbf{X}^*\boldsymbol{\beta}. \tag{4.8}$$

If $p = s$ and $\mathbf{X}^*$ is nonsingular then this is merely a reparametrization. We are interested in the case $p < s$, in which case (4.8) (or equivalently the model (4.6)) imposes a constraint on $\boldsymbol{\mu}$. This constraint is a hypothesis that we can test.

One note of caution as we proceed: here the full model is (4.7), so that in the development at the beginning of Sect. 4.1 we must replace $\mathbf{X}$, p and $\boldsymbol{\beta}$ by $\mathbf{Z}$, s and $\boldsymbol{\mu}$. The hypothesis we are testing is H_0: $\boldsymbol{\mu} = \mathbf{X}^*\boldsymbol{\beta}$ where $\mathbf{X}^*$ is given. As usual, the procedure is to fit $\mathbf{Y}$ to two models:

The full model. The reader has probably noticed that the full model $\mathrm{E}(\mathbf{Y}) = \mathbf{Z}\boldsymbol{\mu}$ is nothing but a one-factor model with s treatments and n_i observations per

[3] The term "lack of fit" has become common in the context of regression models. The test is one of a class of tests that usually go by the name "goodness of fit".

treatment, and so the vector of fitted values $\hat{\mathbf{Y}}$ is given in Example 3.19. Formulas for SSE and df_E in this test are given there as well, with s replacing p. In particular, we see that the test cannot be performed unless $N > s$—that is, *unless we have at least some replication.*

The model under H_0. To find the fitted value $\hat{\mathbf{Y}}_0$ under H_0, we follow the procedure described at the beginning of Sect. 4.1. At this point we may be tempted to write H_0 in the form $\boldsymbol{\mu} \in W$ and then use Theorem 1.36 to rewrite it in the form $\mathrm{E}(\mathbf{Y}) = \mathbf{Z}_0\boldsymbol{\mu}_0$ for some $\mathbf{Z}_0$, as indicated there. But we note that H_0 is already in this form, namely $\mathrm{E}(\mathbf{Y}) = \mathbf{X}\boldsymbol{\beta}$! Here $\mathbf{Z}_0$ and $\boldsymbol{\mu}_0$ are precisely this $\mathbf{X}$ and $\boldsymbol{\beta}$, and so we get $\hat{\mathbf{Y}}_0$ by projecting $\mathbf{Y}$ orthogonally on $V_0 = R(\mathbf{X})$.

Of course, from (4.8) we know that H_0 is indeed of the form $\boldsymbol{\mu} \in W$ if we take W to be the columnspace of $\mathbf{X}^*$, and it is easy and perhaps instructive to see from this that $\mathbf{Z}(W) = R(\mathbf{X})$ (Exercise 4.10).

In the ANOVA equation

$$\|\mathbf{Y} - \hat{\mathbf{Y}}_0\|^2 = \|\mathbf{Y} - \hat{\mathbf{Y}}\|^2 + \|\hat{\mathbf{Y}} - \hat{\mathbf{Y}}_0\|^2,$$

the left hand side is identical to the usual sum of squares for error in fitting the model $\mathrm{E}(\mathbf{Y}) = \mathbf{X}\boldsymbol{\beta}$. The first term on the right, which is the sum of squares for error for the more general model $\mathrm{E}(\mathbf{Y}) = \mathbf{Z}\boldsymbol{\mu}$, is known as the *sum of squares for pure error* since it makes no assumption other than that observations come from s different treatments. The last term is known as the *sum of squares for lack of fit*. With the obvious notation, then, we have

$$SSE = SSPE + SSLF.$$

The corresponding breakdown of the degrees of freedom is

$$N - p = N - s \, + \, s - p.$$

We define $MSPE$ and $MSLF$ in the obvious way. To test for lack of fit, we form the statistics $F = MSLF/MSPE$ and reject good fit (= conclude lack of fit) if $F > F_{s-p,N-s,\alpha}$. If we reject good fit, then we need to consider other models. If not, then we simply ignore this test and use the usual F statistics (with the usual MSE) for the significance tests that we want.

Example 4.6 Table 4.1 displays data to which a simple linear regression model has been fitted. The estimated regression line is $y = 0.9394 + 0.3258x$. In the ANOVA table, the sum of squares and degrees of freedom for error have been broken into those for lack of fit and pure error. The test for lack of fit indicates that the model fits reasonably well, so that we may proceed to test for the significance of the regression model (or, equivalently, of x). The test shows that the coefficient of x is significantly different from zero.

Had we found significant lack of fit, we would typically consider adding other terms to the model.

Table 4.1 Data and ANOVA table for Example 4.6

x	Y	x	Y	x	Y	x	Y
0.0	1.04, 1.17	0.5	1.07	1.1	1.19	1.6	1.38, 1.51
0.1	0.96	0.6	1.15	1.2	1.24, 1.48	1.7	1.51
0.2	0.98, 1.01	0.7	1.05, 1.21	1.3	1.27	1.8	1.62
0.3	1.09, 1.12	0.8	1.06	1.4	1.29	1.9	1.60, 1.75
0.4	1.00, 1.01	0.9	1.08, 1.18	1.5	1.40, 1.52		

Source	SS	df	MS	F	p-value
Regression	1.12137	1	1.12137	111.14	0.000
Error	0.27241	27	0.01009		
Lack of fit	0.18951	17	0.01115	1.34	0.323
Pure error	0.08290	10	0.00829		
Total	1.39379	28			

Remark 4.7 As we have noted, the test for lack of fit of a model $\mathrm{E}(\mathbf{Y}) = \mathbf{X}\boldsymbol{\beta}$ requires two conditions: replication and $p < s$, where p and s are described above. We have assumed that $\mathbf{X}$ is full rank and that $\boldsymbol{\beta}$ is unrestricted.

The lack of fit test is widely used in regression, and is often performed automatically by computer packages when there is replication. In factorial models $p = s$ automatically, as the model is simply the collection of treatment combinations. Testing for lack of fit is not possible here, and would not make sense.

4.2 The Wald Statistic

As we noted above, Corollary 4.5 expresses the degrees of freedom for testing a linear hypothesis directly in terms of the hypothesis: For H_0: $\boldsymbol{\beta} \perp U$ we have

$$\mathrm{df}(H_0) = \dim U$$

when the model has full rank. We seek a similarly direct expression for $SS(H_0)$.

To do this, we write H_0 more concretely[4] as

$$H_0\colon \mathbf{C}'\boldsymbol{\beta} = \mathbf{0} \tag{4.9}$$

where $\mathbf{C}$ is the $p \times d$ matrix

$$\mathbf{C} = (\mathbf{c}_1 \cdots \mathbf{c}_d)$$

and $\mathbf{c}_1, \ldots, \mathbf{c}_d$ is a basis of U (so that $\dim U = d$). As before, $\boldsymbol{\beta}$ is $p \times 1$.

[4] See Lemma 1.33.

Theorem 4.8 *Assume* $\mathbf{Y} = \mathbf{X}\boldsymbol{\beta}$ *where* $\mathbf{X}$ *has full rank, and let* H_0 *be the hypothesis* $\mathbf{C}'\boldsymbol{\beta} = 0$*, where* $\mathbf{C}$ *has full rank. Then*

$$SS(H_0) = (\mathbf{C}'\hat{\boldsymbol{\beta}})'(\mathbf{C}'(\mathbf{X}'\mathbf{X})^{-1}\mathbf{C})^{-1}\mathbf{C}'\hat{\boldsymbol{\beta}} \tag{4.10}$$

where $\hat{\boldsymbol{\beta}}$ *is the least squares estimator of* $\boldsymbol{\beta}$.

Together with Corollaries 4.2 and 4.5, the theorem gives:

Corollary 4.9 *Under the assumptions of Theorem 4.8, the statistic for testing* H_0: $\mathbf{C}'\boldsymbol{\beta} = \mathbf{0}$ *vs.* H_1: $\mathbf{C}'\boldsymbol{\beta} \neq \mathbf{0}$ *is*

$$F = \frac{(\mathbf{C}'\hat{\boldsymbol{\beta}})'(\mathbf{C}'(\mathbf{X}'\mathbf{X})^{-1}\mathbf{C})^{-1}\mathbf{C}'\hat{\boldsymbol{\beta}}}{d \cdot MSE}, \tag{4.11}$$

and we reject H_0 *if* $F > F_{d,N-p,\alpha}$ *where* $d = \text{rank}(\mathbf{C})$ *and* $\mathbf{X}$ *in* $N \times p$.

Remark 4.10 While there are many ways to represent H_0 in the form (4.9), we have required $\mathbf{C}$ to have linearly independent columns. Of course, this is always possible (e.g., by Theorem A.23), and so does not represent a real restriction. We thus are also assuming that $d \leq p$ and that $\mathbf{C}$ has full column rank.

To understand the proof of Theorem 4.8, let $W = U^{\perp}$, so that the null hypothesis says that $\boldsymbol{\beta} \in W$. Viewing $\mathbf{X}$ as a linear transformation, we have the following picture:

$$\begin{array}{ccccc} & & \mathbb{R}^N & & \ni \mathbf{Y} \\ & & \cup & & \\ \boldsymbol{\beta} \in \mathbb{R}^p & \xrightarrow{\mathbf{X}} & V = R(\mathbf{X}) & & \ni \hat{\mathbf{Y}} \\ \cup & & \cup & & \\ W & \longrightarrow & V_0 = \mathbf{X}(W) & & \ni \hat{\mathbf{Y}}_0 \end{array}$$

On the left:	On the right:
$U = \mathbb{R}^p \ominus W$	$\hat{\mathbf{Y}} - \hat{\mathbf{Y}}_0 \in V \ominus V_0$ (Corollary A.96)

Now from this diagram we might hope that $\mathbf{X}(U) = V \ominus V_0$. If this were true, then we could express $\hat{\mathbf{Y}} - \hat{\mathbf{Y}}_0$, and hence its norm, in terms of $\mathbf{X}\mathbf{c}_1, \ldots, \mathbf{X}\mathbf{c}_d$. Unfortunately there is an obstacle: $\mathbf{X}$ doesn't usually preserve orthogonality, and in particular

$$\mathbf{X}(\mathbb{R}^p \ominus W) \neq \mathbf{X}(\mathbb{R}^p) \ominus \mathbf{X}(W).$$

Is there a way to map $\mathbb{R}^p \ominus W$ isomorphically onto $V \ominus V_0$?

Recall the matrix

$$\mathbf{T} = (\mathbf{X}'\mathbf{X})^{-1}\mathbf{X}'$$

defined in Eq. (3.18). ($\mathbf{T}$ is the Moore-Penrose inverse of $\mathbf{X}$. Its transpose $\mathbf{T}'$, like $\mathbf{X}$, maps $\mathbb{R}^p$ one-to-one into $\mathbb{R}^N$. Even better:

Proposition 4.11 *For any subspace $W \subset \mathbb{R}^p$, $\mathbf{T}'(\mathbb{R}^p \ominus W) = \mathbf{X}(\mathbb{R}^p) \ominus \mathbf{X}(W)$. In other words, $\mathbf{T}'$ maps $U = \mathbb{R}^p \ominus W$ isomorphically onto $V \ominus V_0$.*

Let $\mathbf{P}$ and $\mathbf{P}_0$ be the orthogonal projections of $\mathbb{R}^N$ on V and V_0, respectively, so that $\mathbf{Q} = \mathbf{P} - \mathbf{P}_0$ is the orthogonal projection on $V \ominus V_0$. If $\mathbf{c}_1, \ldots, \mathbf{c}_d$ is a basis of U, then

$$\mathbf{Q} = \mathbf{Z}(\mathbf{Z}'\mathbf{Z})^{-1}\mathbf{Z}', \tag{4.12}$$

where $\mathbf{Z} = \mathbf{T}'\mathbf{C}$ and $\mathbf{C}$ is the matrix with columns $\mathbf{c}_i$.

Proof First we claim that $\mathbf{T}'(U) \subset V \ominus V_0$. But since $\mathbf{T}' = \mathbf{X}(\mathbf{X}'\mathbf{X})^{-1}$, we have $R(\mathbf{T}') \subset R(\mathbf{X}) = V$, so on the one hand $\mathbf{T}'(U) \subset V$. On the other hand, Lemma 3.15(d) implies that $\mathbf{T}'(U) \perp \mathbf{X}(W) = V_0$, which proves the claim.

Thus $\mathbf{T}'(U) \subset V \ominus V_0$. To show equality, it suffices to show that the dimensions are equal. But $\mathbf{T}'$ is one-to-one since $\mathbf{X}$ is, so

$$\dim \mathbf{T}'(U) = \dim U = \dim(V \ominus V_0),$$

the latter equality by Corollary 4.5. This establishes the first part of the proposition.

Given the basis $\mathbf{c}_1, \ldots, \mathbf{c}_d$ of U, put $\mathbf{z}_i = \mathbf{T}'\mathbf{c}_i$. By the preceding, $\mathbf{z}_i, \ldots, \mathbf{z}_d$ is a basis of $V \ominus V_0$. Put $\mathbf{Z} = [\mathbf{z}_1 \cdots \mathbf{z}_d] = \mathbf{T}'\mathbf{C}$. Then (4.12) gives the orthogonal projection of $\mathbb{R}^N$ on $V \ominus V_0$, by Proposition 3.3. □

Remark 4.12 If we could show that $\mathbf{T}'(U) = V \ominus V_0$ without using Corollary 4.5, then that corollary would follow immediately from this proposition.

Proof of Theorem 4.8 Let $\mathbf{Q}$ be as in Proposition 4.11. Then, combining the expressions for $\mathbf{Q}$ and $SS(H_0)$ is given by (4.12) and (4.3), we have

$$SS(H_0) = \|\mathbf{QY}\|^2 = \mathbf{Y}'\mathbf{Z}(\mathbf{Z}'\mathbf{Z})^{-1}\mathbf{Z}'\mathbf{Y}.$$

An easy calculation gives

$$\mathbf{Z}'\mathbf{Z} = \mathbf{C}'\mathbf{T}\mathbf{T}'\mathbf{C} = \mathbf{C}'(\mathbf{X}'\mathbf{X})^{-1}\mathbf{C},$$

and moreover,

$$\mathbf{Z}'\mathbf{Y} = \mathbf{C}'\mathbf{T}\mathbf{Y} = \mathbf{C}'(\mathbf{X}'\mathbf{X})^{-1}\mathbf{X}'\mathbf{Y} = \mathbf{C}'\hat{\boldsymbol{\beta}},$$

from which (4.10) follows. □

Example 4.13 Consider the problem of testing H_0: $\mathbf{c}'\boldsymbol{\beta} = 0$ against H_1: $\mathbf{c}'\boldsymbol{\beta} \neq 0$ in a full-rank model $\mathrm{E}(\mathbf{Y}) = \mathbf{X}\boldsymbol{\beta}$. Here formula (4.10) may be written

$$SS(H_0) = (\mathbf{c}'\hat{\boldsymbol{\beta}})'(\mathbf{c}'(\mathbf{X}'\mathbf{X})^{-1}\mathbf{c})^{-1}\mathbf{c}'\hat{\boldsymbol{\beta}} = \frac{(\mathbf{c}'\hat{\boldsymbol{\beta}})^2}{\mathbf{c}'(\mathbf{X}'\mathbf{X})^{-1}\mathbf{c}}, \tag{4.13}$$

and since $\mathrm{df}(H_0) = 1$ this is also $MS(H_0)$. The F-ratio for testing H_0 is therefore

$$F = \frac{(\mathbf{c}'\hat{\boldsymbol{\beta}})^2}{MSE\,\mathbf{c}'(\mathbf{X}'\mathbf{X})^{-1}\mathbf{c}},$$

and we reject H_0 if $F > F_{1,N-p,\alpha}$. From Theorem 3.21 we know that we can also test H_0 with a t-statistic

$$T = \frac{\mathbf{c}'\hat{\boldsymbol{\beta}}}{\sqrt{MSE\,\mathbf{c}'(\mathbf{X}'\mathbf{X})^{-1}\mathbf{c}}},$$

rejecting H_0 if $|T| > t_{N-p,\alpha/2}$. Clearly $F = T^2$, and since $T^2 \sim F(1, N-p)$ (Proposition 1.13), the tests are equivalent.

This is sometimes called a *1-df (1-degree-of-freedom) test*. An example of this is given in Exercise 4.10.

Remark 4.14 The expression (4.11) seems to be widely known as the *Wald statistic*, and the test as the *Wald test* (e.g., [128]), based on an asymptotic test given by Wald [147] for application in much more general circumstances. The statistic (4.11) is simply another form of the "likelihood ratio" statistic given in Corollary 4.1, and its distribution is exact rather than asymptotic. The statistic itself was probably derived several times in the literature, though it does not appear to have been given by Wald himself. Scheffé derived it as a byproduct of finding confidence ellipsoids [121, Sections 2.3–2.4], and in Section 2.5 he showed its equality to the likelihood ratio statistic. A few years later Seber [126] gave another proof of equivalence, and also showed the asymptotic equivalence to the statistic Wald derived in [147].

4.3 The Lattice of Hypotheses

In most situations there are many hypothesis naturally needing to be tested. For example, in a regression model $\mathrm{E}(Y) = \beta_0 + \beta_1 x_1 + \cdots + \beta_k x_k$ we are typically interested in whether any of $\beta_1, \ldots, \beta_k$ is zero. In a factorial experiment we would like to know whether any main effects are absent, and whether the interaction between two or more particular factors is absent as well. In all these cases the hypotheses generate a *lattice*. These problems have a very similar structure, as we see from some examples.

4.3.1 The Two-Predictor Regression Model

In the regression model $\mathrm{E}(Y) = \beta_0 + \beta_1 x_1 + \beta_2 x_2$, the two main hypotheses of interest are $\beta_1 = 0$ and $\beta_2 = 0$, which express the idea that x_1 or x_2, respectively, has no significant effect. The conjunction of these hypotheses is the hypothesis $\beta_1 = \beta_2 = 0$, which says that $\mathrm{E}(Y)$ is constant with respect to x_1 and x_2. Viewing $\boldsymbol{\beta} = (\beta_0, \beta_1, \beta_2)'$ as a point in $\mathbb{R}^3$, we may represent each of these hypotheses in the form $\boldsymbol{\beta} \in W$ for a subspace $W \subset \mathbb{R}^3$, namely

$$W_1 = \text{the } (\beta_0, \beta_2)\text{-plane} \qquad (\beta_1 = 0),$$
$$W_2 = \text{the } (\beta_0, \beta_1)\text{-plane} \qquad (\beta_2 = 0),$$
$$W_0 = \text{the } \beta_0\text{-axis} \qquad (\beta_1 = \beta_2 = 0),$$

and they form an obvious *lattice* given by the *Hasse diagram*

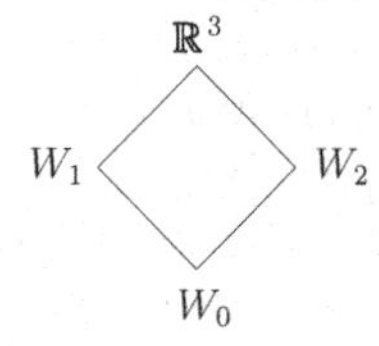

Recall that a lattice is a partially ordered set in which any two elements have a meet or greatest lower bound and a join or least upper bound. The meet of two vector spaces is their intersection and their join is their sum (see the appendix, particularly Sect. A.2.1 and Theorem A.21). In the present case, $W_1 + W_2 = \mathbb{R}^3$ and $W_1 \cap W_2 = W_0$.

4.3.2 The Three-Predictor Regression Model

The corresponding lattice for the regression model $\mathrm{E}(Y) = \beta_0 + \beta_1 x_1 + \beta_2 x_2 + \beta_3 x_3$ is

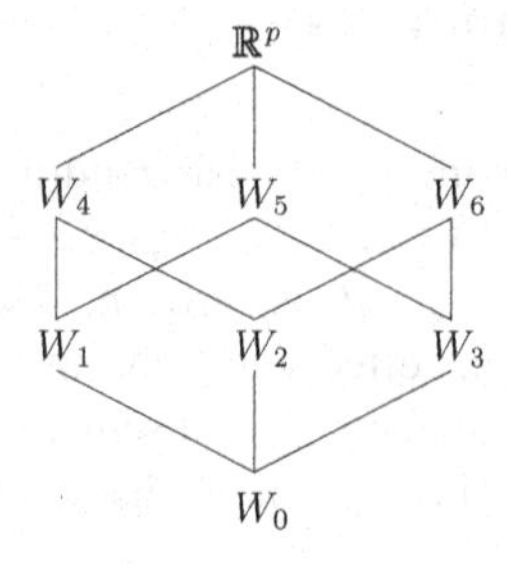

where $p = 4$ and $\boldsymbol{\beta} = (\beta_0, \beta_1, \beta_2, \beta_3)'$. The subspaces W_4, W_5 and W_6 are 3-dimensional subspaces defining the hypotheses $\beta_1 = 0$, $\beta_2 = 0$, and $\beta_3 = 0$, respectively. For example, $W_4 = \{(\beta_0, 0, \beta_2, \beta_3)' \colon \beta_i \in \mathbb{R}, i = 0, 2, 3\}$. The subspaces W_1, W_2 and W_3 are coordinate planes in $\mathbb{R}^4$—for example, $W_1 = W_4 \cap W_5 = \{(\beta_0, 0, 0, \beta_3)' \colon \beta_0, \beta_3 \in \mathbb{R}\}$. Finally, $W_0 = \{(\beta_0, 0, 0, 0)' \colon \beta_0 \in \mathbb{R}\}$, the β_0-axis.

All these subspaces may be expressed in terms of the standard basis vectors $\mathbf{e}_1, \ldots, \mathbf{e}_4$ of $\mathbb{R}^4$. For example, $W_0 = \langle \mathbf{e}_1 \rangle$, where $\mathbf{e}_1 = (1, 0, 0, 0)'$.

The reader may recognize the lattice pictured above as belonging to another important model as well.

4.3.3 The Two-Factor Design

The lattice for the three-predictor regression model has the same Hasse diagram as that in an $a \times b$ factorial experiment, whose hypotheses we displayed in Fig. 2.1 (page 34). The full factorial model contains $p = ab$ parameters μ_{ij}. Comparing with Fig. 2.1, we see that the hypothesis $\boldsymbol{\beta} \in W_4$ is the hypothesis that the A effect is absent, $\boldsymbol{\beta} \in W_5$ means that interactions are absent, and $\boldsymbol{\beta} \in W_6$ means that the B effect is absent. Finally, $\boldsymbol{\beta} \in W_0$ is the hypothesis that all effects are absent, or equivalently that the ab cell means are equal. In this case, $W_0 = \langle \mathbf{1} \rangle$.

We should keep in mind that the main hypotheses in this model were written in the form $\boldsymbol{\beta} \perp U$ in Sect. 2.2, where U is one of three specific subspaces labeled U_1, U_2, and U_{12}. In particular,[5]

$$
\begin{aligned}
W_4 &= U_1^{\perp} \\
W_5 &= U_{12}^{\perp} \\
W_6 &= U_2^{\perp}.
\end{aligned}
$$

The other subspaces are may be written in terms of these. It is easy to see that the seven subspaces form a lattice—for example, $W_1 + W_3 = W_5$ and $W_1 \cap W_3 = W_0$ (Exercise 4.10).

4.3.4 The Hypothesis of No Model Effect

In regression models with more than three predictors, and in factorial models with more than two factors (discussed in Chap. 5), we naturally have a larger lattice of hypotheses of interest. In all these cases, the simplest hypothesis is that there

[5] See Lemma 1.33, page 22.

is no *model effect*. This is the hypothesis that E(Y) is a constant, independent of the predictor variables in regression, or independent of treatment combination in a factorial experiment. In both cases, then, W_0 is one-dimensional, namely $\langle \mathbf{e}_1 \rangle = \{(\beta_0, 0, \ldots, 0) : \beta_0 \in \mathbb{R}\}$ in the regression case, and $\langle \mathbf{1} \rangle = \{(\mu, \ldots, \mu) : \mu \in \mathbb{R}\}$ in the factorial case.

4.3.5 The Lattice in the Observation Space

In order to test a hypothesis $\boldsymbol{\beta} \in W_i$ in a linear model $\mathrm{E}(\mathbf{Y}) = \mathbf{X}\boldsymbol{\beta}$, we consider the subspaces $\mathbf{X}(W_i)$, as we did in Sect. 4.1.

Proposition 4.15 *Let* $\mathbf{X}$ *be* $N \times p$*, viewed as a linear transformation from* $\mathbb{R}^p$ *to* $\mathbb{R}^N$*. Let* W_1 *and* W_2 *be distinct subspaces of* $\mathbb{R}^p$*.*

a. If $W_1 \subset W_2$ *then* $\mathbf{X}(W_1) \subset \mathbf{X}(W_2)$*. If* $\mathbf{X}$ *is one-to-one then the inclusion is proper.*
b. $\mathbf{X}(W_1 + W_2) = \mathbf{X}(W_1) + \mathbf{X}(W_2)$*. (Sums are not necessarily direct.)*
c. $\mathbf{X}(W_1 \cap W_2) \subset \mathbf{X}(W_1) \cap \mathbf{X}(W_2)$*, with equality if* $\mathbf{X}$ *is one-to-one.*

In particular, if $\mathbf{X}$ *is full-rank then it preserves lattice operations.*

The vector spaces $X(W_i)$ in this proposition are subspaces of the observation space $\mathbb{R}^N$. Figure 4.2 illustrates this when applied to the two-predictor regression model and to the three-predictor model and the two-factor design.

The proof of the proposition is left as an exercise.

4.4 Adjusted SS

Following the general approach of Sect. 4.1, we test each hypothesis by comparing the full model to the model restricted by that hypothesis.

As before, let $\boldsymbol{\beta} \in \mathbb{R}^p$ be the parameter vector of the model. Defining the subspaces V and V_i as in Fig. 4.2, let

$$
\begin{aligned}
\mathbf{Y} &= \text{the vector of observations,} \\
\hat{\mathbf{Y}} &= \text{the orthogonal projection of } \mathbf{Y} \text{ on V, and} \\
\hat{\mathbf{Y}}_j &= \text{the orthogonal projection of } \mathbf{Y} \text{ on } V_j \\
&= \text{the fitted value under the hypothesis } H_0^{(j)}: \boldsymbol{\beta} \in W_j.
\end{aligned}
$$

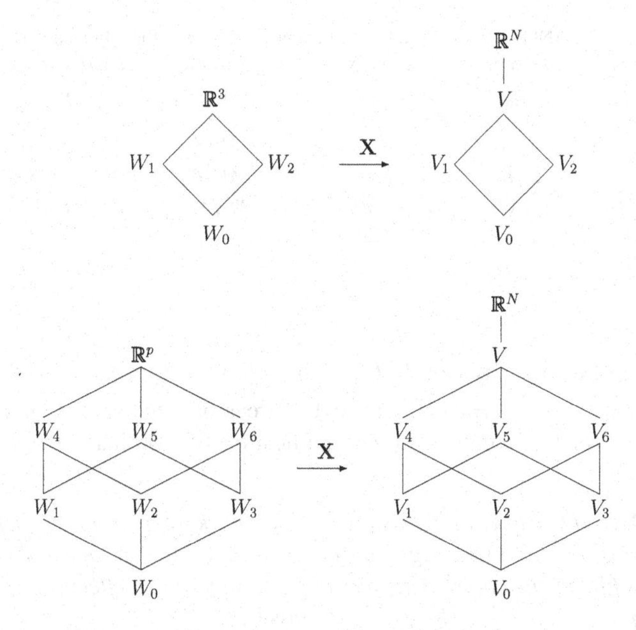

Fig. 4.2 Lattices of subspaces, illustrating Proposition 4.15. Top: 2-predictor regression model. Bottom: a 3-predictor regression model or an $a \times b$ design. $\mathbb{R}^p$ = the parameter space, $\mathbb{R}^N$ = the observation space, $\mathbf{X}$ = the linear transformation given by the regression or design matrix, assumed full rank. $V = R(\mathbf{X})$, $V_i = \mathbf{X}(W_i)$

Then the corresponding sum of squares for testing $H_0^{(j)}$ is

$$SS(H_0^{(j)}) = SS(\boldsymbol{\beta} \in W_j) = \|\hat{\mathbf{Y}} - \hat{\mathbf{Y}}_j\|^2.$$

This is often referred to as the *adjusted sum of squares* for $H_0^{(j)}$. It is "adjusted" in the sense that it assumes that all other terms or effects may be present—that is, it remains agnostic about the validity of the other $H_0^{(i)}$, $i \neq j$. The terminology is not standard—for example, SAS statistical software refers these as being sums of squares *of Type III*. In general, an adjusted sum of squares compares the full model to a model with one effect or term missing.

The hypothesis H_0: $\boldsymbol{\beta} \in W_0$ expresses the absence of an overall model effect. The corresponding sum of squares

$$SS(H_0) = SS(\boldsymbol{\beta} \in W_0) = \|\hat{\mathbf{Y}} - \hat{\mathbf{Y}}_0\|^2$$

is often called the *sum or squares for the model*, and may or may not be included in an ANOVA table. In the regression context it is often called the *sum of squares for regression*, while in the context of factorial experiments it is sometimes called the *sum of squares for treatments*. In the latter case, this sum of squares treats the data as being from a one-factor model with p levels where p is the number of cells.

Table 4.2 ANOVA table for an $a \times b$ experiment, using the adjusted sums of squares. $A \times B$ denotes interaction. Mean squares follow the rule $MS = SS/\text{df}$

Source	SS (adj)	df	MS	F
A	SSA	$a-1$	MSA	MSA/MSE
B	SSB	$b-1$	MSB	MSB/MSE
$A \times B$	$SSAB$	$(a-1)(b-1)$	$MSAB$	$MSAB/MSE$
Error	SSE	$N-p$	MSE	
Total	SST	$N-1$		

In this context, we may call $\text{df}(H_0^{(j)})$ the *adjusted degrees of freedom* for the hypothesis $H_0^{(j)}$, and $\text{df}(H_0)$ the adjusted degrees of freedom for the model, for regression, or for treatments. A direct application of Corollary 4.5 gives us the following:

Corollary 4.16 *In a linear regression model with k regressors, each regression coefficient carries 1 adjusted degree of freedom. In an $a \times b$ factorial experiment with all cells filled,*[6] *the adjusted degrees of freedom for main effects and interaction are $a-1, b-1$ and $(a-1)(b-1)$, respectively.*

The adjusted degrees of freedom for the model is k in the regression model and $ab-1$ in the factorial model.

Proof In a linear regression model with $\boldsymbol{\beta} = (\beta_0 \beta_1, \ldots)'$, the hypothesis H_0: $\beta_i = 0$ is of the form $\boldsymbol{\beta} \perp \mathbf{e}_i$, so by Corollary 4.5 $\text{df}(H_0) = \dim\langle\, \mathbf{e}_i \,\rangle = 1$.

In an $a \times b$ experiment with $\boldsymbol{\beta}$ = the vector of cell means, the result follows from Theorem 2.7 and Corollary 4.5. □

This corollary extends to factorial designs with more than two factors (see Corollary 5.19). For two-factor designs, the ANOVA table has the form given in Table 4.2. The F values have denominators MSE, based on Theorem 4.22.[7] Note that in both regression and factorial experiments the adjusted sums of squares do not necessarily add up to SST. Conditions under which they do are discussed in Sects. 4.5 and 4.6.

Example 4.17 Searle [124, Chapter 4] presents and analyzes the following data for a hypothetical 2×3 experiment:

		Variety		
		1	2	3
Soil	1	6, 10, 11	13, 15	14, 22
	2	12, 15, 19, 18	31	18, 9, 12

[6] All cells are filled if there is at least one observation in each cell.

[7] This assumes that no factors are random. See Sect. 4.9.

The responses are "the number of days to first germination of three varieties of carrot seed grown in two different potting soils". An analysis of variance may look like this:

Source	SS (adj)	df	MS	F	p-value
Soil	123.77	1	123.77	9.28	0.014
Variety	192.13	2	96.06	7.20	0.014
Interaction	222.77	2	111.38	8.35	0.009
Error	120.00	9	13.33		
Total	520.00	14			

With this analysis, we see that each effect is rather significant. Note that while the degrees of freedom add to the total, the sums of squares do not.

We also reject the hypothesis that the cell means are equal (that is, that there is no model effect at all), as indicated in the following table:

Source	SS (adj)	df	MS	F	p-value
Model	400.00	5	80.00	6.00	0.0103
Error	120.00	9	13.33		
Total	520.00	14			

The fact that in this case the model and error sums of squares add up to the total comes from the basic ANOVA equation (4.2).

Example 4.18 Table 4.3 gives data and an ANOVA table for a polynomial regression model

$$E(Y) = \beta_0 + \beta_1 x + \beta_2 x^2 + \beta_3 x^3.$$

The reader can verify (Exercise 4.10) that the adjusted sums of squares for x, x^2 and x^3 are indeed those given by equation (4.13) for β_1, β_2 and β_3—that is, it assumes that each term is the "last term added".

We see that the linear and quadratic terms are highly significant, while the x^3 term is not. We should keep in mind that the F-tests compare the full model with the model with only that term missing. We also note that while the degrees of freedom are additive, the sums of squares for these three terms do not add up to the sum of squares for regression. An alternate way of breaking down the regression sum of squares is given in Sect. 4.5.

Table 4.3 Data and ANOVA table for Example 4.18 using the adjusted sums of squares

x	Y	x	Y	x	Y	x	Y	x	Y
0.0	1.031	0.4	0.333	0.8	0.099	1.2	0.064	1.6	0.272
0.1	0.655	0.5	0.165	0.9	0.056	1.3	0.007	1.7	0.544
0.2	0.401	0.6	0.043	1.0	-0.024	1.4	0.307	1.8	0.503
0.3	0.360	0.7	-0.122	1.1	-0.081	1.5	0.271	1.9	0.858

Source	SS (adj)	df	MS	F	p-value
Regression	1.68890	3	0.56297	60.1923	0.000000
x	0.41138	1	0.41138	43.9843	0.000006
x^2	0.11367	1	0.11367	12.1531	0.003052
x^3	0.01324	1	0.01324	1.4155	0.251506
Error	0.14965	16	0.00935		
Total	1.83855	19			

4.5 Nested Hypotheses. Sequential SS.

In this section we extend the basic ANOVA equation (4.1) to situations involving a chain of hypotheses.

We say that hypothesis $H^{(1)}$ is *nested* in hypothesis $H^{(2)}$ if $H^{(1)}$ implies $H^{(2)}$. If $H^{(i)}$ is of the form $\boldsymbol{\beta} \in W_i$, then $H^{(1)}$ is nested in $H^{(2)}$ iff $W_1 \subset W_2$. If $H^{(i)}$ is written in the form $\boldsymbol{\beta} \perp U_i$, then $H^{(1)}$ is nested in $H^{(2)}$ iff $U_1 \supset U_2$ (note the reversal of inclusion!). In this section we consider *chains* of hypothesis, that is, hypotheses

$$H^{(i)}\colon \boldsymbol{\beta} \in W_i$$

where $W_0 \subset W_1 \subset \cdots \subset W_k \subset \mathbb{R}^p$ and the W_i are distinct. These can also be described in the form H_0: $\boldsymbol{\beta} \perp U_i$ where $U_0 \supset U_1 \supset \cdots \supset U_k$.

In the following, *we will typically use the superscript* 0 *(as in* $H^{(0)}$*) to denote the "smallest" hypothesis under consideration*—typically denoting the simplest possible model.

In the two-predictor regression model discussed above there are two chains of hypotheses, corresponding to $W_0 \subset W_1 \subset \mathbb{R}^3$ and $W_0 \subset W_2 \subset \mathbb{R}^3$. In the models described by Fig. 4.2 one can find six chains, such as the one corresponding to $W_0 \subset W_1 \subset W_5 \subset \mathbb{R}^p$. Sometimes one chain will arise more naturally, as in the following example.

Example 4.19 Consider the polynomial regression model $\mathrm{E}(Y) = \beta_0 + \beta_1 x + \beta_2 x^2$. Here the two natural hypotheses are

$$H^{(0)}\text{: E}(Y) \text{ is a constant function of } x\text{:} \qquad \beta_1 = \beta_2 = 0$$

$$\text{and} \quad H^{(1)}\text{: E}(Y) \text{ is a linear function of } x\text{:} \qquad \beta_2 = 0.$$

Clearly $H^{(0)}$ is nested in $H^{(1)}$. The parameter of interest is $\boldsymbol{\beta} = (\beta_0, \beta_1, \beta_2)' \in \mathbb{R}^3$, and the hypotheses may be written in the form $\boldsymbol{\beta} \in W_i$ where

$$W_0 = \{(\beta_0, 0, 0)' \colon \beta_0 \in \mathbb{R}\}$$
$$\text{and} \quad W_1 = \{(\beta_0, \beta_1, 0)' \colon \beta_0, \beta_1 \in \mathbb{R}\}.$$

If we let the standard basis vectors of $\mathbb{R}^3$ be $\mathbf{e}_1 = (1, 0, 0)'$, $\mathbf{e}_2 = (0, 1, 0)'$, and $\mathbf{e}_3 = (0, 0, 1)'$, then $W_0 = \langle \mathbf{e}_1 \rangle$ and $W_1 = \langle \mathbf{e}_1, \mathbf{e}_2 \rangle$. Note that we can also represent the hypotheses $\boldsymbol{\beta} \in W_i$ as $\boldsymbol{\beta} \perp U_i$ where $U_0 = \langle \mathbf{e}_2, \mathbf{e}_3 \rangle$ and $U_1 = \langle \mathbf{e}_3 \rangle$.

As before, we let $\mathbf{X}$ be the $N \times p$ regression or design matrix, considered as a linear transformation from $\mathbb{R}^p$ to $\mathbb{R}^N$. We consider a chain of subspaces

$$W_0 \subset W_1 \subset \cdots \subset W_k \subset \mathbb{R}^p,$$

and again let $V_j = \mathbf{X}(W_j)$ (the image of W_j) and $V = R(\mathbf{X})$. We denote by $\hat{\mathbf{Y}}$ the orthogonal projection of $\mathbf{Y}$ on V, and by $\hat{\mathbf{Y}}_j$ the orthogonal projection of $\mathbb{R}^N$ on V_j—that is, the fitted value under the hypothesis $H^{(j)}$: $\boldsymbol{\beta} \in W_j$.

Proposition 4.20 *Under the above assumptions,*

a. we have the orthogonal sum

$$V \ominus V_0 = (V \ominus V_k) \oplus (V_k \ominus V_{k-1}) \oplus \cdots \oplus (V_1 \ominus V_0). \tag{4.14}$$

b. $\hat{\mathbf{Y}} - \hat{\mathbf{Y}}_k \in V \ominus V_k$ *and* $\hat{\mathbf{Y}}_j - \hat{\mathbf{Y}}_{j-1} \in V_j \ominus V_{j-1}$.
c. The expressions $\mathbf{Y} - \hat{\mathbf{Y}}$, $\hat{\mathbf{Y}} - \hat{\mathbf{Y}}_k$, $\hat{\mathbf{Y}}_k - \hat{\mathbf{Y}}_{k-1}, \ldots, \hat{\mathbf{Y}}_1 - \hat{\mathbf{Y}}_0$ *are mutually orthogonal.*

Proof Property (a) follows from property (A.16) of Corollary A.71 by induction. Now for simplicity, let $V_{k+1} = V$. Let $\mathbf{P}_i$ be the orthogonal projections of $\mathbb{R}^N$ on $V_i, i = 0, \ldots, k+1$. Then $\hat{\mathbf{Y}}_i - \hat{\mathbf{Y}}_{i-1} = (\mathbf{P}_i - \mathbf{P}_{i-1})\mathbf{Y} \in V_i \ominus V_{i-1}$ by Corollary A.96, which proves (b). Property (c) follows from this and the orthogonality in (a). □

From this and the extended Pythagorean Theorem (Theorem A.57a) we have an extended form of Eq. (4.1) promised at the beginning of this section:

$$\|\mathbf{Y} - \hat{\mathbf{Y}}_0\|^2 = \|\mathbf{Y} - \hat{\mathbf{Y}}\|^2 + \|\hat{\mathbf{Y}} - \hat{\mathbf{Y}}_k\|^2 + \|\hat{\mathbf{Y}}_k - \hat{\mathbf{Y}}_{k-1}\|^2 + \cdots + \|\hat{\mathbf{Y}}_1 - \hat{\mathbf{Y}}_0\|^2. \tag{4.15}$$

As before, the left-hand member is usually referred to as the *total sum of squares*, *SST*, and the first term on the right is the *sum of squares for error*, *SSE*. The other terms are *sequential sums of squares*.[8] The second term, $\|\hat{\mathbf{Y}} - \hat{\mathbf{Y}}_k\|^2$, is the sum of squares for testing H_0: $\boldsymbol{\beta} \in W_k$, as in Sect. 4.1, and so is also the adjusted sum of

[8] In SAS, sequential sums of squares are said to be *of Type I*.

squares for that hypothesis. The term

$$SS(\boldsymbol{\beta} \in W_{j-1}|\boldsymbol{\beta} \in W_j) = \|\hat{\mathbf{Y}}_j - \hat{\mathbf{Y}}_{j-1}\|^2 \tag{4.16}$$

is the sum of squares for testing that $\boldsymbol{\beta} \in W_{j-1}$, given that $\boldsymbol{\beta} \in W_j$. When the specific sequence of hypotheses is given, it is usually just called the *sequential sum of squares for testing* H_0: $\boldsymbol{\beta} \in W_{j-1}$. Equation (4.15) may now be written

$$\begin{aligned} SST &= SSE+ \\ &SS(\boldsymbol{\beta} \in W_k) + SS(\boldsymbol{\beta} \in W_{k-1}|\boldsymbol{\beta} \in W_k) + \cdots + SS(\boldsymbol{\beta} \in W_0|\boldsymbol{\beta} \in W_1). \end{aligned} \tag{4.17}$$

The quantity

$$SS(\boldsymbol{\beta} \in W_0) = \|\hat{\mathbf{Y}} - \hat{\mathbf{Y}}_0\|^2,$$

not explicitly shown in Eq. (4.15), is the *sum of squares for the model* that we introduced in Sect. 4.4. Proposition 4.20 shows that

$$\begin{aligned} &SS(\text{model}) \; (= SS(\boldsymbol{\beta} \in W_0)) \\ &= SS(\boldsymbol{\beta} \in W_k) + SS(\boldsymbol{\beta} \in W_{k-1}|\boldsymbol{\beta} \in W_k) + \cdots + SS(\boldsymbol{\beta} \in W_0|\boldsymbol{\beta} \in W_1). \end{aligned} \tag{4.18}$$

Equations (4.17) and (4.18) express the *additivity* of sequential sums of squares.[9]

Finally, an application of Proposition 4.20 shows that

$$SS(\boldsymbol{\beta} \in W_{j-1}|\boldsymbol{\beta} \in W_j) = SS(\boldsymbol{\beta} \in W_{j-1}) - SS(\boldsymbol{\beta} \in W_j). \tag{4.19}$$

Because of this, $SS(\boldsymbol{\beta} \in W_{j-1}|\boldsymbol{\beta} \in W_j)$ is also known as a *reduction in sum of squares* [123] or as an *extra sum of squares* [51]. The reduction is due to the addition of a term in the model.

Example 4.21 Consider a regression model

$$\mathrm{E}(Y) = \beta_0 + \beta_1 x_1 + \cdots + +\beta_k x_k, \tag{4.20}$$

and let $\boldsymbol{\beta} = (\beta_0, \ldots, \beta_k)'$. Suppose that the indexing indicates the order in which we want to consider the regressors for inclusion. (In a polynomial model, for example, $x_i = x^i$, and the regressors are naturally ordered by degree.) We may then consider the hypotheses

$$\begin{aligned} \beta_k &= 0, \quad (\boldsymbol{\beta} \in W_{k-1}) \quad (x_k \text{ has no effect}) \\ \beta_{k-1} = \beta_k &= 0, \quad (\boldsymbol{\beta} \in W_{k-2}) \quad (x_{k-1} \text{ and } x_k \text{ have no effect}) \end{aligned}$$

---

[9] This should not be confused with *additivity of factors* in a factorial experiment.

$$\begin{array}{lll} \vdots & \vdots & \vdots \\ \beta_2 = \cdots = \beta_k = 0, & (\boldsymbol{\beta} \in W_1) & \text{(only } x_1 \text{ has an effect)} \\ \beta_1 = \beta_2 = \cdots = \beta_k = 0. & (\boldsymbol{\beta} \in W_0) & \text{(no regression effect)} \end{array}$$

Here $p = k + 1$ and $W_j = \{\boldsymbol{\beta} \in \mathbb{R}^p : \boldsymbol{\beta} = (\beta_0, \ldots, \beta_j, 0, \ldots, 0)'\}$, so that $W_0 \subset \cdots \subset W_{k-1} \subset \mathbb{R}^p$.

The *sum of squares for regression*, $SS(\boldsymbol{\beta} \in W_0)$, tests the hypothesis that the explanatory variables have no effect at all. The term $SS(\boldsymbol{\beta} \in W_{j-1} | \boldsymbol{\beta} \in W_j)$ is used to test whether β_j is significantly different from zero, given that the model includes all x_i for $i < j$.

Notation The quantity $SS(\boldsymbol{\beta} \in W_{j-1} | \boldsymbol{\beta} \in W_j)$ is often written $R(\beta_j | \beta_0, \ldots, \beta_{j-1})$, where R stands for "reduction sum of squares" [37, 123], or $SS(\beta_j | \beta_0, \ldots, \beta_{j-1})$, the extra sum of squares due to the term β_j [51]. Notation such as $SSR(x_j | x_1, \ldots, x_{j-1})$ is also used [37, 83].

The traditional notation emphasizes the building of a model from the bottom up, where terms are *added* sequentially. The notation we have introduced, $SS(H^{(0)})$ and $SS(H^{(0)} | H^{(1)})$, works from the top down and emphasizes the terms that are *missing*.

Our notation:	Applied to the model (4.20):	Traditional notation:
$SS(\boldsymbol{\beta} \in W_0)$	$SS(\beta_1 = \cdots = \beta_k = 0)$	$R(\text{regression} \vert \beta_0)$
$SS(\boldsymbol{\beta} \in W_0 \vert \boldsymbol{\beta} \in W_1)$	$SS(\beta_1 = 0 \vert \beta_2 = \cdots = \beta_k = 0)$	$R(\beta_1 \vert \beta_0)$
$SS(\boldsymbol{\beta} \in W_{j-1} \vert \boldsymbol{\beta} \in W_j)$	$SS(\beta_j = 0 \vert \beta_{j+1} = \cdots = \beta_k = 0)$	$R(\beta_j \vert \beta_0, \ldots, \beta_{j-1})$
$SS(\boldsymbol{\beta} \in W_{k-1})$	$SS(\beta_k = 0)$	$R(\beta_k \vert \beta_0, \ldots, \beta_{k-1})$

Some authors (e.g., [123, Section 6.3]) also use $R(\cdot)$-notation for sequential sums of squares in factorial experiments, using the notation of the factor-effects model (Sect. 2.5) to indicate terms being added. Thus, for example, $R(\alpha | \mu, \beta)$ is the reduction sum of squares for fitting a model with only a B (or β) effect compared with an additive model having both A and B effects.

In ANOVA tables it is standard to list sequential sums of squares in order from the simplest model (having the fewest terms) to the most complex. Thus the last sequential sum of squares corresponds to the "last term added to the model," and is also therefore the adjusted sum of squares for that term.

We now take up the distribution theory for the sums of squares we have developed.

Theorem 4.22 *Assume that* $\mathbf{Y} \sim N(\mathbf{X}\boldsymbol{\beta}, \sigma^2\mathbf{I})$. *Consider a chain of linear hypotheses* H_0: $\boldsymbol{\beta} \in W_i$ *where* $W_0 \subset W_1 \subset \cdots \subset W_k \subset \mathbb{R}^p$. *Put* $V = R(\mathbf{X})$ *and* $V_i = \mathbf{X}(W_i)$, *with* $r = \dim(V)$ *and* $r_i = \dim(V_i)$, *and assume* $0 < r_0 < \cdots < r_k < r$. *Let* $\mathbf{P}$ *and* $\mathbf{P}_i$ *be the orthogonal projections of* $\mathbb{R}^N$ *on* V *and* V_i. *Then:*

a. $SS(\boldsymbol{\beta} \in W_k)/\sigma^2 \sim \chi^2(r - r_k, \delta/\sigma^2)$ *where* $\delta = \boldsymbol{\beta}'\mathbf{X}'(\mathbf{P} - \mathbf{P}_k)\mathbf{X}\boldsymbol{\beta}$. *If* $\boldsymbol{\beta} \in W_k$, *then* $SS(\boldsymbol{\beta} \in W_k)/\sigma^2 \sim \chi^2(r - r_k)$.
b. $SS(\boldsymbol{\beta} \in W_{j-1}|\boldsymbol{\beta} \in W_j)/\sigma^2 \sim \chi^2(r_j - r_{j-1}, \delta_j/\sigma^2)$ *where* $\delta_j = \boldsymbol{\beta}'\mathbf{X}'(\mathbf{P}_j - \mathbf{P}_{j-1})\mathbf{X}\boldsymbol{\beta}$. *If* $\boldsymbol{\beta} \in W_{j-1}$, *then* $SS(\boldsymbol{\beta} \in W_{j-1}|\boldsymbol{\beta} \in W_j)/\sigma^2 \sim \chi^2(r_j - r_{j-1})$.
c. $SS(\boldsymbol{\beta} \in W_k)$, $SS(\boldsymbol{\beta} \in W_{j-1}|\boldsymbol{\beta} \in W_j)$ *and* SSE *are independent.*

The proof of this theorem is left as an exercise. The quantity $r_j - r_{j-1}$ may be called the *sequential degrees of freedom* and denoted by $\text{df}(\boldsymbol{\beta} \in W_{j-1}|\boldsymbol{\beta} \in W_j)$ or $\text{df}(\boldsymbol{\beta} \perp U_{j-1}|\boldsymbol{\beta} \perp U_j)$.

As with Theorem 4.1, when $\mathbf{X}$ has full rank we may describe the sequential degrees of freedom in terms of the corresponding hypotheses.

Corollary 4.23 *Under the assumptions of Theorem 4.22, if* $\mathbf{X}$ *has full rank, then*

$$\text{df}(\boldsymbol{\beta} \in W_{j-1}|\boldsymbol{\beta} \in W_j) = \dim(W_j) - \dim(W_{j-1}).$$

Alternatively,

$$\text{df}(\boldsymbol{\beta} \perp U_{j-1}|\boldsymbol{\beta} \perp U_j) = \dim(U_{j-1}) - \dim(U_j).$$

Proof By Proposition 4.11 the vector spaces $\mathbb{R}^p \ominus W_i$ and $V \ominus V_i$ are isomorphic, so that their dimensions are equal. Now it is not hard to show (see exercises) that

$$\mathbb{R}^p \ominus W_{j-1} = (\mathbb{R}^p \ominus W_j) \oplus (W_j \ominus W_{j-1}) \tag{4.21}$$

and

$$V \ominus V_{j-1} = (V \ominus V_j) \oplus (V_j \ominus V_{j-1}), \tag{4.22}$$

from which it follows easily that $\dim(W_j) - \dim(W_{j-1}) = \dim(W_j \ominus W_{j-1}) = \dim(V_j \ominus V_{j-1}) = r_j - r_{j-1}$.

Finally, we note that

$$W_j \ominus W_{j-1} = W_j \cap W^{\perp}{}_{j-1} = U^{\perp}{}_j \cap U_{j-1} = U_{j-1} \ominus U_j,$$

so that we also have $r_j - r_{j-1} = \dim(U_{j-1}) - \dim(U_j)$, as claimed. □

As an application of Corollary 4.23 we have the following:

Corollary 4.24 *In a linear regression model, each regression coefficient contributes 1 sequential df to the degrees of freedom for regression. In an* $a \times b$ *factorial* *experiment with all cells filled, the sequential degrees of freedom for main effects and interaction are* $a - 1, b - 1$ *and* $(a - 1)(b - 1)$*, respectively.*

In particular, the sequential degrees of freedom are the same as the corresponding adjusted degrees of freedom.

As with adjusted degrees of freedom, this result extends to multifactor designs (Corollary 5.19).

Table 4.4 illustrates one way of displaying the analysis of variance. For $a \times b$ designs (with no random factors) the ANOVA table looks much the same as Table 4.2, with sequential sums of squares replacing adjusted ones. The following examples will illustrate the theorem.

Example 4.25 Table 4.5 reanalyzes the data in Table 4.3 using the sequential sum of squares. The first four sums of squares in the table are, in a different order, the four terms in the equation

$$\begin{aligned} & SS(\beta_1 = \beta_2 = \beta_3 = 0) \\ & = SS(\beta_3 = 0) + SS(\beta_2 = 0|\beta_3 = 0) + SS(\beta_1 = 0|\beta_2 = \beta_3 = 0), \end{aligned} \tag{4.23}$$

which is Eq. (4.18) with $k = 2$. In traditional notation, this equation reads

$$R(\beta_1, \beta_2, \beta_3|\beta_0) = R(\beta_3|\beta_0, \beta_1, \beta_2) + R(\beta_2|\beta_0, \beta_1) + R(\beta_1|\beta_0).$$

Table 4.4 ANOVA table for nested hypotheses. The sum of squares for the model is labeled SSR since it is generally included only for regression problems, in which case "Model" is labeled "Regression". The sequential sums of squares add up to SSR; degrees of freedom add up correspondingly. Each mean square is computed by $MS = SS/\text{df}$. $SS(\boldsymbol{\beta} \in W_k)$ has been abbreviated $SS(W_k)$, and so on

Source	SS (seq)	df	MS	F
Model	SSR	$r - r_0$	$SSR/(r - r_0)$	MSR/MSE
$\boldsymbol{\beta} \in W_0$	$SS(W_0\|W_1)$	$r_1 - r_0$		$MS(W_0\|W_1)/MSE$
$\vdots$	$\vdots$	$\vdots$	$\vdots$	$\vdots$
$\boldsymbol{\beta} \in W_{k-1}$	$SS(W_{k-1}\|W_k)$	$r_k - r_{k-1}$		$MS(W_{k-1}\|W_k)/MSE$
$\boldsymbol{\beta} \in W_k$	$SS(W_k)$	$r - r_k$	$SS(W_k)/(r - r_k)$	$MS(W_k)/MSE$
Error	SSE	$N - r$	$SSE/(N - r)$	
Total	SST	$N - r_0$		

Table 4.5 ANOVA table for $E(Y) = \beta_0 + \beta_1 x + \beta_2 x^2 + \beta_3 x^3$ using the sequential sums of squares, as in Example 4.25

Source	SS (seq)	df	MS	F	p-value
Regression	1.68890	3	0.56297	60.192	0.000
x	0.00670	1	0.00670	0.716	0.410
x^2	1.66896	1	1.66896	178.445	0.000
x^3	0.01324	1	0.01324	1.415	0.252
Error	0.14965	16	0.00935		
Total	1.83855	19			

The left-hand side of (4.23) is the regression sum of squares, and is the same as in Table 4.3. The three terms on the right are the sequential sums of squares, listed in the ANOVA table in the order in which terms were added, starting with x. In practice, the order in which terms are added to a regression model is generally specified by the user. We can verify that these three terms are as claimed by making the following observations:

- The sequential sum of squares for x^3 is the same as its adjusted sum of squares (Table 4.3), indicating that the x^3 term was fitted last. The sum of squares is therefore $R(\beta_3|\beta_0, \beta_1, \beta_2)$.
- The term $R(\beta_1|\beta_0)$ is the regression sum of squares for the model

$$E(Y) = \beta_0 + \beta_1 x \tag{4.24}$$

as we may verify by running a regression analysis for this smaller model:

Source	SS	df
Regression	**0.0067**	1
Error	1.8318	18
Total	1.8385	19

In that sense, we say that β_1 (or x) has been "fitted first". (In this ANOVA table, the label "Regression" refers to the model (4.24), not to the original model.)
- We may similarly calculate $R(\beta_2|\beta_0, \beta_1)$ by noting that the regression sum of squares for the model $E(Y) = \beta_0 + \beta_1 x + \beta_2 x^2$ is

$$R(\beta_1, \beta_2|\beta_0) = R(\beta_2|\beta_0, \beta_1) + R(\beta_1|\beta_0). \tag{4.25}$$

A regression analysis for this model gives the numerical value of this sum of squares:

Source	SS	df
Regression	**1.67566**	2
Error	0.16288	17
Total	1.83855	19

The value of $R(\beta_2|\beta_0, \beta_1)$, which is the sequential sum of squares for the term x^2, can thus be gotten by subtraction:

$$1.67566 - 0.0067 = \mathbf{1.66896}.$$

The p-values for the sequential ANOVA seem to indicate that the linear (x) term has very little significance, and that the quadratic term is the only essential one. One possibility is not that the linear term is unimportant, but that a linear model has too little explanatory power, which therefore inflates the MSE and consequently lowers the F-value for that simple model. Certainly the adjusted ANOVA tells a different story, where the addition of the linear term *at the end* is highly significant. In practice one might want to examine a variety of models in which the terms enter in different orders. Finally, a scatterplot of the data does indeed show a pronounced convex curve, and we see that the addition of a cubic term is not significant, so a quadratic model is probably the right one.

Example 4.26 Let us reanalyze the data from Example 4.17 using sequential sums of squares.

Source	SS (seq)	df	MS	F	p-value
Soil	52.50	1	52.50	3.94	0.079
Variety	124.73	2	62.37	4.68	0.040
Interaction	222.77	2	111.38	8.35	0.009
Error	120.00	9	13.33		
Total	520.00	14			

The order of entry of terms in the model—in this case, Soil, then Variety, then Interaction—determines the sequence of the sums of squares. It appears that Soil by itself is not very significant, but that the additional effect of Variety is, and that the interaction of these factors is highly significant.

Equation (4.18) would look something like this:

$$\begin{aligned} SS(\text{model}) &= SS(\text{no interaction}) + SS(\text{only soil}|\text{no interaction}) \\ &\quad + SS(\text{no effects}|\text{only soil}) \end{aligned}$$

("only soil" means "only soil present"). In R-notation this might be written

$$R(\mu, \alpha, \beta, \gamma) = R(\gamma|\mu, \alpha, \beta) + R(\beta|\mu, \alpha) + R(\alpha|\mu),$$

where γ represents interaction and α and β represent soil and variety effects, respectively. In this rather artificial example, $SS(\text{model}) = 400$, which is the sum of the three sequential sums of squares.

We can verify the sequence of models used in this example by examining some smaller ANOVA tables:

- The sequential sum of squares for Soil corresponds to what we would have called a "soil-only" model in Sect. 2.2.1. That is, the Soil effect was added first. Indeed, the analysis of variance and the fitted values (estimated cell means) for this model looks like this:

Source	SS (seq)	df
Soil	**52.50**	1
Error	467.50	13
Total	520.00	14

		Variety		
		1	2	3
Soil	1	13	13	13
	2	16.75	16.75	16.75

Note how the fitted values follow the pattern of display (2.4).

- We generate the sequential sum of squares for Variety by fitting a no-interaction model, since that is the model we get by adding the effect of Variety:

Source	SS (seq)	df
Soil	52.50	1
Variety	**124.73**	2
Error	342.77	11
Total	520.00	14

		Variety		
		1	2	3
Soil	1	10.23	18.05	12.10
	2	15.07	22.89	16.94

Now the fitted values, shown in the right-hand array, satisfy an additive (no-interaction) model. The quantity 124.73, the sequential sum of squares for Variety given that Soil is already in the model, is said by Searle [124, Table 4.10] to be due to "Columns, adjusted for rows", and 52.50 as due to "Rows, adjusted for mean". As in Example 4.25, changing the order of entry of terms into the model will change the sequential sums of squares (Exercise 4.10).

- Finally, we note that the sequential and adjusted sums of squares for interaction are equal, indicating that interaction is fitted last.[10]

4.5.1 Adjusted or Sequential?

There are several aspects to this question. We will explore some answers in Sects. 4.5.2 and 4.6.

1. Which sequence of nested hypotheses should we use for the analysis of variance?

There is no single answer to this question. In the case of factorial models, it is typical to fit main effects first, then first-order (two-factor) interactions,[11] and so

[10] Searle [123, pp. 301–302] claims that in a two-factor experiment it is impossible to fit interactions first. More precisely, he claims to show that the sequential sum of squares $SS(\text{no } B \text{ effect}|\text{no interaction})$ $(= R(\beta|\mu, \alpha, \gamma))$ is identically zero, but the argument appears to be in error.

on if there are more factors. Even this leaves open some choices—for example, the order in which main effects should enter. A polynomial regression model such as that in Example 4.25 is unusual in that among all the possible chains of nested hypotheses there is a unique "natural" one, ordered by the exponent on x.

In regression models the various possible sequences of submodels give rise to methods of model-building based on *sequential F-tests.* Given an overall initial model with a large set of regressors, the procedure can begin with a small initial set of regressors and add new ones one-by-one (forward selection), begin with the overall model and remove regressors one-by-one (backward elimination), or alternately add and remove regressors from an initial set (a stepwise procedure). At each step one compares two regression submodels that differ only in the presence or absence of a given term, the smaller model always treated as the "null" model. The "extra sum of squares" is used for the numerator of the F-statistic, and the error mean square for the larger model—*not necessarily that of the overall model*—is the denominator. Such tests are often called *partial F tests*—see, for example, [100] or [151].

Connected with this question is the following:

2. Which sum of squares is most appropriate to test for the presence or absence of a given effect?

This is more than just a choice between "adjusted" and "sequential", since typically any given effect can be represented by *many* choices of sequential sum of squares, depending on the order in which effects enter into a model.

Of course, one advantage of using the adjusted sum of squares is that it avoids this problem. In addition, it is in some ways a natural choice. For example, the sum of squares (4.13) for testing $\mathbf{c}'\boldsymbol{\beta} = 0$ is an adjusted sum of squares. We saw in Example 4.13 that the test of this hypothesis is equivalent to the t-test. If one accepts the t-test as a "natural" one, then this argues for the appropriateness of the "topmost" or adjusted sum of squares.

On the other hand, one important argument in favor of using sequential sums of squares is their additivity. The most basic meaning of "analysis of variance" is separation of variance into parts, and sequential sums of squares do separate a total sum of squares into a sum of smaller ones. The use of sequential sums of squares in regression is pervasive, where it has been called the *extra sum of squares principle* [51].

We should note that sequential sums of squares are *not* of the form $SS(H)$ that we described in Sect. 4.1, and while we could give a reasonably satisfactory justification for the definition and use of $SS(H)$ in testing a hypothesis H, we have not provided a similar development for using $SS(H^{(1)}|H^{(2)})$. There is actually an argument that a sequential sum of squares tests a hypothesis different from the one intended. We will take this up in Sect. 4.5.2.

[11] See Sect. 5.3 for a discussion of the *order* of an interaction.

These observations lead us to ask the following:

3. When do the sequential sums of squares have values that are independent of the order of nesting of hypotheses? When do the adjusted sums of squares add up to the sum of squares for the model?

As it turns out, these two questions have the same answer, as we will see in Sect. 4.6. When we have independence of order, every sequential sum of squares is also an adjusted sum of squares, and so the adjusted sums of squares add up to the sum of squares for the model. When this holds, of course, the preceding questions become moot.

Remark 4.27 If the analysis of variance for an $a \times b$ design shows significant interaction, should one test for main effects? Many authors say no. Presumably it would make no sense to keep open the possibility that, say, the A effect is absent if one already knows there is significant $A \times B$ interaction. Instead, they suggest simply examining various contrasts in the ab cell means, as though dealing with a one-factor model. In fact, one also finds the suggestion that when interactions are *not* significant one should re-analyze the data as coming from an additive model.

The problem, as we discussed in Remark 2.9, may be that we attribute too much to the meaning of "interaction", which is actually defined in a very narrow and specific way. From this point of view, the significance of interaction is quite separate from that of main effects, and there is no necessary reason to avoid testing for main effects when interaction is significant. Scheffé [121, pp. 94 and 116] agrees, and gives an alternate explanation for his position.

4.5.2 Associated Hypotheses

In his analysis of the data in Example 4.26, Searle asserts that the sequential sum of squares for Soils actually tests the hypothesis

$$\frac{1}{7}(3\mu_{11} + 2\mu_{12} + 2\mu_{13}) = \frac{1}{8}(4\mu_{21} + \mu_{22} + 3\mu_{23}), \tag{4.26}$$

and refers to this and similar hypotheses as "a sorry lot." What does he mean, and where did he get (4.26)?

Searle's objection to testing a hypothesis like (4.26) is that the coefficients 3, 2, etc., are precisely the sample sizes for the six treatment combinations (and the denominators are their sums). But *hypotheses ought to be framed independent of the data.* Of course, our description of sequential sums of squares involved a comparison of two hypotheses, neither of which involved the sample sizes, so how did they creep in? We need to look at this more carefully.

What accounts for the equality of these two sums of squares, the sequential sum of squares for Soil and the sum of squares for testing the hypothesis (4.26)? Of course, we can compute the latter, namely the sum of squares for the contrast

$$\frac{1}{7}(3\mu_{11} + 2\mu_{12} + 2\mu_{13}) - \frac{1}{8}(4\mu_{21} + \mu_{22} + 3\mu_{23}) = 0,$$

and verify that it is equal to 52.50, but what Searle is asserting is that the two sums of squares are equal for *any* data $\mathbf{Y}$.

As we noted above, the usual sum of squares for testing a hypothesis like (4.26) is actually an adjusted sum of squares. So Searle has found a hypothesis whose adjusted sum of squares is the same as the sequential sum of squares he started with.

Without loss of generality, we consider the nested hypotheses $\boldsymbol{\beta} \in W_j$, $j = 1, 2$, where $W_1 \subset W_2$, and the corresponding sequential sum of squares. The *hypothesis tested by the sequential sum of squares* $SS(\boldsymbol{\beta} \in W_1 | \boldsymbol{\beta} \in W_2)$ is defined to be the hypothesis H^*: $\boldsymbol{\beta} \in W^*$ whose adjusted sum of squares equals the sequential one, that is, such that

$$SS(\boldsymbol{\beta} \in W^*) = SS(\boldsymbol{\beta} \in W_1 | \boldsymbol{\beta} \in W_2). \tag{4.27}$$

Searle [124, p. 40] refers to H^* as the *associated hypothesis* for the sequential sum of squares.

It is not entirely clear that such a hypothesis must exist, but the following theorem shows that it does and outlines a general method for finding it, assuming that $\mathbf{X}$ is full-rank.

Theorem 4.28 *Consider the model* $\mathrm{E}(\mathbf{Y}) = \mathbf{X}\boldsymbol{\beta}$, *where* $\mathbf{X}$ *(*$N \times p$*) has full rank, and let* $W_1 \subset W_2 \subset \mathbb{R}^p$. *Then there is a unique subspace* W^* *satisfying (4.27), and we have*

$$\mathrm{df}(\boldsymbol{\beta} \in W^*) = \mathrm{df}(\boldsymbol{\beta} \in W_1 | \boldsymbol{\beta} \in W_2). \tag{4.28}$$

The subspace is given by $W^* = R(\mathbf{TP}^*)$, *where* $\mathbf{T} = (\mathbf{X}'\mathbf{X})^{-1}\mathbf{X}'$ *and* $\mathbf{P}^*$ *is defined as follows.*

Let $V_i = \mathbf{X}(W_i)$, *let* $V = R(\mathbf{X})$ *be the range (columnspace) of* $\mathbf{X}$, *and let* $\mathbf{P}$ *and* $\mathbf{P}_i$ *be the orthogonal projections of* $\mathbb{R}^N$ *on* V *and on* V_i, *respectively. Then* $\mathbf{P}^* = \mathbf{P} - \mathbf{P}_2 + \mathbf{P}_1$.

We are writing the orthogonal projections as matrices for convenience. This is no restriction. The matrix $\mathbf{T}$ is the Moore-Penrose inverse of $\mathbf{X}$, defined in (3.18).

The proof of this theorem relies on the following lemma. We state it for $\mathbb{R}^N$, but it applies more generally in any inner product space.

Lemma 4.29 *Let* $\mathbf{Q}_1$ *and* $\mathbf{Q}_2$ *be orthogonal projections of* $\mathbb{R}^N$ *on subspaces* V_1 *and* V_2, *respectively. If* $\|\mathbf{Q}_1\mathbf{y}\| = \|\mathbf{Q}_2\mathbf{y}\|$ *for all* $\mathbf{y} \in \mathbb{R}^N$, *then* $\mathbf{Q}_1 = \mathbf{Q}_2$.

Proof It suffices to show that $V_1 = V_2$.

For any projection $\mathbf{Q}$ and any $\mathbf{y} \in \mathbb{R}^N$ we have the orthogonal decomposition

$$\mathbf{y} = \mathbf{Q}\mathbf{y} + (\mathbf{I} - \mathbf{Q})\mathbf{y}$$

(Corollary A.91). Thus for all $\mathbf{y} \in \mathbb{R}^N$

$$\begin{aligned}\|(\mathbf{I} - \mathbf{Q}_1)\mathbf{y}\|^2 &= \|\mathbf{y}\|^2 - \|\mathbf{Q}_1\mathbf{y}\|^2 \\ &= \|\mathbf{y}\|^2 - \|\mathbf{Q}_2\mathbf{y}\|^2 = \|(\mathbf{I} - \mathbf{Q}_2)\mathbf{y}\|^2,\end{aligned}$$

so for all $\mathbf{y} \in \mathbb{R}^N$

$$\|(\mathbf{I} - \mathbf{Q}_1)\mathbf{y}\| = \|(\mathbf{I} - \mathbf{Q}_2)\mathbf{y}\|.$$

In particular, let $\mathbf{y} \in V_1$. We have $\|(\mathbf{I} - \mathbf{Q}_1)\mathbf{y}\| = 0$, so $\|(\mathbf{I} - \mathbf{Q}_2)\mathbf{y}\| = 0$, and so

$$\mathbf{y} = \mathbf{Q}_2\mathbf{y}.$$

But then $\mathbf{y} \in V_2$. This shows that $V_1 \subset V_2$. Similarly, $V_2 \subset V_1$, so $V_1 = V_2$. □

Proof of Theorem 4.28 First, let $W^* \subset \mathbb{R}^p$ be an arbitrary subspace, and consider testing H^*: $\boldsymbol{\beta} \in W^*$. Let $V^* = \mathbf{X}(W^*)$, and let $\mathbf{P}^*$ be the orthogonal projection of $\mathbb{R}^N$ on V^*. Given $\mathbf{Y} = \mathbf{y}$, $\hat{\mathbf{y}}^* = \mathbf{P}^*\mathbf{y}$ is the fitted value for $\boldsymbol{\beta} \in W^*$. We first determine $\mathbf{P}^*$ and V^* to satisfy (4.27).

Let $\hat{\mathbf{y}}$ and $\hat{\mathbf{y}}_j$ be the usual fitted values corresponding to $\boldsymbol{\beta} \in \mathbb{R}^p$ and $\boldsymbol{\beta} \in W_j$. Then (4.27) is the condition

$$\|\hat{\mathbf{y}} - \hat{\mathbf{y}}^*\|^2 = \|\hat{\mathbf{y}}_2 - \hat{\mathbf{y}}_1\|^2 \quad \text{for all } \mathbf{y} \in \mathbb{R}^N.$$

Letting $\mathbf{P}$ and $\mathbf{P}_j$ be the orthogonal projections on V and V_j, respectively, we may rewrite this in the form

$$\|\mathbf{P}\mathbf{y} - \mathbf{P}^*\mathbf{y}\|^2 = \|\mathbf{P}_2\mathbf{y} - \mathbf{P}_1\mathbf{y}\|^2$$

for all $\mathbf{y} \in R^N$. Now $V^* \subset V$ and $V_1 \subset V_2$, so $\mathbf{P} - \mathbf{P}^*$ and $\mathbf{P}_2 - \mathbf{P}_1$ are orthogonal projections (Corollary A.96). We may thus apply Lemma 4.29 and conclude that $\mathbf{P} - \mathbf{P}^* = \mathbf{P}_2 - \mathbf{P}_1$. Thus we set

$$\mathbf{P}^* = \mathbf{P} - \mathbf{P}_2 + \mathbf{P}_1$$

and

$$V^* = R(\mathbf{P}^*).$$

Since $\mathbf{P} - \mathbf{P}^* = \mathbf{P}_2 - \mathbf{P}_1$, their ranges must be equal, i.e.,

$$V \ominus V^* = V_2 \ominus V_1. \tag{4.29}$$

If W^* is such that $V^* = \mathbf{X}(W^*)$, then (4.28) follows immediately from (4.29) by taking dimensions of both sides.

Thus we need to solve $V^* = \mathbf{X}(W^*)$ for W^*. But applying $\mathbf{T}$ to both sides of this equation and using the fact that $\mathbf{TX} = \mathbf{I}$ (Lemma 3.15(a)) gives us $W^* = \mathbf{T}(V^*) = \mathbf{TP}^*(\mathbb{R}^N) = R(\mathbf{TP}^*)$, as claimed. The construction makes it clear that W^* exists and is unique. □

Of course, we may put the associated hypothesis $\boldsymbol{\beta} \in W^*$ in the form $\boldsymbol{\beta} \perp U^*$ by letting $U^* = (W^*)^\perp$. In this form we are asking for the relations between cell means.

Corollary 4.30 *Given the assumptions and notation of Theorem 4.28, the subspace U^* is given by $U^* = N(\mathbf{P}^*\mathbf{T}')$.*

Proof From Theorem A.79(c) and the symmetry of $\mathbf{P}^*$ we have $U^* = (R(\mathbf{TP}^*))^\perp = N((\mathbf{TP}^*)') = N(\mathbf{P}^*\mathbf{T}')$. □

In Example 4.26, $\boldsymbol{\beta} \in W_2$ is the hypothesis "only the Soil effect is present" while $\boldsymbol{\beta} \in W_1$ is the hypothesis "no effects are present" (i.e., the cell means are equal). (We would normally denote these W_1 and W_0; the numbering in Theorem 4.28 was generic.) Exercise 4.10 invites the reader to use this to show that (4.26), with arbitrary cell counts, is indeed the hypothesis being tested by the sequential sum of squares for Soil.

We can now answer a question we posed earlier: the cell counts n_{ij} enter the associated hypothesis $\boldsymbol{\beta} \in W^*$ because $W^* = \mathbf{T}(V^*)$ and $\mathbf{T}$ itself depends on the n_{ij}. In fact, this seems almost inevitable, no matter what $V^* \subset R(\mathbf{T})$ we consider. It certainly is true in Example 4.26.

Perhaps a more fundamental question is whether this does argue against the use of sequential sums of squares in hypothesis tests. We must grant that a sequential sum of squares will always equal an adjusted one. But what is the implication of this? In either case we are making a comparison: that between two nested hypotheses (in the sequential case), or that between a hypothesis and the full model (in the adjusted one). If the latter hypothesis is inappropriate, does that invalidate the use of the sum of squares for the former? Searle would say yes. (A less polemical discussion is given by Hocking [73, pp. 150–152], based on the paper [75].[12]) Comparison of a hypothesis with the full model—a kind of top-down analysis—seems to have a privileged place.

[12] This is based in turn on the dissertation [67] of Olga Hackney.

4.6 Orthogonal Hypotheses

In the last section we raised several questions concerning a model having a lattice of hypotheses such as those given in Fig. 4.2. Using the notation of that section, Question 3 asks for conditions such that

$$\|\hat{\mathbf{Y}} - \hat{\mathbf{Y}}_4\|^2 = \|\hat{\mathbf{Y}}_5 - \hat{\mathbf{Y}}_1\|^2 = \|\hat{\mathbf{Y}}_6 - \hat{\mathbf{Y}}_2\|^2 = \|\hat{\mathbf{Y}}_3 - \hat{\mathbf{Y}}_0\|^2. \tag{4.30}$$

These correspond to "parallel" lines in Fig. 4.2. Similar equations hold for $\|\hat{\mathbf{Y}} - \hat{\mathbf{Y}}_5\|^2$ and for $\|\hat{\mathbf{Y}} - \hat{\mathbf{Y}}_6\|^2$. We referred to this as the *independence of order of nesting*. We also noted that this represents the *equality of adjusted and sequential sums of squares*: in (4.30) the first term is an adjusted sum of squares, while the others are sequential. Finally, it implies that the adjusted sums of squares inherit the additivity of sequential ones (Eq. (4.15)).

Since $\hat{\mathbf{Y}}$ and $\hat{\mathbf{Y}}_i$ are the orthogonal projections of $\mathbf{Y}$ in V and in V_i, respectively, it is easy to see that (4.30) holds for all $\mathbf{Y}$ if and only if

$$V \ominus V_4 = V_5 \ominus V_1 = V_6 \ominus V_2 = V_3 \ominus V_0. \tag{4.31}$$

Finally, (4.31) can be rewritten

$$V \ominus V_4 = V_5 \ominus (V_4 \cap V_5) = V_6 \ominus (V_4 \cap V_6) = (V_5 \cap V_6) \ominus (V_4 \cap V_5 \cap V_6). \tag{4.32}$$

The reader can fill in the corresponding statements for $V \ominus V_5$ and $V \ominus V_6$. We seek conditions on the subspaces V_i that give us the desired equalities.

If we move beyond a two-factor design or a three-regressor model, we must consider more than 3 subspaces V_i lying just below V in our lattice, so we generalize our problem as follows. Let V be a subspace of $\mathbb{R}^N$, and suppose V itself has subspaces $V_1, \ldots, V_k$.[13] We seek a condition on these subspaces such that for every $J \subset \{1, \ldots, k\}$ and every $i \in J^c$ we have

$$V \ominus V_i = (\cap_{j \in J} V_j) \ominus (\cap_{j \in J} V_j \ \cap \ V_i).$$

For ease of reading, let us put

$$V_J = \cap_{j \in J} V_j.$$

The condition we seek is thus one that guarantees that

$$V \ominus V_i = V_J \ominus (V_J \cap V_i) \tag{4.33}$$

[13] At this point we are ignoring the role of $\mathbf{X}$. Note that we are numbering the subspaces V_i differently from those in Fig. 4.2.

for all $J \subset \{1, \ldots, k\}$ and every $i \in J^c$. Equation (4.33) is the generalization of (4.32) to k subspaces V_i. The hatch marks in the diagram below indicate the equality in Eq. (4.33).

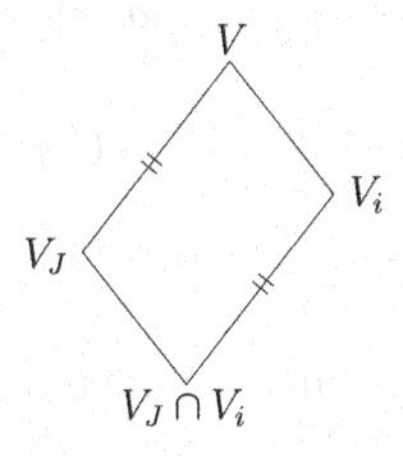

Theorem 4.31 (Orthogonality Theorem [128, Theorem 6.2.1]) *Let $V, V_1, \ldots, V_k$ be subspaces of $\mathbb{R}^N$, $V_i \subset V$. Then (4.33) holds for all $J \subset \{1, \ldots, k\}$ and every $i \in J^c$ if and only if*

$$V \ominus V_i \perp V \ominus V_j \tag{4.34}$$

for all distinct i and j.

Seber [128, p. 42] remarks that we can recast the condition (4.34) in another form that will be useful to us. We formulate this as a lemma:

Lemma 4.32 *Under the assumptions of Theorem 4.31, (4.34) holds if and only if $V \ominus V_i \subset V_j$, $i \neq j$.*

Proof Clearly (4.34) holds iff $V \ominus V_i \subset (V \ominus V_j)^{\perp}$. But using a De Morgan law (A.20) and the involutory property of $^{\perp}$ (Theorem A.70) we see that

$$\begin{aligned}(V \ominus V_j)^{\perp} &= (V \cap V^{\perp}{}_j)^{\perp} \\ &= V^{\perp} + V_j \\ &= V^{\perp} \oplus V_j \qquad \text{(orthogonal sum)},\end{aligned}$$

the last equality holding since $V_j \subset V$. That is, (4.34) holds iff

$$V \ominus V_i \subset V^{\perp} \oplus V_j, \tag{4.35}$$

so we claim that *this* holds if and only if $V \ominus V_i \subset V_j$. One direction is immediate: Clearly $V_j \subset V^{\perp} \oplus V_j$, so if $V \ominus V_i \subset V_j$ then (4.35) holds.

Conversely, assume (4.35) and let $\mathbf{v} \in V \ominus V_i$. We must show that $\mathbf{v} \in V_j$. Using (4.35) we may write

$$\mathbf{v} = \mathbf{v}_1 + \mathbf{v}_2, \quad \mathbf{v}_1 \in V^{\perp}, \mathbf{v}_2 \in V_j.$$

Of course, $\mathbf{v} \in V$, so $\mathbf{v}_1 = \mathbf{v} - \mathbf{v}_2 \in V$. But we also have $\mathbf{v}_1 \in V^\perp$, so $\mathbf{v}_1 = \mathbf{0}$. Thus $\mathbf{v} = \mathbf{v}_2 \in V_j$. □

Proof of Theorem 4.31 Assume (4.34), and fix $J \subset \{1, \ldots, k\}$ and $i \in J^c$.

Applying a De Morgan law, the right-hand side of (4.33) is

$$\begin{aligned} V_J \ominus (V_J \cap V_i) &= V_J \cap (V_J \cap V_i)^\perp \\ &= V_J \cap (V^\perp{}_J + V^\perp{}_i). \end{aligned} \tag{4.36}$$

We would like to "distribute" V_J, but the lattice of subspaces of $\mathbb{R}^N$ only satisfies the modular law (A.6), so we need to re-write the sum in (4.36) so that this law applies.

But Eq. (A.17) (itself an application of the modular law) says that

$$V^\perp{}_i = (V \ominus V_i) + V^\perp \tag{4.37}$$

(the sum is actually orthogonal, but we don't need this). Replacing $V^\perp{}_i$ in (4.36) by the expression given in (4.37), we have

$$\begin{aligned} V_J \ominus (V_J \cap V_i) &= V_J \cap (V^\perp{}_J + (V \ominus V_i) + V^\perp) \\ &= V_J \cap (V^\perp{}_J + V^\perp + V \ominus V_i) \\ &= V_J \cap ((V_J \cap V)^\perp + V \ominus V_i) \\ &= V_J \cap (V^\perp{}_J + V \ominus V_i). \end{aligned}$$

Now it follows from the lemma and the definition of V_J that $V_J \supset V \ominus V_i$, so by the modular law this

$$\begin{aligned} &= (V_J \cap V^\perp{}_J) + V \ominus V_i \\ &= V \ominus V_i, \end{aligned}$$

which establishes (4.33).

Conversely, assume Eq. (4.33) for $J \subset \{1, \ldots, k\}$ and $i \in J^c$. When $J = \{j\}$ this becomes

$$V \ominus V_i = V_j \ominus (V_j \cap V_i),$$

which implies

$$V \ominus V_i \subset V_j.$$

But by the lemma, this is equivalent to (4.34). □

Remark 4.33 Darroch and Silvey [39, p. 564] define an experimental design to be *orthogonal* relative to hypotheses $H^{(1)}, \ldots, H^{(k)}$ if condition (4.34) holds (their subspaces ω_i^p are our $V \ominus V_i$). As we noted in Remark 1.38, they generally treat a linear hypothesis as a constraint on $\mathrm{E}(\mathbf{Y})$ rather than on $\boldsymbol{\beta}$. For them, the hypotheses are of the form $\mathrm{E}(\mathbf{Y}) \in V_i$.

Actually, the Orthogonality Theorem (Theorem 4.31) makes no reference to hypotheses or indeed to a linear model. We will make that connection now.

The first order of business is to restate the Orthogonality Theorem in the language of testing a family of hypotheses $\boldsymbol{\beta} \perp U_i$. Let $W_i = U^{\perp}{}_i$, so that $V_i = \mathbf{X}(W_i)$, and let $V = R(\mathbf{X})$ as before.

Corollary 4.34 *Given a finite set of hypotheses $\boldsymbol{\beta} \perp U_i$ (or $\boldsymbol{\beta} \in W_i$), their sequential sums of squares are independent of order of nesting if and only if (4.34) holds.*

How does the condition (4.34) apply to the original hypotheses? The picture looks something like this:

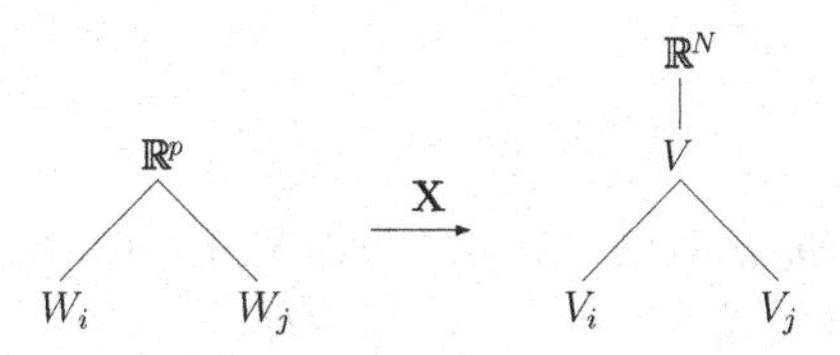

Let $\mathbf{T} = (\mathbf{X}'\mathbf{X})^{-1}\mathbf{X}'$ be the Moore-Penrose inverse of $\mathbf{X}$. Recall that $\mathbf{T}'$ (like $\mathbf{T}$) is full rank if $\mathbf{X}$ is, and that it maps U_i isomorphically onto $V \ominus V_i$ (Proposition 4.11):

$\mathbb{R}^p$: U_i, U_j $\xrightarrow{\mathbf{T}'}$ V: $V \ominus V_i$, $V \ominus V_j$

We want conditions on $\mathbf{T}'$—that is, on $\mathbf{X}$—and on U_i and U_j that guarantee a right angle on the right-hand side of this picture. Thus two questions naturally arise:

1. Given $\mathbf{X}$, what is the relation of U_i and U_j that guarantees that $V \ominus V_i \perp V \ominus V_j$?

In other words, what kind of hypotheses of form $\boldsymbol{\beta} \perp U$ lead to sequential sums of squares that are independent of order of nesting? A companion question arises when we are given "orthogonal" hypotheses, such as in a factorial design:

2. Given that $U_i \perp U_j$, what conditions on $\mathbf{X}$ imply that $V \ominus V_i \perp V \ominus V_j$?
   This is a "design" question, and is perhaps of more direct practical interest.

We begin by defining[14]

$$\langle \mathbf{x}, \mathbf{y} \rangle = \mathbf{x}'(\mathbf{X}'\mathbf{X})^{-1}\mathbf{y}, \tag{4.38}$$

assuming that $\mathbf{X}$ has full rank, and writing

$$\mathbf{x} \perp_* \mathbf{y}$$

if $\langle \mathbf{x}, \mathbf{y} \rangle = 0$. The following corollary to Theorem 4.31 answers the first question:

Corollary 4.35 *Given a finite set of hypotheses $\boldsymbol{\beta} \perp U_i$ (or $\boldsymbol{\beta} \in W_i$), their sequential sums of squares are independent of the order of nesting if and only if $U_i \perp_* U_j$ for all distinct i and j.*

The corollary depends on the following result; the proof of both is left as an exercise.

Lemma 4.36 *Equation (4.38) defines an inner product on $\mathbb{R}^p$. Letting $\mathbf{T} = (\mathbf{X}'\mathbf{X})^{-1}\mathbf{X}'$, we have*

$$(\mathbf{T}'\mathbf{x}) \cdot (\mathbf{T}'\mathbf{y}) = \langle \mathbf{x}, \mathbf{y} \rangle. \tag{4.39}$$

(The left-hand side is the usual dot product in $\mathbb{R}^N$.) Letting U_i, U_j, V, V_i and V_j be defined as above, $V \ominus V_i \perp V \ominus V_j$ iff $U_i \perp_* U_j$.

Our answer to the second question will be restricted to certain models. Corollary 4.35—in particular the inner product (4.38)—shows that the desired orthogonality depends directly on the matrix $\mathbf{X}'\mathbf{X}$, which in turn depends on the structure of $\mathbf{X}$ since the ijth entry of $\mathbf{X}'\mathbf{X}$ is the dot product of columns i and j of $\mathbf{X}$. We consider three possibilities:

- $\mathbf{X}'\mathbf{X}$ is a *scalar matrix*, that is, a multiple of the identity matrix. This clearly holds iff the columns of $\mathbf{X}$ are mutually orthogonal and have the same (Euclidean) length.
- $\mathbf{X}'\mathbf{X}$ is diagonal. This holds iff the columns of $\mathbf{X}$ are mutually orthogonal.
- $\mathbf{X}'\mathbf{X}$ is *block diagonal*: that is, it is of the form

$$\begin{pmatrix} \mathbf{B}_1 & & & \\ & \mathbf{B}_2 & & \\ & & \ddots & \\ & & & \mathbf{B}_k \end{pmatrix}$$

[14] We have also used $\langle \cdots \rangle$ to denote the span of a set of vectors. With two vectors, we will have to distinguish from context whether we mean their span or their special inner product (4.38).

where $\mathbf{B}_i$ are square blocks of entries, not necessarily of the same size, and entries outside of the blocks are zero. This holds iff the columns of $\mathbf{X}$ can be partitioned into blocks $B_1, \ldots, B_k$ such that the submatrix $\mathbf{B}_i$ has order $|B_i| \times |B_i|$ and blocks B_i and B_j are mutually orthogonal for $i \neq j$.

We leave it as an exercise to show that a matrix $\mathbf{M}$ has any of these properties iff $\mathbf{M}^{-1}$ does. Thus we may state our results in terms of $\mathbf{X}'\mathbf{X}$ rather than its inverse. We start with the simplest case, where we will need the following lemma. Again let $\perp_*$ denote perpendicularity with respect to the new inner product (4.38).

Lemma 4.37 *If, for all* $\mathbf{x}$ *and* $\mathbf{y}$ *in* $\mathbb{R}^p$, $\mathbf{x} \perp \mathbf{y}$ *implies* $\mathbf{x} \perp_* \mathbf{y}$, *then* $\mathbf{X}'\mathbf{X}$ *is a scalar matrix.*

Proof Let $\mathbf{e}_1, \ldots, \mathbf{e}_p$ be the standard basis vectors of $\mathbb{R}^p$:

$$\mathbf{e}_i = (0, \ldots, 0, \overset{\substack{i \\ |}}{1}, 0, \ldots, 0)'. \tag{4.40}$$

Since $\mathbf{e}_i \perp \mathbf{e}_j$, we have $\mathbf{e}_i \perp_* \mathbf{e}_j$ by assumption, so that

$$0 = \mathbf{e}_i'(\mathbf{X}'\mathbf{X})^{-1}\mathbf{e}_j = \text{the } ij\text{th element of } (\mathbf{X}'\mathbf{X})^{-1}.$$

Thus the off-diagonal elements of $(\mathbf{X}'\mathbf{X})^{-1}$ are zero, so that $\mathbf{X}'\mathbf{X}$ itself is diagonal. Letting $\mathbf{x} = \mathbf{e}_1 + \mathbf{e}_i$ and $\mathbf{y} = \mathbf{e}_1 - \mathbf{e}_i$, we easily see that $\mathbf{x} \perp \mathbf{y}$, so we similarly must have

$$\begin{aligned}
0 = \langle \mathbf{x}, \mathbf{y} \rangle &= \langle \mathbf{e}_1 + \mathbf{e}_i, \mathbf{e}_1 - \mathbf{e}_i \rangle \\
&= \langle \mathbf{e}_1, \mathbf{e}_1 \rangle - \langle \mathbf{e}_1, \mathbf{e}_i \rangle + \langle \mathbf{e}_1, \mathbf{e}_i \rangle - \langle \mathbf{e}_i, \mathbf{e}_i \rangle \\
&= \langle \mathbf{e}_1, \mathbf{e}_1 \rangle - \langle \mathbf{e}_i, \mathbf{e}_i \rangle,
\end{aligned}$$

the difference of the first and ith diagonal entries of $(\mathbf{X}'\mathbf{X})^{-1}$. Since i is arbitrary, the diagonal entries are equal, and so $\mathbf{X}'\mathbf{X} = c\mathbf{I}$ for some c, as claimed. □

We can now begin to answer the second question above.

Theorem 4.38 *If* $\mathbf{X}'\mathbf{X}$ *is a scalar matrix, then for any* $U_1, \ldots, U_k$ *with* $U_i \perp U_j$, *the sequential sums of squares for testing the hypotheses* $\boldsymbol{\beta} \perp U_1, \ldots, \boldsymbol{\beta} \perp U_k$ *is independent of order of nesting. Conversely, if for any* U_1 *and* U_2 *with* $U_1 \perp U_2$ *the sequential sums of squares for testing* $\boldsymbol{\beta} \perp U_1$ *and* $\boldsymbol{\beta} \perp U_2$ *are independent of order, then* $\mathbf{X}'\mathbf{X}$ *is a scalar matrix.*

Proof If $\mathbf{X}'\mathbf{X}$ is scalar then the inner product (4.38) is simply a scalar multiple of the dot product, and so if $U_i \perp U_j$ then $U_i \perp_* U_j$. The conclusion follows from Corollary 4.35.

On the other hand, if for all orthogonal subspaces U_1 and U_2 of $\mathbb{R}^p$ we have independence of order of the sequential sums of squares for testing $\boldsymbol{\beta} \perp U_1$ and

$\boldsymbol{\beta} \perp U_2$, then by Corollary 4.35 it follows that $U_1 \perp_* U_2$. In particular, letting $\mathbf{u}_1$ and $\mathbf{u}_2$ be arbitrary vectors and putting $U_i = \langle \mathbf{u}_i \rangle$, we see that $\mathbf{u}_1 \perp \mathbf{u}_2$ implies that $\mathbf{u}_1 \perp_* \mathbf{u}_2$. Now Lemma 4.37 implies that $\mathbf{X}'\mathbf{X}$ is scalar. □

The assumption in the converse part of Theorem 4.38 can be weakened, although one needs to investigate to what extent. Of particular interest is the case of a small number of hypotheses known to be orthogonal—for example, the usual main effects and interactions hypotheses in a factorial design. (See Theorem 4.44 below.)

Now consider the case that $\mathbf{X}'\mathbf{X}$ is a diagonal matrix. While not all sets of hypotheses have independence of order of nesting, certain ones still do. This is based on the following lemma. Let $\mathbf{e}_1, \ldots, \mathbf{e}_p$ be the standard orthonormal basis vectors of $\mathbb{R}^p$ given by (4.40).

Lemma 4.39 *Let* $\mathbf{D}$ *be* $p \times p$. *Then* $\mathbf{D}$ *is diagonal if and only if* $\mathbf{e}_i'\mathbf{D}\mathbf{e}_j = 0$ *for all* $i \neq j$.

Proof We simply observe that $\mathbf{e}_i'\mathbf{D}\mathbf{e}_j = d_{ij}$, the ijth entry of $\mathbf{D}$. □

Now consider $\mathrm{E}(\mathbf{Y}) = \mathbf{X}\boldsymbol{\beta}$, and let the components of $\boldsymbol{\beta}$ be β_i.

Theorem 4.40 *The sequential sums of squares for the hypotheses* H_0: $\beta_i = 0$ *are independent of the order of nesting iff* $\mathbf{X}'\mathbf{X}$ *is diagonal, that is, iff the columns of* $\mathbf{X}$ *are orthogonal.*

Proof The hypotheses H_0 may be written $\boldsymbol{\beta} \perp \mathbf{e}_i$ (or $\boldsymbol{\beta} \perp U_i$ where U_i is the subspace spanned by $\mathbf{e}_i$). Then by Corollary 4.35 we have independence of order of nesting iff $\langle \mathbf{e}_i, \mathbf{e}_j \rangle = 0$ for all distinct i and j, where $\langle \cdot, \cdot \rangle$ is given by (4.38), and this holds according to the lemma if and only if $(\mathbf{X}'\mathbf{X})^{-1}$, and therefore $\mathbf{X}'\mathbf{X}$, is diagonal. □

We may generalize this as follows. Partition and $\mathbf{X}$ and $\boldsymbol{\beta}$ correspondingly as

$$\mathbf{X} = \begin{pmatrix} \mathbf{X}_1 & \vdots & \cdots & \vdots & \mathbf{X}_k \end{pmatrix} \quad \text{and} \quad \boldsymbol{\beta} = \begin{pmatrix} \boldsymbol{\beta}_1 \\ \cdots \\ \vdots \\ \cdots \\ \boldsymbol{\beta}_k \end{pmatrix}.$$

By appropriately generalizing Lemma 4.39, we arrive at this result:

Theorem 4.41 *The sequential sums of squares for the hypotheses* H_0: $\boldsymbol{\beta}_i = \mathbf{0}$ *are independent of the order of nesting iff* $\mathbf{X}'\mathbf{X}$ *is block diagonal with the same partition as* $\mathbf{X}$, *that is, iff the columns of* $\mathbf{X}_i$ *are orthogonal to those of* $\mathbf{X}_j$ *for* $i \neq j$.

We leave the proof of this as an exercise.

4.6.1 Application: Factorial Designs

Consider a factorial experiment with n_t observations on treatment combination t, and write its cell-means model in the form (1.18) where $\mathbf{X}$ is an $N \times p$ matrix with the vectors $\mathbf{1}_{n_t}$ down the "diagonal", as in (1.19). (We assume that we have imposed a fixed order on the set T of treatment combinations.) Here the columns of $\mathbf{X}$ are orthogonal, and in fact we see that $\mathbf{X}'\mathbf{X}$ *is a diagonal matrix with the sample sizes* $n_t, t \in T$, *down the diagonal.*[15]

In particular, $\mathbf{X}'\mathbf{X}$ is a scalar matrix iff the design is *equireplicate*, that is, iff the sample sizes n_t are equal (the data is *balanced*).

$\mathbf{X}'\mathbf{X}$ Scalar

We saw in Sect. 2.2 that the subspaces representing main effects and interactions in a two-factor design are mutually orthogonal, and in Sect. 5.3 we will see[16] that this holds true as well in a design with more than two factors. (We defined these subspaces for three-factor designs in Sect. 2.3.) The first part of Theorem 4.38 now has this easy consequences.

Corollary 4.42 *In an equireplicate factorial experiment, the sequential sums of squares for main effects and interactions are independent of the order of nesting. A sequential sum of squares for testing a main effect or interaction is equal to its adjusted sum of squares.*

Example 4.43 Table 4.6 gives a simulated data set and ANOVA table for a balanced 3×3 experiment. The adjusted and sequential sums of squares are equal, and are simply indicated by the SS column heading.

Here both main effects and interactions are statistically significant. We will refine this example at the end of Sect. 5.6, where we will split the interaction sum of squares into two components.

We are of course interested in the converse of Corollary 4.42. At this point we will only take up the case of a two-factor design. If the factors are A and B, then the hypotheses of interest here are $\boldsymbol{\beta} \perp U_1$ (no A effect), $\boldsymbol{\beta} \perp U_2$ (no B effect), and $\boldsymbol{\beta} \perp U_{12}$ (no interaction), where U_1, U_2 and U_{12} are defined in Sect. 2.2.

Theorem 4.44 *If, in a two-factor experiment, the sequential sums of squares for main effects and interactions are independent of the order of nesting, then the design is equireplicate.*

---

[15] Our ability to write $\mathbf{X}'\mathbf{X}$ in diagonal form depends on our willingness to use the cell-means model, and in particular the form (1.18) for $\mathbf{X}$.

[16] Theorem 5.18.

Table 4.6 Data and ANOVA table for an equireplicate 3 × 3 experiment, from Example 4.43

cell	Y	cell	Y	cell	Y
00	2.61, 1.66	10	4.16, 2.20	20	2.55, 2.33
01	0.03, 2.29	11	−3.54, −3.57	21	−3.76, −4.63
02	1.29, 2.76	12	−2.06, −2.79	22	1.35, −1.18

Source	SS	df	MS	F	p-value
A	25.794	2	12.897	11.75	0.003
B	68.951	2	34.476	31.42	0.000
$A \times B$	29.483	4	7.371	6.72	0.009
Error	9.876	9	1.097		
Total	134.104	17			

Proof Let factor A have a levels, and factor B, b levels. We assume that the $p = ab$ treatment combinations have been given a fixed order.

Because of independence of nesting, Corollary 4.35 implies that the subspaces U_1, U_2 and U_{12} are orthogonal with respect to the inner product (4.38). This orthogonality means that for arbitrary vectors $\mathbf{c} \in U_1, \mathbf{d} \in U_2$ and $\mathbf{e} \in U_{12}$ we have $\langle \mathbf{c}, \mathbf{d} \rangle = 0$, $\langle \mathbf{c}, \mathbf{e} \rangle = 0$, and $\langle \mathbf{d}, \mathbf{e} \rangle = 0$. We must show that this implies that the sample sizes n_{ij} are equal.

As we have noted above, our cell-means parametrization gives the matrix $\mathbf{X}'\mathbf{X}$ a diagonal form with diagonal elements n_{ij}. Thus $(\mathbf{X}'\mathbf{X})^{-1}$ has the same form with diagonal elements

$$m_{ij} = n_{ij}{}^{-1}.$$

On the other hand, the subspace $U_1 \subset \mathbb{R}^p$ consists of those contrast vectors $\mathbf{c}$ whose components c_{ij} have values independent of j. Thus there are constants $c_1, \ldots, c_a$ such that

$$c_{ij} \equiv c_i \text{ for all } i \text{ and } j$$

and such that $\sum_i c_i = 0$. Similarly, $\mathbf{d} \in U_2$ iff the components d_{ij} of $\mathbf{d}$ satisfy

$$d_{ij} \equiv d_j \text{ for all } i \text{ and } j$$

where $\sum_j d_j = 0$. Finally, a basis of U_{12} is given by vectors $\mathbf{e} = \mathbf{e}_{k\ell}$, $k = 2, \ldots, a$, $\ell = 2, \ldots, b$, where for fixed k and ℓ, the ijth component of $\mathbf{e}$ is

$$e_{ij} = \begin{cases} 1, \ (i, j) = (1, 1), (k, \ell), \\ -1, \ (i, j) = (1, \ell), (k, 1), \\ 0 \text{ otherwise.} \end{cases} \tag{4.41}$$

(Caution: these are *not* the standard basis vectors in $\mathbb{R}^p$. The vectors **c** and **e** are depicted in displays (2.12) and (2.9), where the cells are listed lexicographically.)

The components of **c**, **d** and **e** and the diagonal elements of $(\mathbf{X}'\mathbf{X})^{-1}$ are all listed consistently according to the order of the cells (i, j), so we have

$$\begin{aligned}\langle \mathbf{c}, \mathbf{d} \rangle &= \mathbf{c}'(\mathbf{X}'\mathbf{X})^{-1}\mathbf{d} \\ &= \sum_i \sum_j c_{ij} d_{ij} m_{ij} \\ &= \sum_i \sum_j c_i d_j m_{ij}.\end{aligned}$$

If we take, in particular,

$$(c_1, \ldots, c_a) = (1, \ldots, \overset{\overset{i}{|}}{-1} \ldots) \quad \text{and} \quad (d_1, \ldots, d_b) = (1, \ldots, \overset{\overset{j}{|}}{-1}, \ldots)$$

(omitted elements being zero), then

$$\langle \mathbf{c}, \mathbf{d} \rangle = m_{11} - m_{1j} - m_{i1} + m_{ij}.$$

Thus we are assuming that

$$m_{11} - m_{i1} - m_{1j} + m_{ij} = 0 \quad \text{for all } i, j. \tag{4.42}$$

Similarly, in order for U_1 and U_{12} to be orthogonal with respect to $\langle \cdot, \cdot \rangle$ it is necessary (and sufficient) that this hold for each $\mathbf{c} \in U_1$ and each basis element **e** of U_{12} given by (4.41). Now

$$\begin{aligned}\langle \mathbf{c}, \mathbf{e} \rangle &= \sum_i \sum_j c_{ij} e_{ij} m_{ij} \\ &= \sum_i c_i \sum_j e_{ij} m_{ij}.\end{aligned}$$

Fixing k and ℓ in the formula for e_{ij} and letting $c_1 = 1$, $c_k = -1$, and $c_i = 0$ otherwise, this

$$\begin{aligned}&= \sum_j e_{1j} m_{1j} - \sum_j e_{kj} m_{kj} \\ &= (m_{11} - m_{1\ell}) - (-m_{k1} + m_{k\ell}) \\ &= m_{11} + m_{k1} - m_{1\ell} - m_{k\ell}.\end{aligned}$$

Since k and ℓ are arbitrary, we are thus also assuming that

$$m_{11} + m_{i1} - m_{1j} - m_{ij} = 0 \quad \text{for all } i, j. \tag{4.43}$$

Adding Eqs. (4.42) and (4.43), we have $m_{1j} = m_{11}$ for all j, while subtracting the equations gives $m_{ij} = m_{1j}$ for all i and j. Together these imply that the quantities m_{ij}, and consequently n_{ij}, are equal. □

Remark 4.45 A quick way to see this argument is to consider the vector $\mathbf{m} \in \mathbb{R}^p$ whose components are the quantities m_{ij} in the given order. Equations (4.42) and (4.43) are contrasts in the m_{ij}. The coefficient vectors in Eq. (4.42) belong to U_{12}, while those in Eq. (4.43) are easily seen to be perpendicular to U_{12}, so belong to $U_1 \oplus U_2$, according to equation (2.14). Thus Eqs. (4.42) and (4.43) show that $\mathbf{m} \perp U_{12}$ and $\mathbf{m} \perp U_1 \oplus U_2$. According to (2.14), then, $\mathbf{m} \in \langle \mathbf{1} \rangle$, which means that the components of are equal.

Note that we could not rely on Theorem 4.38, which requires that sums of squares be independent of order of testing for *any* pair of hypotheses $\boldsymbol{\beta} \perp U_i$ for which $U_i \perp U_j$.

As we saw in Sect. 4.6, when the levels of a factor are quantitative, the main effect for that factor can be broken down orthogonally into various polynomial effects—linear, quadratic, and so on—each represented by a single contrast. Each contrast, of course, carries one degree of freedom. As those contrasts form an orthogonal basis of the effect, their individual sums of squares add up, in the equireplicate case, to the sum of squares for the main effect of that factor. To see examples of such output, the reader is referred to standard introductory texts such as [81], [96] or [151].

We developed those contrasts in a one-factor experiment, but we noted (page 41) that in a multifactor experiment the contrasts must be written with a pattern of repetition. In Sect. 5.4 we will learn a simple method to determine this pattern, and also how to compute interaction contrasts for so-called linear-by-linear, linear-by-quadratic, and other effects. Again, additivity of these sums of squares will hold in equireplicate experiments.

X′X Diagonal: Proportional Counts

One further result, something of a curiosity, concerns *factor-effects models* that we studied in Sect. 2.5. Consider the $a \times b$ design, and let U_1^*, U_2^*, and U_{12}^* be the subspaces of $\mathbb{R}^p$ ($p = ab$) spanned by the contrasts representing α's, β's, and γ's, respectively. We know (Theorem 2.18(d)) that U_1^*, U_2^*, and U_{12}^* are not mutually orthogonal with respect to the usual dot product except when uniform weights are used, in which case they coincide with U_1, U_2, and U_{12}. It is interesting to note, then, that there are sets of sample sizes n_{ij} for which U_1^*, U_2^*, and U_{12}^* are mutually orthogonal with respect to the inner product (4.38), as we now see.

Suppose we display the cell counts n_{ij} in an $a \times b$ matrix. We say that the counts are *proportional* if the counts in any row are a multiple of the counts in any other row. This holds iff we compare any row with row 1 as follows: For all i and j,

$$\frac{n_{i1}}{n_{11}} = \frac{n_{ij}}{n_{1j}}. \tag{4.44}$$

Since this equation is symmetric if we replace $n_{k\ell}$ by $n_{\ell k}$, it holds iff the counts in columns are proportional as well. Moreover, it is an easy exercise to show that (4.44) holds iff

$$n_{ij} = \frac{n_{i.}n_{.j}}{N}, \tag{4.45}$$

where as usual $n_{i.}$ and $n_{.j}$ are row and column totals and $N = n_{..}$ is the grand total. Equireplicate data is of course a special case of proportional counts.

The proof of the following theorem proceeds in the same way as that of Theorem 2.18(d), and is left as an exercise.

Theorem 4.46 *Suppose the counts* n_{ij} *are proportional, and consider the factor-effects parametrization* $\mathrm{E}(Y_{ijk}) = \mu + \alpha_i + \beta_j + \gamma_{ij}$ *with identifiability constraints (2.28). Then the contrast vectors for* α_i, β_j, *and* γ_{ij} *are mutually orthogonal with respect to the inner product (4.38) if and only if we use weights*

$$u_i = \frac{n_{i.}}{N} \quad \textit{and} \quad v_j = \frac{n_{.j}}{N}. \tag{4.46}$$

The orthogonality in this theorem is of course equivalent to that of U_1^*, U_2^*, and U_{12}^*. When in fact the n_{ij} are equal, the inner product (4.38) is a multiple of the ordinary dot product, and we recover Theorem 2.18(d).

Seber [128, Theorem 6.3.1] shows that the conditions (4.45) and (4.46) together characterize the independence of order of nesting $\boldsymbol{\mu} \perp U_1^*$, $\boldsymbol{\mu} \perp U_2^*$, and $\boldsymbol{\mu} \perp U_{12}^*$, but under the assumption that the model satisfies the added constraint $\mu = 0$ (which he states as a fourth hypothesis). As one can see from simple examples, though, these hypotheses depend on the sample sizes n_{ij}. Aside from independence of the order of nesting, then, it is not clear why one would want to test them.

4.6.2 Application: Regression Models

Consider the regression model $\mathrm{E}(Y) = \beta_0 + \beta_1 x_1 + \cdots + \beta_{p-1} x_{p-1}$. We are interested in hypotheses of the form $\beta_i = 0$, or perhaps $\beta_i = \cdots = \beta_j = 0$. Based on a sample of size N, we write $\mathrm{E}(\mathbf{Y}) = \mathbf{X}\boldsymbol{\beta}$ as usual.

According to Theorem 4.40, the sums of squares for $\beta_i = 0$ are independent of the order of nesting if and only if the columns of $\mathbf{X}$ are mutually orthogonal, that is, if $\mathbf{X}'\mathbf{X}$ is diagonal. This is a design problem, and it is not always possible to accommodate this requirement. For example, if regressor x_2 is the square of x_1, it may not be possible to design $\mathbf{x}_1$ a priori so that $\mathbf{x}_2$ is orthogonal to it. Note also that $\mathbf{1}$ must be a column of $\mathbf{X}$ if the regression model has a constant term, and so orthogonality implies that the other columns must add to zero.

One possibility is to *redesign* $\mathbf{X}$ by using the Gram-Schmidt process, replacing the columns $\mathbf{x}_1, \ldots, \mathbf{x}_p$ by orthogonal columns $\mathbf{z}_1, \ldots, \mathbf{z}_p$. One needs to keep in mind that this involves reparametrizing the model. For

$$\mathbf{z}_k = \sum_{j=1}^{k} a_{kj}\mathbf{x}_j = \mathbf{X}\begin{pmatrix} a_{k1} \\ \vdots \\ a_{kk} \\ 0 \\ \vdots \\ 0 \end{pmatrix},$$

so putting $\mathbf{Z} = (\mathbf{z}_1, \ldots, \mathbf{z}_p)$ and $\mathbf{A} = (a_{kj})$ we have $\mathbf{Z} = \mathbf{X}\mathbf{A}$. The matrix $\mathbf{A}$ is triangular and its diagonal elements a_{kk} are nonzero, so $\mathbf{A}$ is invertible, and so

$$\mathbf{X}\boldsymbol{\beta} = \mathbf{Z}\mathbf{A}^{-1}\boldsymbol{\beta} = \mathbf{Z}\boldsymbol{\gamma}$$

where $\boldsymbol{\gamma} = \mathbf{A}^{-1}\boldsymbol{\beta}$ is the new parameter vector. While the sums of squares for the hypotheses $\gamma_i = 0$ are independent of the order of nesting (and add up to the regression sum of squares), each γ_i is a sum of regression coefficients β_j, and so one must deal with the issue of interpretation. A similar problem of interpretation confronts the use of principal component analysis.

When the regressors are powers of x, as in a polynomial model, the resulting columns are polynomials in $\mathbf{x}$, and are known as *orthogonal polynomials*. Various schemes exist for computing these, including methods not equivalent to the Gram-Schmidt process, and for analyzing the results; see, for example, [106, Section 6.3–6.5] and [127, Section 8.2].

If the columns of $\mathbf{X}$ may be partitioned into mutually orthogonal sets of columns, and if the vector $\boldsymbol{\beta}$ may be partitioned in corresponding subvectors $\boldsymbol{\beta}_i$ of the same size, then Theorem 4.41 says that the sums of squares for the hypotheses $\boldsymbol{\beta}_i = \mathbf{0}$ are independent of the order of nesting. See [51, Appendix 6A].

4.7 Affine Hypotheses. Confidence Sets

Let $\mathbf{Y} \sim N(\mathbf{X}\boldsymbol{\beta}, \sigma^2 I)$, $\boldsymbol{\beta} \in \mathbb{R}^p$. In order to develop confidence sets for $\boldsymbol{\beta}$, it's necessary to broaden the notion of a linear hypothesis.

An *affine constraint* about $\boldsymbol{\beta}$ is a system of equations

$$\begin{cases} \mathbf{c}_1'\boldsymbol{\beta} = a_1 \\ \quad\vdots \\ \mathbf{c}_d'\boldsymbol{\beta} = a_d. \end{cases} \tag{4.47}$$

An *affine hypothesis* is an affine constraint that is subject to a statistical test. Like a linear hypothesis, an affine hypothesis may be written in several equivalent forms:

Lemma 4.47 *Let $U \subset \mathbb{R}^p$ be spanned by $\mathbf{c}_1, \ldots, \mathbf{c}_d$, and let these be the columns of a matrix $\mathbf{C}$. Let $W = U^\perp$, the orthocomplement of U. Fix $a_1, \ldots, a_d$, and let $\mathbf{a} = (a_1, \ldots, a_d)'$. Then the following are equivalent:*

a. $\boldsymbol{\beta}$ satisfies (4.47).
b. $\boldsymbol{\beta}$ satisfies

$$\mathbf{C}'\boldsymbol{\beta} = \mathbf{a}. \tag{4.48}$$

c. If $\boldsymbol{\beta}_0$ is any solution of (4.48) then

$$\boldsymbol{\beta} - \boldsymbol{\beta}_0 \perp U. \tag{4.49}$$

d. If $\boldsymbol{\beta}_0$ is any solution of (4.48) then

$$\boldsymbol{\beta} - \boldsymbol{\beta}_0 \in W. \tag{4.50}$$

Proof The equivalences (a) $\Leftrightarrow$ (b) and (c) $\Leftrightarrow$ (d) follow as in the proof of Lemma 1.33.

(b) $\Rightarrow$ (c): Since $\mathbf{C}'(\boldsymbol{\beta} - \boldsymbol{\beta}_0) = \mathbf{0}$, we may take $U = N(\mathbf{C}')$.

(c) $\Rightarrow$ (a): Let $\mathbf{c}_1, \ldots, \mathbf{c}_d$ be a basis of U. Then for each i, $\boldsymbol{\beta} - \boldsymbol{\beta}_0 \perp \mathbf{c}_i$, so that $\mathbf{c}_i'(\boldsymbol{\beta} - \boldsymbol{\beta}_0) = 0$, and so $\mathbf{c}_i'\boldsymbol{\beta} = \mathbf{c}_i'\boldsymbol{\beta}_0 = a_i$. □

As usual, we may always assume that the equations in (4.47) are linearly independent, so that the matrix $\mathbf{C}$ in (4.48) has d linearly independent columns and the subspace U in (4.49) has dimension d. As we noted in Remark 4.10, we must then have $d \leq p$. Condition (4.50) asserts that $\boldsymbol{\beta}$ belongs to the affine set $W + \boldsymbol{\beta}_0$ in $\mathbb{R}^p$, so it makes sense to refer to the hypotheses in Lemma 4.47 as *affine*.[17]

Unlike a linear hypothesis, an affine hypothesis can be empty, e.g., if Eqs. (4.47) are inconsistent. This is usually due to misspecification.

[17] *Caution*: The vector $\boldsymbol{\beta}_0$ is *not* analogous to the vector $\boldsymbol{\beta}_0$ in Lemma 1.33.

For testing, the form (4.48) turns out to be the most convenient. The test of

$$H_0\colon \mathbf{C}'\boldsymbol{\beta} = \mathbf{a} \tag{4.51}$$

is the natural modification of the test of the linear hypothesis $\mathbf{C}'\mathbf{a} = \mathbf{0}$ given in Corollary 4.9. It is given in the following theorem, whose proof is left as an exercise.

Theorem 4.48 *Let* $\mathbf{Y} \sim N(\mathbf{X}\boldsymbol{\beta}, \sigma^2 I)$*, where* $\mathbf{X}$ *has full rank. Let* H_0 *be given by (4.51), and assume that* H_0 *is nonempty and that* $\mathbf{C}$ *has full rank* $d \leq p$*. The Wald statistic for testing* H_0 *vs.* $H_1\colon \mathbf{C}'\boldsymbol{\beta} \neq \mathbf{a}$ *is*

$$F = \frac{(\mathbf{C}'\hat{\boldsymbol{\beta}} - \mathbf{a})'(\mathbf{C}'(\mathbf{X}'\mathbf{X})^{-1}\mathbf{C})^{-1}(\mathbf{C}'\hat{\boldsymbol{\beta}} - \mathbf{a})}{d \cdot MSE}, \tag{4.52}$$

where $\hat{\boldsymbol{\beta}} = (\mathbf{X}'\mathbf{X})^{-1}\mathbf{X}'\mathbf{Y}$*, the usual least-squares estimate, and we reject* H_0 *if* $F > F_{d,N-p,\alpha}$*.*

A $(1-\alpha)$-level *confidence set* for $\mathbf{C}'\boldsymbol{\beta}$ is the set of all values $\mathbf{a} \in \mathbb{R}^d$ which would not be rejected by the test in this theorem. (As noted in Sect. 1.2.3, we say we are *inverting the test*.) Thus we seek the set of $\mathbf{a}$ satisfying

$$(\mathbf{C}'\hat{\boldsymbol{\beta}} - \mathbf{a})'(\mathbf{C}'(\mathbf{X}'\mathbf{X})^{-1}\mathbf{C})^{-1}(\mathbf{C}'\hat{\boldsymbol{\beta}} - \mathbf{a}) \leq d \cdot MSE \cdot F_{\alpha,d,N-r}. \tag{4.53}$$

This is a solid ellipsoid in $\mathbb{R}^d$ with center at $\mathbf{C}'\hat{\boldsymbol{\beta}}$, known naturally enough as a *confidence ellipsoid*. Some important special cases are the following:

$d = 1$: The statistic (4.52) is the square of the t-statistic (3.25), and the F-test in Theorem 4.48 is therefore equivalent to the t-test for testing $H_0\colon \mathbf{c}'\boldsymbol{\beta} = a$ *vs.* $H_1\colon \mathbf{c}'\boldsymbol{\beta} \neq a$ given in Sect. 3.4 (a special case is given in Example 4.13, page 91). The confidence ellipsoid (4.53) reduces to the t-interval (3.26).

$d = 2$: The ellipsoid (4.53) is an ellipse in $\mathbb{R}^2$.

$d = p$, $\mathbf{C} = \mathbf{I}$: The ellipsoid (4.53) takes the form

$$(\hat{\boldsymbol{\beta}} - \boldsymbol{\beta})\mathbf{X}'\mathbf{X}(\hat{\boldsymbol{\beta}} - \boldsymbol{\beta}) \leq p \cdot MSE \cdot F_{p,N-p,\alpha}.$$

This gives us a level $1 - \alpha$ confidence ellipsoid in $\mathbb{R}^p$ for the vector $\boldsymbol{\beta}$.

A confidence ellipsoid for a vector-valued parameter may also regard as a simultaneous confidence set for its components. For example, the confidence ellipsoid for $\boldsymbol{\beta}$ given above is a simultaneous confidence set for the parameters $\beta_1, \ldots, \beta_p$. This is the topic to which we now turn.

4.8 Simultaneous Inference

Section 4.7 has anticipated a key question: How do we make inference *simultaneously* concerning several parameters—for example, the components $\beta_1, \ldots, \beta_p$ of $\boldsymbol{\beta}$, or more generally the values of the parametric functions

$$\mathbf{c}_1'\boldsymbol{\beta}, \ldots, \mathbf{c}_k'\boldsymbol{\beta}\ ?$$

One may pose the question even more generally with regard to arbitrary statistical hypotheses.

In the simultaneous testing of k null hypotheses $H_{01}, \ldots, H_{0k}$, we form an overall null hypotheses declaring that all are true:

$$H_0 = H_{01} \wedge \cdots \wedge H_{0k}$$

($\wedge$ = "and"). The alternate hypothesis H_1 states that H_{0i} is false for at least one i. If $\mathscr{P} = \{P_\theta : \theta \in \Theta\}$, and if the ith null hypothesis is $H_{0i}\colon \theta \in \Theta_{0i}$, then the overall null hypothesis is

$$H_0\colon \theta \in \Theta_0 = \Theta_{01} \cap \cdots \cap \Theta_{0k}. \tag{4.54}$$

We assume that each hypothesis has its own test, and define an overall test of H_0 in the natural way: reject H_0 if we reject at least one of the individual hypotheses. Thus if R_i is the rejection region of H_{0i}, then the rejection region for testing H_0 against H_1 is

$$R = R_1 \cup \cdots \cup R_k. \tag{4.55}$$

The number k may be very large, as in some applications (for example, in the analysis of microarray data). In fact, there are many cases where we need to deal with an arbitrary collection of null hypotheses H_{0i}, $i \in I$, where I may be infinite and even uncountable. Here we are testing

$$H_0\colon\ H_{0i} \text{ is true for all } i$$

against

$$H_1\colon\ H_{0i} \text{ is false for at least one } i.$$

When expressing H_0 in a parametrized model, the finite union in (4.54) is replaced by an arbitrary union, and likewise the rejection region (4.55).

The significance level for testing H_0 is known as the *experimentwise* or *familywise error rate (FWER)* of this test, while the significance level of the test of H_{0i} is called an *individual* or *comparisonwise error rate*. (The term "comparisonwise" is used when the hypotheses H_{0i} deal with comparisons between parameters, e.g., statements like $\theta_1 = \theta_2$.)

The *problem of multiple comparisons* is to construct the individual tests so that the FWER does not exceed a preassigned level. A similar problem arises by duality with respect to confidence intervals. Many methods have been devised to deal with this. We shall consider two, one based on the Bonferroni inequality, the other due to Scheffé.

4.8.1 The Bonferroni Method

The *Bonferroni test* applies to a finite number of hypotheses, which may be of arbitrary form.

The *Boole inequality* (sometimes called the *Bonferroni inequality*[18]) says that for any probability measure P and any sets $R_1, \ldots, R_k$,

$$\mathrm{P}(R) \le \mathrm{P}(R_1) + \cdots + \mathrm{P}(R_k), \tag{4.56}$$

where $R = \cup_i R_i$. It is a straightforward exercise to show that if $\Theta_0 = \Theta_{01} \cap \cdots \cap \Theta_{0k}$ then

$$\sup_{\theta \in \Theta_0} \mathrm{P}_\theta(R) \le \sup_{\theta \in \Theta_{01}} \mathrm{P}_\theta(R_1) + \cdots + \sup_{\theta \in \Theta_{0k}} \mathrm{P}_\theta(R_k). \tag{4.57}$$

In our application the left-hand side of (4.57) is by definition the significance level of the test of H_0—that is, the FWER. The ith term on the right-hand side is the significance level of the ith individual test.

If we want the FWER to be $\le \alpha$, then we may require each individual error rate to be $\le \alpha/k$. For example, if we want to test five hypotheses with overall significance level 0.05, then we should test each hypothesis at level 0.01. Note that this procedure is conservative in the sense that we have made it harder to reject any individual null hypothesis. The replacement of α by α/k is known as the *Bonferroni correction.*[19]

A similar principle applies to confidence intervals. Suppose $\theta_1, \ldots, \theta_k$ are functions of θ. If I_i is a confidence interval for θ_i of level $1 - \alpha'$, then (prior to observing data) we have $\mathrm{P}_\theta(\theta_i \in I_i) \ge 1 - \alpha'$. We would like to guarantee that

$$\mathrm{P}_\theta(\theta_1 \in I_1 \text{ and} \cdots \text{and } \theta_k \in I_k) \ge 1 - \alpha, \tag{4.58}$$

[18] The name Bonferroni is attached to a family of inequalities extending Boole's original result.

[19] Of course, we could set $\sup_{\theta \in \Theta_{0i}} \mathrm{P}_\theta(R_i) \le \alpha_i$ as long as α_i are chosen so that $\sum_i \alpha_i \le \alpha$. But there is usually no reason to use different individual error rates.

where α is a pre-assigned value. But the Boole inequality implies that

$$P(S_1 \cap \cdots \cap S_k) \geq 1 - \sum_{i=1}^{k} P(S_i^c). \tag{4.59}$$

If S_i is the event $\theta_i \in I_i$, then this says that we satisfy (4.58) if we again choose $\alpha' = \alpha/k$. For example, in forming 5 simultaneous intervals with overall (or "familywise") confidence 95%, we should arrange that each interval have confidence 99%. Wider intervals sacrifice precision, and so again we see that the Bonferroni procedure is conservative.

Note that this procedure produces a level $1 - \alpha$ *confidence rectangle* for $\boldsymbol{\theta} = (\theta_1, \ldots, \theta_k)$ in $\mathbb{R}^k$.

The Bonferroni method is useful because it can be applied very generally—for example, H_0 need not be limited to linear parametric functions. A weakness of the method is that it only produces bounds—upper bounds for significance levels, lower bounds for confidence levels. Moreover, the bounds are somewhat crude. For example, it is not unusual to create an *uncountable* set of confidence intervals—for example, in forming *confidence bands* in a regression (see below). If the interval S_r has confidence level $1 - \alpha_r$, then the Bonferroni inequality asserts merely that the familywise confidence level is 0, since it only asserts that $P(\cap_r S_r) \geq 0$ (Exercise 4.27)!

Example 4.49 In Example 4.6 we fitted a simple linear model to a data set, and estimated the expected response at x by the equation $\widehat{E(Y)} = 0.9394 + 0.3258x$. Suppose that we want simultaneous confidence intervals for the expected response at $x = 0.0, 0.3, 1.0$ and 1.7 with overall confidence level $1 - \alpha$. The endpoints of the intervals would be given by (3.28) with $\alpha/8$ replacing $\alpha/2$:

$$\hat{\beta}_0 + \hat{\beta}_1 x \pm t_{N-2,\,\alpha/8}\sqrt{MSE\left(\frac{1}{N} + \frac{(x - \bar{x})^2}{S_{xx}}\right)}. \tag{4.60}$$

For a 95% familywise confidence level ($\alpha = 0.05$) we would use the value $t_{27,0.00625} = 2.6763$ $(0.05/8 = 0.00625)$. In this example we also have $\bar{x} = 0.9207$, $S_{xx} = \sum_i (x_i - \bar{x})^2 = 10.5676$, and $MSE = 0.01009$. This gives the following:

x	Point est. of $E(Y)$	Confidence interval
0.0	0.9394	[0.8484, 1.0304]
0.3	1.0371	[0.9655, 1.1087]
1.0	1.2652	[1.2149, 1.3155]
1.7	1.4932	[1.4117, 1.5747]

Had we not used the Bonferroni correction, these intervals would have been smaller, since $t_{27,0.025} = 2.0518$. For example, a 95% confidence interval for the mean response at $x = 0.3$ is $[0.9822, 1.0920]$. Of course, the *familywise* confidence level for the four intervals would then have been less than 95%.

For intervals at k different values of x with overall confidence level $1 - \alpha$, we would use formula (3.28), replacing α by α/k and x by the specific values of interest, say $z_1, \ldots, z_k$. If we plot the estimated regression line and the endpoints of each interval, we will end up with a graph that looks something like this:

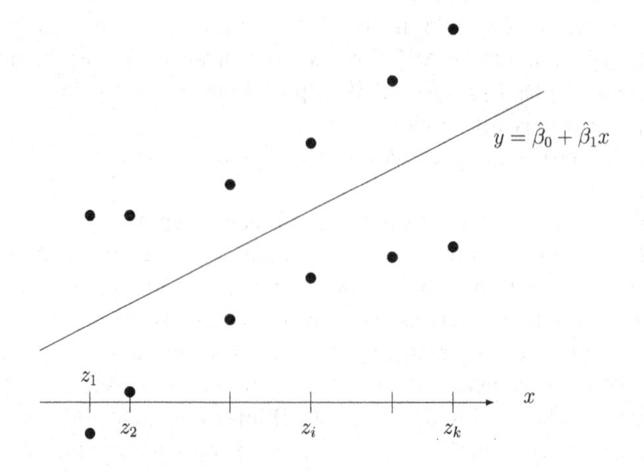

If we increase k while maintaining the same level of confidence, the Bonferroni method would move the upper endpoints higher and the lower ones lower.

It is tempting to connect the dots such a way as to create curves above and below the estimated line, but such "confidence bands" would represent *uncountably many* simultaneous confidence intervals, and the Bonferroni method would assert merely that the simultaneous confidence level is at least 0. It may come as a surprise that there actually is a method for drawing confidence bands with any prescribed (positive) overall confidence level. This was accomplished by Working and Hotelling [150], a method later generalized by Scheffé [118].[20]

4.8.2 The Scheffé Method

In making simultaneous inference about a large number of linear parametric functions $\mathbf{c}_i'\boldsymbol{\beta}$, the Bonferroni method produces tests which have either a high FWER or poor power of detecting individual departures from null hypotheses. Similarly, Bonferroni confidence intervals either have low confidence level or poor precision (because they are very wide).

[20] Curiously, Scheffé's paper does not mention that of Working and Hotelling. Scheffé makes that connection in [121, p. 68].

We seek a method of making inference about an *arbitrary* (possibly infinite) set of quantities $\mathbf{c}'\boldsymbol{\beta}$. For testing, the method is to guarantee a preassigned FWER α, and for confidence intervals, a preassigned familywise confidence level $1-\alpha$.

Thus let $S \subset \mathbb{R}^p$, and consider testing

$$H_0\colon \mathbf{c}'\boldsymbol{\beta} = 0 \quad \text{for all } \mathbf{c} \in S \qquad (4.61)$$
$$vs.\ H_1\colon \mathbf{c}'\boldsymbol{\beta} \neq 0 \quad \text{for some } \mathbf{c} \in S.$$

Let us write $SS_{\mathbf{c}}$ for the sum of squares for testing $\mathbf{c}'\boldsymbol{\beta} = 0$, as given in Example 4.13:

$$SS_{\mathbf{c}} = (\mathbf{c}'\hat{\boldsymbol{\beta}})^2/\mathbf{c}'(\mathbf{X}'\mathbf{X})^{-1}\mathbf{c}.$$

For each $\mathbf{c}$ we seek a test of $\mathbf{c}'\boldsymbol{\beta} = 0$ with a rejection rule of the form

$$\frac{SS_{\mathbf{c}}}{MSE} > K, \qquad (4.62)$$

where K is independent of $\mathbf{c}$ and is chosen so that the FWER does not exceed the prescribed α. Of course, the t-test of $\mathbf{c}'\boldsymbol{\beta} = 0$ is already of the form (4.62) with $K = F_{1,N-p,\alpha}$, as we saw in Example 4.13. But rather than "correcting" α, as the Bonferroni method does, *the Scheffé method will modify the numerator degrees of freedom.*

We begin by noting that the hypothesis (4.61) is equivalent to

$$H_0\colon \boldsymbol{\beta} \perp U \qquad (4.63)$$

where $U = \langle S \rangle$, the span of S in $\mathbb{R}^p$ (Theorem A.57(c)). If we instead test the hypothesis (4.63), we arrive at the form of the *Scheffé test*:

$$\text{Reject } H_0 \text{ if } \quad \frac{SS_{\mathbf{c}}}{MSE} > K \text{ for at least one } \mathbf{c} \in U. \qquad (4.64)$$

Given α, we must find K so that the probability of this event is at most α when H_0 is true. In fact, we do even better. Recall that we already have an F-test of H_0 given by Corollary 4.9:

$$\text{Reject } H_0 \text{ if } \quad \frac{SS(H_0)}{MSE} > d \cdot F_{d,N-p,\alpha} \qquad (4.65)$$

where

$$SS(H_0) = (\mathbf{C}'\hat{\boldsymbol{\beta}})'(\mathbf{C}'(\mathbf{X}'\mathbf{X})^{-1}\mathbf{C})^{-1}\mathbf{C}'\hat{\boldsymbol{\beta}},$$

and d, $\mathbf{c}$ and $\hat{\boldsymbol{\beta}}$ are described in the following theorem.

Theorem 4.50 *Let $\hat{\boldsymbol{\beta}}$ be the least squares estimator of $\boldsymbol{\beta}$. In the problem of testing $H_0 : \boldsymbol{\beta} \perp U$, let $d = \dim U$ and let $\mathbf{C}$ be any full-rank matrix such that H_0 may be written $\mathbf{C}'\boldsymbol{\beta} = \mathbf{0}$.*[21] *With the choice*

$$K = d \cdot F_{d,N-p,\alpha},$$

the following tests are equivalent:

- *the F-test (4.65).*
- *the Scheffé test (4.64).*
- *the test which reject H_0 if $\dfrac{SS_{\mathbf{c}}}{MSE} > K$, where $\mathbf{c}$ is any scalar multiple of the vector*

$$\hat{\mathbf{c}} = \mathbf{C}(\mathbf{C}'(\mathbf{X}'\mathbf{X})^{-1}\mathbf{C})^{-1}\mathbf{C}'\hat{\boldsymbol{\beta}}. \tag{4.66}$$

In particular, the FWER of the Scheffé test is exactly α.

Note that while the vector $\hat{\mathbf{c}}$ is determined by data, it is treated as a constant vector in the test. Theorem 4.50 is almost an immediate consequence of the following result, which may be viewed as something of a minor miracle:

Proposition 4.51 *We have*

$$\max_{\mathbf{c} \in U} SS_{\mathbf{c}} = SS(H_0),$$

the sum of squares for testing H_0: $\boldsymbol{\beta} \perp U$. Moreover, the maximum is attained when $\mathbf{c}$ is a scalar multiple of $\hat{\mathbf{c}} \in U$ given by (4.66).

The proof of Proposition 4.51 relies on the Maximization Lemma A.116 and is left as an exercise.

Proof of Theorem 4.50 For any K we have

$$\frac{SS_{\mathbf{c}}}{MSE} > K \text{ for some } \mathbf{c} \in U \quad \text{iff} \quad \max_{\mathbf{c} \in U} \frac{SS_{\mathbf{c}}}{MSE} > K.$$

Proposition 4.51 now shows that the three tests are equivalent. The power of these tests at a given $\boldsymbol{\beta}$ is thus

$$\mathrm{P}_{\boldsymbol{\beta}}\left(\frac{SS(H_0)}{MSE} > K\right), \tag{4.67}$$

which $= \alpha$ for all $\boldsymbol{\beta} \perp U$ when $K = d \cdot F_{d,N-p,\alpha}$, according to Corollary 4.2. □

[21] That is, the columns of $\mathbf{C}$ are a basis of U (Lemma 1.33).

We can now test as many hypotheses $\mathbf{c}'\boldsymbol{\beta} = 0$ as we like, over $\mathbf{c} \in U$, with overall significance level (FWER) α. We simply make this comparison:

$$\text{If } SS_{\mathbf{c}} > d \cdot F_{d,N-p,\alpha} \cdot MSE, \text{ reject } \mathbf{c}'\boldsymbol{\beta} = 0.$$

This process has been termed *data snooping* [121, p. 80] or *post hoc analysis*. Of course, if the F-test does not reject the overall hypothesis H_0: $\boldsymbol{\beta} \perp U$ at level α, then the Scheffé test will not reject any of the individual hypotheses either.

While the experimenter may be interested in certain linear functions $\mathbf{c}'\boldsymbol{\beta}$ a priori, hunting for functions that are significantly different from zero is somewhat hit-or-miss. Assuming that the overall F-test rejects H_0, Theorem 4.50 gives us a way of pinpointing a vector $\mathbf{c} = \hat{\mathbf{c}} \in U$ (determined only up to scalar multiple) for which we would definitely have rejected $\mathbf{c}'\boldsymbol{\beta} = 0$. The parametric function $\hat{\mathbf{c}}'\boldsymbol{\beta}$ is denoted $\hat{\psi}_{\max}$ by Scheffé [121, Section 3.5], who gives a different formula for it. For want of a better term, we may call $\hat{\mathbf{c}}'\boldsymbol{\beta}$ the linear parametric function *most responsible for rejecting* H_0.

Example 4.52 In [81, Example 6.2] Kuehl discusses a 2×4 factorial experiment which measured the effect of aggregate type and compaction method on the tensile strength (psi) of asphaltic concrete. The two aggregate types were basalt and silicious rock; the compaction methods included static compaction and three types of kneading (regular, low and very low). Three samples were prepared for each of the eight treatment combinations. The eight cell averages and the ANOVA table were as follows:

		Compaction Method			
			Kneading		
		Static	Regular	Low	Very Low
Agg. type	Basalt	65.333	129.000	97.333	57.333
	Silicious	67.667	111.000	60.667	41.667

Source	SS	df	MS	F
Compaction	16,243.50	3	5,414.50	596.05
Aggregate	1734.00	1	1.734.00	182.53
Interaction	1,145.00	3	381.67	40.18
Error	152.00	16	9.50	
Total	19.274.50	23		

(Since the design is balanced, the sums of squares are both adjusted and sequential.) To apply the Scheffé method to examine all possible contrasts in Compaction method, one would use the $F_{3,16,\alpha}$ significance point in the Scheffé test.

The reader can verify (Exercise 4.29) that the contrast most responsible for rejecting the hypothesis of no Compaction effect is proportional to

$$\hat{\mathbf{c}} = (-49, 165, 1, -117, -49, 165, 1, -117)'$$

where the eight cells have been listed row by row, and that the sum of squares for this contrast equals the sum of squares for Compaction. This is primarily a contrast between "regular kneading" and a weighted average of "static compaction" and "very low kneading". Evidently "low kneading" plays little role in giving a significant Compaction effect.

Remark 4.53 Let $S \subset \mathbb{R}^p$ and let $U = \langle S \rangle$. Although the hypotheses (4.61) and (4.63) are equivalent, the Scheffé test (4.64) is not equivalent to the test

$$\text{Reject } H_0 \text{ if } \frac{SS_{\mathbf{c}}}{MSE} > K \text{ for at least one } \mathbf{c} \in S \tag{4.68}$$

since it is possible to reject $\mathbf{c}'\boldsymbol{\beta} = 0$ for some $\mathbf{c} \in U$ but not for any $\mathbf{c} \in S$. That is, extending S to its span U results in a test that is more likely to reject H_0. On the other hand, when applied to any one hypothesis $\mathbf{c}'\boldsymbol{\beta} = 0$, the Scheffé test is less powerful than the usual t-test, as $F_{1,N-p,\alpha} < F_{d,N-p,\alpha}$.

While the test (4.64) has an FWER exactly equal to α, one can only say that the FWER of the test (4.68) is at most α.

Affine Hypotheses and Scheffé Confidence Intervals

Consider a null hypothesis

$$\mathbf{C}'\boldsymbol{\beta} = \mathbf{a}. \tag{4.69}$$

It may be written H_0: $\boldsymbol{\beta} - \boldsymbol{\beta}_0 \perp U$ if $\boldsymbol{\beta}_0$ is any solution of (4.69), according to Lemma 4.47. Thus we are indexing H_0 by $\boldsymbol{\beta}_0$, and we might write it $H_0(\boldsymbol{\beta}_0)$. As before, we can test this with a modified F-statistic (4.52), which we may rewrite as

$$\frac{SS(\boldsymbol{\beta}_0)}{d \cdot MSE}$$

where

$$SS(\boldsymbol{\beta}_0) = (\mathbf{C}'(\hat{\boldsymbol{\beta}} - \boldsymbol{\beta}_0))'(\mathbf{C}'(\mathbf{X}'\mathbf{X})^{-1}\mathbf{C})^{-1}(\mathbf{C}'(\hat{\boldsymbol{\beta}} - \boldsymbol{\beta}_0)).$$

Here $SS(\boldsymbol{\beta}_0)$ is an abbreviation for $SS(H_0(\boldsymbol{\beta}_0))$. We *fail* to reject H_0 at level α if

$$\frac{SS(\boldsymbol{\beta}_0)}{d \cdot MSE} \leq F_{d,N-p,\alpha}.$$

But by Proposition 4.51, and with the obvious notation,

$$SS(\boldsymbol{\beta}_0) = \max_{\mathbf{c} \in U} SS_{\mathbf{c}}(\boldsymbol{\beta}_0)$$
$$= \max_{\mathbf{c} \in U} \frac{(\mathbf{c}'(\hat{\boldsymbol{\beta}} - \boldsymbol{\beta}_0))^2}{\mathbf{c}'(\mathbf{X}'\mathbf{X})^{-1}\mathbf{c}}.$$

Setting this

$$\leq d \cdot MSE \cdot F_{d,N-p,\alpha}$$

and solving for $\mathbf{c}'\boldsymbol{\beta}_0$ gives a confidence interval for $\mathbf{c}'\boldsymbol{\beta}$ with endpoints

$$\mathbf{c}'\hat{\boldsymbol{\beta}} \pm \sqrt{\mathbf{c}'(\mathbf{X}'\mathbf{X})^{-1}\mathbf{c} \cdot d \cdot F_{d,N-p,\alpha} \cdot MSE}. \tag{4.70}$$

Call this interval $I_{\mathbf{c}}$. Then for all $\boldsymbol{\beta}$,

$$\mathrm{P}_{\boldsymbol{\beta}}(\mathbf{c}'\boldsymbol{\beta} \in I_{\mathbf{c}} \text{ for all } \mathbf{c} \in U) = 1 - \alpha.$$

The intervals $I_{\mathbf{c}}$ are Scheffé intervals. They are wider than the usual t-interval (3.26) of level α, the price we pay for having a FWER of α.

Application: Confidence Bands

Consider the regression model $\mathrm{E}(Y) = \beta_0 + \beta_1 x_1 + \cdots + \beta_k x_k$. Suppose we want a confidence interval for $\mathrm{E}(Y)$ at *all* values of $x_1, \ldots, x_k$ simultaneously:

$$L(x_1, \ldots, x_k) \leq \beta_0 + \beta_1 x_1 + \cdots + \beta_k x_k \leq M(x_1, \ldots, x_k).$$

This means that we seek simultaneous confidence intervals for $\mathbf{c}'\boldsymbol{\beta}$ where

$$\mathbf{c} = (1, x_1, \ldots, x_k)' \quad \text{and} \quad \boldsymbol{\beta} = (\beta_0, \ldots, \beta_k)'.$$

The vectors $\mathbf{c}$ span all of $\mathbb{R}^p$, where $p = k+1$, so $U = \mathbb{R}^p$, and in particular $d = p$. The endpoints L and M are given by (4.70).

In particular, if $x_i = x^i$, $\mathrm{E}(Y)$ is given by a *polynomial regression model* in x, and we may assert that

$$L(x) \leq \beta_0 + \beta_1 x + \cdots + \beta_k x^k \leq M(x)$$

with confidence $1 - \alpha$, so that L and U are now functions of x. Here $\mathbf{c} = (1, x, x^2, \ldots, x^k)'$. Note that for each x, $L(x)$ and $M(x)$ are random variables due to the presence of $\hat{\boldsymbol{\beta}}$ and MSE in (4.70). The graphs of $y = L(x)$ and $y = M(x)$

form lower and upper boundaries for a $1-\alpha$-level *confidence band* for the regression line. That is, for all $\boldsymbol{\beta}$

$$\mathrm{P}_{\boldsymbol{\beta}}(L(x) \leq \beta_0 + \beta_1 x + \cdots + \beta_k x^k \leq M(x) \text{ for all } x) = 1 - \alpha.$$

The dependence of L and M on x comes through the quadratic form $\mathbf{c}'(\mathbf{X}'\mathbf{X})^{-1}\mathbf{c}$ in (4.70) with

$$\mathbf{c} = (1, x, x^2, \ldots, x^k)',$$

so that the form is a polynomial of degree $2k$. Thus the actual formulas for $L(x)$ and $M(x)$ are not very tractable except in the simplest case of simple linear regression ($k = 1$), where the form is a quadratic function of x and the bands are hyperbolas. This special case is originally due to Working and Hotelling [150].

Example 4.54 In Example 4.49 we used the Bonferroni method to compute confidence intervals for the expected response in a simple linear regression with familywise confidence level 0.95. For Scheffé intervals in this context, formula (4.70) may be written

$$\hat{\beta}_0 + \hat{\beta}_1 x \pm \sqrt{2F_{2,27,.05} MSE\left(\frac{1}{N} + \frac{(x - \bar{x})^2}{S_{xx}}\right)}, \tag{4.71}$$

where, as before, $S_{xx} = \sum_i (x_i - \bar{x})^2$. Comparing this with the Bonferroni formula (4.60), we see that (4.71) replaces $t_{27,0.00625} = 2.6763$ with $\sqrt{2F_{2,27,0.05}} = 2.5900$, so that the Scheffé intervals will all be shorter than the Bonferroni intervals in that example, viz.:

x	Point est. of E(Y)	Confidence interval
0.0	0.9394	[0.8513, 1.0275]
0.3	1.0371	[0.9678, 1.1064]
1.0	1.2652	[1.2164, 1.3139]
1.7	1.4932	[1.4143, 1.5721]

Of course, the Scheffé method would allow us to add confidence intervals at arbitrarily many other values of x without changing the 95% familywise confidence level.

It is not uncommon for textbooks to form a confidence band for a regression by simply connecting the endpoints of t-intervals given by (3.26), without the Bonferroni correction. As we've seen, the Bonferroni inequality can only assert that the confidence level for the resulting band is at least 0. But the Scheffé method allows us to calculate the exact confidence level for this procedure in particular cases—and the news isn't good. Exercise 4.30 gives an example.

4.9 Inference for Variance Components Models

Section 2.7 introduced the idea of a random effect and the standard way of modeling experiments having such effects. We saw that such models automatically create correlated observations, and that the variance of an observation is the sum of terms that are naturally called *variance components*. We will only give a brief introduction to inference concerning these components, concentrating on the case of *balanced data*. This allows us to use Kronecker products to represent matrices, which greatly facilitates computation. The reader should review the rules for Kronecker products, which are covered in Sect. A.4.8 of the Appendix. The mixed-product rule is especially useful here.

We will emphasize the one-factor model (2.43), whose analysis contains many of the essential ideas, and include a brief introduction to the analysis of two-factor models. An extensive treatment is in the literature mentioned earlier. Our approach follows [125].

In forming the observation vector $\mathbf{Y}$, the observations within each cell are listed consecutively, as usual. The design matrix $\mathbf{X}$ then has a "diagonal" form (1.19), with vectors $\mathbf{1}$ down the "diagonal", one for each cell (treatment or treatment combination). For balanced data, all these vectors have length n, so that we may write

$$\mathbf{X} = \mathbf{I}_p \otimes \mathbf{1}_n \tag{4.72}$$

where

$$p = \text{the number of cells.}$$

As before, $\mathbf{I}$ is an identity matrix, $\mathbf{1}$ is a vector of 1's, $\mathbf{J}$ is a square matrix of 1's, and subscripts denote dimensions. For ease of reading, we will omit subscripts when dimensions are obvious. We note that

$$\mathbf{J}_n = \mathbf{1}_n\mathbf{1}_n' \text{ and so } \mathbf{J}_n^2 = n\mathbf{J}_n.$$

In Sect. 2.7 we described the typical hypotheses that we test in variance components models. Although these differ markedly from the linear hypotheses we test in fixed-effects models, *the standard tests are still based on the usual sums of squares*, and it is to these that we turn our attention.

4.9.1 The One-Factor Design

The usual sum of squares for error is

$$SSE = \|(\mathbf{I} - \mathbf{P})\mathbf{Y}\|^2 = \mathbf{Y}'(\mathbf{I} - \mathbf{P})\mathbf{Y}, \tag{4.73}$$

where $\mathbf{P} = \mathbf{X}(\mathbf{X}'\mathbf{X})^{-1}\mathbf{X}'$. Here $\mathbf{X}'\mathbf{X} = n\mathbf{I}_p$ while $\mathbf{X}\mathbf{X}' = (\mathbf{I}_p \otimes \mathbf{1}_n)(\mathbf{I}_p' \otimes \mathbf{1}_n') = \mathbf{I}_p \otimes \mathbf{J}_n$, so that

$$\mathbf{P} = (1/n)\mathbf{I}_p \otimes \mathbf{J}_n. \tag{4.74}$$

In the one-factor fixed-effects model with p treatments, the usual sum of squares for treatment is

$$SSTr = \|(\mathbf{P} - \mathbf{P}_0)\mathbf{Y}\|^2 = \mathbf{Y}'(\mathbf{P} - \mathbf{P}_0)\mathbf{Y},$$

where from Eq. (4.5) we have

$$\mathbf{P}_0 = (1/N)\mathbf{1}_N\mathbf{1}_N' = (1/N)\mathbf{J}_N\,, \tag{4.75}$$

where $N = np$ is the total sample size.

The degrees of freedom attached to these sums of squares are the same as in the fixed effects case. (A rigorous justification will be given later.) Thus, as before, the mean squares are

$$MSTr = SSTr/(p-1) \text{ and } MSE = SSE/(N-p).$$

Our first step is to calculate the expected value of these mean squares.

As we saw in Sect. 2.7, under the assumption that the sole factor is random, $\mathbf{Y}$ has mean vector[22]

$$\boldsymbol{\mu} = \mu\mathbf{1}_N, \tag{4.76}$$

and covariance matrix

$$\boldsymbol{\Sigma} = \mathbf{I}_p \otimes (\sigma_\tau^2\mathbf{J}_n + \sigma_e^2\mathbf{I}_n). \tag{4.77}$$

Theorem 4.55 *In the one-factor random-effects model,*

$$\mathrm{E}(MSTr) = n\sigma_\tau^2 + \sigma_e^2 \tag{4.78}$$

and

$$\mathrm{E}(MSE) = \sigma_e^2. \tag{4.79}$$

[22] The fact that the mean vector in (4.76) is the same as that in the null one-way fixed-effects model is pure coincidence.

Proof In both cases, we make use of the formula

$$\mathrm{E}(\mathbf{Y}'\mathbf{A}\mathbf{Y}) = \mathrm{tr}(\mathbf{A}\boldsymbol{\Sigma}) + \boldsymbol{\mu}'\mathbf{A}\boldsymbol{\mu} \tag{4.80}$$

(Proposition 1.5). Our sums of squares are of this form, with $\mathbf{A} = \mathbf{P} - \mathbf{P}_0$ for $SSTr$ and $= \mathbf{I} - \mathbf{P}$ for SSE.

Now $(\mathbf{P} - \mathbf{P}_0)\mathbf{1} = \mathbf{0}$ and $(\mathbf{I} - \mathbf{P})\mathbf{1} = \mathbf{0}$ (either by direct computation or by geometry), and because of (4.76) it follows that $(\mathbf{P} - \mathbf{P}_0)\boldsymbol{\mu} = \mathbf{0}$ and $(\mathbf{I} - \mathbf{P})\boldsymbol{\mu} = \mathbf{0}$. But then

$$\boldsymbol{\mu}'(\mathbf{P} - \mathbf{P}_0)\boldsymbol{\mu} = 0 \quad \text{and} \quad \boldsymbol{\mu}'(\mathbf{I} - \mathbf{P})\boldsymbol{\mu} = 0,$$

so that

$$\mathrm{E}(SSTr) = \mathrm{tr}[(\mathbf{P} - \mathbf{P}_0)\boldsymbol{\Sigma}] \quad \text{and} \quad \mathrm{E}(SSE) = \mathrm{tr}[(\mathbf{I} - \mathbf{P})\boldsymbol{\Sigma}].$$

From (4.74) and (4.75) and using the properties of the Kronecker product, we may write

$$\mathbf{P} - \mathbf{P}_0 = (\mathbf{I}_p - (1/p)\mathbf{J}_p) \otimes (1/n)\mathbf{J}_n \tag{4.81}$$

and

$$\mathbf{I} - \mathbf{P} = \mathbf{I}_p \otimes (\mathbf{I}_n - (1/n)\mathbf{J}_n), \tag{4.82}$$

as $\mathbf{I}\ (= \mathbf{I}_N) = \mathbf{I}_p \otimes \mathbf{I}_n$ and $\mathbf{J}_N = \mathbf{J}_p \otimes \mathbf{J}_n$. Now using (4.77) and the mixed-product rule we have

$$(\mathbf{P} - \mathbf{P}_0)\boldsymbol{\Sigma} = (\mathbf{I}_p - (1/p)\mathbf{J}_p) \otimes (\sigma_\tau^2 + \sigma_e^2/n)\mathbf{J}_n, \tag{4.83}$$

so that

$$\begin{aligned}\mathrm{E}(SSTr) &= \mathrm{tr}(\mathbf{I}_p - (1/p)\mathbf{J}_p)\,\mathrm{tr}(\sigma_\tau^2 + \sigma_e^2/n)\mathbf{J}_n \\ &= (p-1)(n\sigma_\tau^2 + \sigma_e^2),\end{aligned}$$

from which (4.78) follows. Similarly,

$$(\mathbf{I} - \mathbf{P})\boldsymbol{\Sigma} = \sigma_e^2(\mathbf{I}_p \otimes (\mathbf{I}_n - (1/n)\mathbf{J}_n)), \tag{4.84}$$

from which it follows that $\mathrm{E}(MSE) = \sigma_e^2$. Verification of this along with (4.81), (4.82) (4.83) and (4.84) is left as an exercise. □

Theorem 4.55 has two consequences. First, it tells us that

$$\hat{\sigma}_\tau^2 = (MSTr - MSE)/n \tag{4.85}$$

is an unbiased estimator of σ_τ^2. Second, it suggests that the ratio

$$F = MSTr/MSE \tag{4.86}$$

would be a reasonable test statistic for the random-effect hypothesis H_0: $\sigma_\tau^2 = 0$, since this ratio would be tend to be small under H_0 but large under H_1, as is true of $\mathrm{E}(MSTr)/\mathrm{E}(MSE)$. That is, we should reject H_0 if F is sufficiently large. Of course, this is the same test that is used in the fixed-effects model, but the reasoning is quite different.

To get the distributions of $SSTr$, SSE, and F, we must quote another result [123, Section 2.5, Theorem 2]:

Theorem 4.56 *Let* $\mathbf{Y} \sim N(\boldsymbol{\mu}, \boldsymbol{\Sigma})$ *and let* $\mathbf{A}$ *be symmetric. Then* $\mathbf{Y}'\mathbf{A}\mathbf{Y} \sim \chi^2(\mathrm{rank}(\mathbf{A}), (1/2)\boldsymbol{\mu}'\mathbf{A}\boldsymbol{\mu})$ *iff* $\mathbf{A}\boldsymbol{\Sigma}$ *is idempotent.*

The proof of Theorem 4.56 in [123] is a moment-generating function argument.

Theorem 4.57 *Suppose that in the one-factor random-effects model (2.43) with balanced data we assume in addition that* τ_i *and* e_{ij} *are normally distributed. Then* $SSTr$ *and* SSE *are independent,*

$$\frac{SSTr}{n\sigma_\tau^2 + \sigma_e^2} \sim \chi^2(p-1) \tag{4.87}$$

and

$$\frac{SSE}{\sigma_e^2} \sim \chi^2(N-p), \tag{4.88}$$

where $N = np$. *We have*

$$F \sim \frac{n\sigma_\tau^2 + \sigma_e^2}{\sigma_e^2} F(p-1, N-p). \tag{4.89}$$

In particular, $F \sim F(p-1, N-p)$ *under* H_0: $\sigma_\tau^2 = 0$.

Proof From (4.82) and (4.83) we see that $(\mathbf{P} - \mathbf{P}_0)\boldsymbol{\Sigma}(\mathbf{I} - \mathbf{P})' = \mathbf{0}$, so Corollary 1.8 implies that $(\mathbf{P} - \mathbf{P}_0)\mathbf{Y}$ and $(\mathbf{I} - \mathbf{P})\mathbf{Y}$ are independent. But since $SSTr = \|(\mathbf{P} - \mathbf{P}_0)\mathbf{Y}\|^2$ and $SSE = \|(\mathbf{I} - \mathbf{P})\mathbf{Y}\|^2$, we see that $SSTr$ and SSE are also independent (Theorem 1.1).

The products $(\mathbf{P} - \mathbf{P}_0)\mathbf{\Sigma}$ and $(\mathbf{I} - \mathbf{P})\mathbf{\Sigma}$ are given in equations (4.83) and (4.84). While these are not quite idempotent, it is easy to verify the idempotence of

$$(n\sigma_\tau^2 + \sigma_e^2)^{-1}(\mathbf{P} - \mathbf{P}_0)\mathbf{\Sigma} = (\mathbf{I}_p - (1/p)\mathbf{J}_p) \otimes \mathbf{J}_n$$

and

$$\sigma_e^{-2}(\mathbf{I} - \mathbf{P})\mathbf{\Sigma} = \mathbf{I}_p \otimes (\mathbf{I}_n - (1/n)\mathbf{J}_n),$$

so Theorem 4.56 applies with $\mathbf{A} = (n\sigma_\tau^2 + \sigma_e^2)^{-1}(\mathbf{P} - \mathbf{P}_0)$ and $\mathbf{A} = \sigma_e^{-2}(\mathbf{I} - \mathbf{P})$, respectively. This gives us (4.87) and (4.88). From this and independence, (4.89) follows easily. The null distribution of F is then obvious. □

Thus the null distribution of F is the same as in the one-way fixed-effects model, and the test procedure is the same as well (rejecting H_0 if $F > F_{p-1,N-p,\alpha}$). However, the alternative distribution of F is different: In the fixed-effects model it is noncentral, while in the random-effects model it is that of constant times a central-F statistic. Rewriting that constant shows that it depends on the ratio σ_τ^2/σ_e^2.

Much ink has been spilled over the fact that the estimator (4.85) can be negative. Theorem 4.57 allows us to calculate the probability of this, and shows that it can be a rather common outcome in data sets of typical size (as in Exercise 4.32). The probability of this occurrence depends on the value of σ_τ^2/σ_e^2, and one can easily see that this probability is a decreasing function of this ratio. In particular, it is highest when $\sigma_\tau^2 = 0$. The possibility of a negative estimate of a variance is an obvious practical problem. Discussions of this problem may be found in [123] and [125].

4.9.2 The Two-Factor Design

The divergence of test procedures from the fixed-effects case becomes more obvious with more than one factor, and we will examine this briefly in the case of two-factor ($a \times b$) experiments, where $p = ab$. As before, we list cells in lexicographic order ("row by row", as in Sect. 2.2). The model is given by (2.46), and we consider the case that factor A is random and B is fixed.

The analysis of variance is summarized in Table 4.7, which includes an $\mathrm{E}(MS)$ column to explain the F-ratios. These ratios are the main difference between this ANOVA table and Table 4.2. Following the principle we observed in the one-factor model, we define F-ratios by comparing the expected mean squares of two sources that differ only in the parameter of interest. For example, the F-ratio for testing H_0: $\sigma_\alpha^2 = 0$ is $MSA/MSAB$ because $\mathrm{E}(MSA)$ has just one more term than $\mathrm{E}(MSAB)$, namely the term involving σ_α^2.

The F-distributions in this table follow the degrees of freedom. For example, under the hypothesis that $\sigma_\alpha^2 = 0$, $MSA/MSAB \sim F(a-1, (a-1)(b-1))$.

To prove all of these requires several things:

Table 4.7 ANOVA table for an $a \times b$ experiment, with A random and B fixed. $\theta_\beta^2 = \sum_{j=1}^b (\bar{\mu}_{\cdot j} - \bar{\mu}_{\cdot\cdot})^2/(b-1) = \sum_j (\beta_j - \bar{\beta}_\cdot)^2/(b-1)$. Mean squares follow the rule $MS = SS/\,\text{df}$

Source	SS	df	MS	$E(MS)$	F
A	SSA	$a-1$	MSA	$\sigma_e^2 + n\sigma_\gamma^2 + bn\sigma_\alpha^2$	$MSA/MSAB$
B	SSB	$b-1$	MSB	$\sigma_e^2 + n\sigma_\gamma^2 + an\theta_\beta^2$	$MSB/MSAB$
$A \times B$	$SSAB$	$(a-1)(b-1)$	$MSAB$	$\sigma_e^2 + n\sigma_\gamma^2$	$MSAB/MSE$
Error	SSE	$N-p$	MSE	σ_e^2	
Total	SST	$N-1$			

- using Eq. (4.80) to derive expected mean squares (this doesn't depend on normality),
- proving independence of the sums of squares, as needed, and
- applying Theorem 4.56 to get the appropriate χ^2 distributions for sums of squares.

The various F distributions follow naturally. Verifications of all these follow the same steps as in the one-factor model, but are more laborious. We illustrate this by determining $E(MSA)$.

The observation vector $\mathbf{Y}$ now has mean vector $\boldsymbol{\mu}$ and covariance matrix $\boldsymbol{\Sigma}$ given by (2.48) and (2.49). (These involve the vector $\boldsymbol{\nu}$ and the matrices $\mathbf{B}$ and $\mathbf{D}$ defined there.) The design matrix $\mathbf{X}$ is still of the form (4.72), but with $p = ab$. Thus $\mathbf{X}'\mathbf{X} = n\mathbf{I}_p$. Rather than writing SSA in the form $\mathbf{Y}'(\mathbf{P}-\mathbf{P}_0)\mathbf{Y}$ for appropriate $\mathbf{P}$ and $\mathbf{P}_0$, we will write it in the form $\mathbf{Y}'\mathbf{Q}\mathbf{Y}$ where $\mathbf{Q}$ is given by (4.12) (Proposition 4.11). This equation expresses $\mathbf{Q}$ in terms of two other matrices, $\mathbf{T}$ and $\mathbf{C}$, which we now describe.

The matrix $\mathbf{T} = (\mathbf{X}'\mathbf{X})^{-1}\mathbf{X}'$, the Moore-Penrose inverse of $\mathbf{X}$, was introduced in (3.18). We have $\mathbf{T} = (1/n)\mathbf{X}'$ and $\mathbf{T}\mathbf{T}' = (\mathbf{X}'\mathbf{X})^{-1} = (1/n)\mathbf{I}_{ab}$, as is easily verified. Let $\mathbf{c}_1, \ldots, \mathbf{c}_{a-1}$ be linearly independent contrast vectors in $\mathbb{R}^a$. Then $\mathbf{c}_1 \otimes \mathbf{1}_b, \ldots, \mathbf{c}_{a-1} \otimes \mathbf{1}_b$ form the basis of U_1 given in (2.12).[23] If we put $\mathbf{C}_0 = [\mathbf{c}_1, \ldots, \mathbf{c}_{a-1}]$, then the desired matrix is

$$\mathbf{C} = \mathbf{C}_0 \otimes \mathbf{1}_b.$$

We now calculate:

$$\begin{aligned}
\mathbf{Z} = \mathbf{T}'\mathbf{C} &= (1/n)(\mathbf{I}_{ab} \otimes \mathbf{1}_n)(\mathbf{C}_0 \otimes \mathbf{1}_b) \\
&= (1/n)(\mathbf{I}_a \otimes (\mathbf{I}_b \otimes \mathbf{1}_n))(\mathbf{C}_0 \otimes \mathbf{1}_b) \\
&= (1/n)(\mathbf{C}_0 \otimes \mathbf{1}_{bn}). \\
\mathbf{Z}'\mathbf{Z} &= (1/n^2)(\mathbf{C}_0' \otimes \mathbf{1}_{bn}')(\mathbf{C}_0 \otimes \mathbf{1}_{bn})
\end{aligned}$$

[23] This is a special case of the multilinear algebra presented in Sect. 5.4.

$$= (1/n^2)\, \mathbf{C}_0'\mathbf{C}_0 \otimes bn$$
$$= (b/n)\, \mathbf{C}_0'\mathbf{C}_0 \otimes 1.$$
$$\mathbf{Q} = \mathbf{Z}(\mathbf{Z}'\mathbf{Z})^{-1}\mathbf{Z}' = (1/n)(\mathbf{C}_0 \otimes \mathbf{1}_{bn})\,(n/b)((\mathbf{C}_0'\mathbf{C}_0)^{-1} \otimes 1)\,(1/n)(\mathbf{C}_0' \otimes \mathbf{1}_{bn}')$$
$$= (1/bn)\, \mathbf{C}_0(\mathbf{C}_0'\mathbf{C}_0)^{-1}\mathbf{C}_0' \otimes \mathbf{J}_{bn}.$$

Now in $\mathbb{R}^a$,

$$\mathbf{C}_0(\mathbf{C}_0'\mathbf{C}_0)^{-1}\mathbf{C}_0' = \text{the orthogonal projection on } \mathbf{1}_a^{\perp} \text{ (Proposition 3.3)}$$
$$= \mathbf{I}_a - (1/a)\mathbf{J}_a,$$

so

$$\mathbf{Q} = (1/bn)(\mathbf{I}_a - (1/a)\mathbf{J}_a) \otimes \mathbf{J}_{bn}.$$

Since $SSA = \mathbf{Y}'\mathbf{Q}\mathbf{Y}$, we have

$$\mathrm{E}(SSA) = \mathrm{tr}(\mathbf{Q}\boldsymbol{\Sigma}) + \boldsymbol{\mu}'\mathbf{Q}\boldsymbol{\mu}$$

as before. Now

$$\mathbf{Q}\boldsymbol{\mu} = [(1/bn)(\mathbf{I}_a - (1/a)\mathbf{J}_a) \otimes \mathbf{J}_{bn}][\mathbf{1}_a \otimes (\boldsymbol{\nu} \otimes \mathbf{1}_n)] = \mathbf{0}$$

as $(\mathbf{I}_a - (1/a)\mathbf{J}_a)\mathbf{1}_a = \mathbf{0}$. Therefore,

$$\boldsymbol{\mu}'\mathbf{Q}\boldsymbol{\mu} = 0.$$

On the other hand,

$$\mathbf{Q}\boldsymbol{\Sigma} = (1/bn)[(\mathbf{I}_a - (1/a)\mathbf{J}_a) \otimes \mathbf{J}_{bn}]\,[\mathbf{I}_a \otimes (\mathbf{J}_b \otimes \mathbf{B} + \mathbf{I}_b \otimes \mathbf{D})]$$
$$= (1/bn)(\mathbf{I}_a - (1/a)\mathbf{J}_a) \otimes \mathbf{J}_{bn}(\mathbf{J}_b \otimes \mathbf{B} + \mathbf{I}_b \otimes \mathbf{D})]$$

Now $\mathbf{J}_n\mathbf{B} = \mathbf{J}_n(\sigma_\alpha^2\mathbf{J}_n) = n\sigma_\alpha^2\mathbf{J}_n$ and $\mathbf{J}_n\mathbf{D} = \mathbf{J}_n(\sigma_e^2\mathbf{I}_n + \sigma_\gamma^2\mathbf{J}_n) = (\sigma_e^2 + n\sigma_\gamma^2)\mathbf{J}_n$, so

$$\mathbf{J}_{bn}(\mathbf{J}_b \otimes \mathbf{B} + \mathbf{I}_b \otimes \mathbf{D}) = (\mathbf{J}_b \otimes \mathbf{J}_n)(\mathbf{J}_b \otimes \mathbf{B} + \mathbf{I}_b \otimes \mathbf{D})$$
$$= b\mathbf{J}_b \otimes n\sigma_\alpha^2\mathbf{J}_n + \mathbf{J}_b \otimes (\sigma_e^2 + n\sigma_\gamma^2)\mathbf{J}_n$$
$$= (bn\sigma_\alpha^2 + n\sigma_\gamma^2 + \sigma_e^2)\mathbf{J}_b \otimes \mathbf{J}_n = (bn\sigma_\alpha^2 + n\sigma_\gamma^2 + \sigma_e^2)\mathbf{J}_{bn},$$

and so

$$\mathbf{Q}\boldsymbol{\Sigma} = \frac{bn\sigma_\alpha^2 + n\sigma_\gamma^2 + \sigma_e^2}{bn}[(\mathbf{I}_a - (1/a)\mathbf{J}_a) \otimes \mathbf{J}_{bn}].$$

Hence, finally,

$$\begin{aligned} \mathrm{E}(SSA) = \mathrm{tr}(\mathbf{Q}\boldsymbol{\Sigma}) &= \frac{bn\sigma_\alpha^2 + n\sigma_\gamma^2 + \sigma_e^2}{bn}\, \mathrm{tr}(\mathbf{I}_a - (1/a)\mathbf{J}_a)\,\mathrm{tr}\,\mathbf{J}_{bn} \\ &= (bn\sigma_\alpha^2 + n\sigma_\gamma^2 + \sigma_e^2)(a-1) \end{aligned}$$

and so

$$\mathrm{E}(MSA) = bn\sigma_\alpha^2 + n\sigma_\gamma^2 + \sigma_e^2.$$

Clearly the calculation of expected mean squares can be rather arduous. Algorithms for computing them can be found in many introductory texts, such as [81], [96] and [100].

4.9.3 Some Challenges

The present text is concerned primarily with fixed-effects models, and our treatment of variance-components models is meant only as a brief introduction to the topic. The reader is encouraged to consult the literature for more information—a good source (to which we have repeatedly referred) is [125].

Variance components models present challenges not encountered with fixed effects models. These issues arise from model formulation and from methodology.

- We have already noted the problem of negative estimates of variance components. It is not hard to find examples where unbiasedness produces poor or even absurd results,[24] so perhaps we shouldn't be surprised at this. In dealing with negative estimates, Searle et al. describe several "courses of action" in Section 4.4 of [125], "few of them satisfactory".[25]
- A related problem sometimes arises from the use of expected mean squares to form F-ratios. For example, in a 3-factor model with all factors random, there is no obvious choice for the denominator of an F-ratio to test for a main effect, as the expected mean squares for interactions differ from those for main effects by two components (see, e.g., [81, Table 7.3]).

[24] In estimating the positive quantity $e^{-2\lambda}$ from an observation $X \sim \text{Poisson}(\lambda)$, the estimator $\phi(X) = (-1)^X$ is easily seen to be unbiased, but has a high probability of being negative.

[25] Earlier, in [123, Section 9.8b], Searle wrote, "none" rather than "few".

The usual approach is to use a linear combination of mean squares in place of a single one. Note that there can be more than one way to do this. In any case, this naturally results in a ratio that no longer has an exact F distribution, and one uses a procedure due to Satterthwaite to get an approximate F distribution (see [63] for results of simulation studies of this method). The result is sometimes called a *pseudo-F-test.*

- Both of these problems raise a far more basic question: the use of the usual mean squares as a basis for inference. After all, the usual sums of squares arise from least-squares fitting of fixed-effects models, as in Sect. 4.1. Their use with variance components models may be convenient—standard statistical packages compute these quantities automatically—but the basic justification is lost.
  Maximum likelihood estimation and Bayesian methods have been developed for these models, and provide estimates that are more model-driven. Both methods, of course, require specifying distributions at the outset, whereas the least squares approach does not require distributional assumptions until the point at which one must test hypotheses. Except in special cases, maximum likelihood does not give closed-form solutions. Bayesian methods require additional assumptions about prior distributions, as well as a choice of estimator: in [125, pp. 100 and 316], both the posterior mode and the posterior mean are suggested. That text gives an extensive discussion of Bayesian methods. Maximum likelihood is discussed in [73] and [125].
- On the face of it, we should have an easy way to test whether, say, $\sigma_\alpha^2 = 0$ in the $a \times b$ model where A is random: If $\alpha_i = 0$ for all i, then we conclude that $\sigma_\alpha^2 = 0$, while if $\alpha_i \neq 0$ for some i, then we conclude that $\sigma_\alpha^2 > 0$. Moreover, the probabilities of type I and type II errors are both zero.[26] But such a test cannot be used, since α_i are *not observable* random variables. Of course, our methods end up only involving actual observations.
  Hocking [73, Chapters 8 and 9] offers an approach that considers only the actual observations $\mathbf{Y}$ and assumes a covariance structure $\mathbf{\Sigma} = \sum_i \phi_i \mathbf{V}_i$, where the matrices $\mathbf{V}_i$ are fixed (known) and symmetric and the parameters ϕ_i are constrained so that $\mathbf{\Sigma}$ is positive definite. This includes the covariance matrices (4.77) and (2.49) for the one-random-factor and the mixed two-factor models; for example,

$$\mathbf{\Sigma} = \sigma_\alpha^2 \mathbf{I}_a \otimes \mathbf{J}_{bn} + \sigma_\gamma^2 \mathbf{I}_{ab} \otimes \mathbf{J}_n + \sigma_e^2 \mathbf{I}_{abn}$$

  in the $a \times b$ mixed model with A random, as can be seen by multiplying out the Kronecker products in (2.49). Here the quantities ϕ_i are variance components, necessarily all nonnegative, which is a stronger constraint than requiring positive-definiteness of $\mathbf{\Sigma}$.

[26] For example, if H_0: $\sigma_\alpha^2 = 0$ holds then the probability of a type I error is P(reject H_0) = P($\alpha_i \neq 0$ for some i) = 0. The distributions specified by $\sigma_\alpha^2 = 0$ and $\sigma_\alpha^2 > 0$ are said to be *mutually singular*.

This approach is similar in spirit to the cell-means philosophy, of which Hocking is also a key exponent. In dispensing with the factor-effects model of E(**Y**), it allows the parameters ϕ_i to be negative, thus avoiding the potential problem of negative estimates. On the other hand, by dispensing with that model it is less clear just how to specify the appropriate covariance structure $\mathbf{\Sigma}$.

4.10 Exercises

Section 4.1

4.1. Given the model $E(\mathbf{Y}) = \mathbf{X}\boldsymbol{\beta}$ and $\mathbf{\Sigma}_{\mathbf{Y}} = \sigma^2\mathbf{I}$, let $\hat{\mathbf{Y}}$ be the vector of fitted values, and let $\hat{\mathbf{Y}}_0$ be the vector of fitted values for the model subject to a linear constraint. Using Corollary A.93, for example,

(i) show that $\mathbf{Y} - \hat{\mathbf{Y}}$ and $\mathbf{Y} - \hat{\mathbf{Y}}_0$ are correlated.
(ii) show that $\mathbf{Y} - \hat{\mathbf{Y}}$ and $\hat{\mathbf{Y}} - \hat{\mathbf{Y}}_0$ are uncorrelated.

4.2. In a linear model $\mathbf{Y} = \mathbf{X}\boldsymbol{\beta}$, what constraint or hypothesis on $\boldsymbol{\beta}$ results in a restricted sum of squares $SSE_R = \|\mathbf{Y}\|^2$? (This known as the "uncorrected" total sum of squares.)

Section 4.1.1

4.3. Consider a linear model $E(\mathbf{Y}) = \mathbf{X}\boldsymbol{\beta}$ under the constraint $\boldsymbol{\beta} \in W_1$, and assume that we wish to test the hypothesis $H_0 : \boldsymbol{\beta} \in W_0$ for some $W_0 \subset W_1$.

(i) Using (1.31) to rewrite the model with parameter $\boldsymbol{\beta}_0 \in \mathbb{R}^k$ as in Theorem 1.36, show that H_0 can be rewritten as $\boldsymbol{\beta}_0 \in W_0^*$ for some subspace $W_0^* \subset \mathbb{R}^k$.
(ii) Show that the parametrization by $\boldsymbol{\beta}_0 = (b_1, \ldots, b_k)'$ can be chosen so that, for some j, H_0 has the form $b_{j+1} = \cdots = b_k = 0$.

Section 4.1.2

4.4. Let $\mathbf{X}^*$ be an $s \times p$ matrix. Let $\mathbf{Z}$ be $N \times s$ having rows $\mathbf{e}_1' = (1, 0, \ldots, 0)$, $\mathbf{e}_2' = (0, 1, 0, \ldots, 0), \ldots, \mathbf{e}_s' = (0, \ldots, 0, 1)$, where $\mathbf{e}_i'$ is repeated n_i times. (Thus $\mathbf{Z}$ has the form (1.19).) Let $\mathbf{X} = \mathbf{Z}\mathbf{X}^*$. Show that $\mathbf{X}$ has the same rows of $\mathbf{X}^*$ with row i repeated n_i times. Deduce that if $W = R(\mathbf{X}^*)$ then $\mathbf{Z}(W) = R(\mathbf{X})$. (Recall that $R(\mathbf{M})$ denotes the columnspace of $\mathbf{M}$.)

Section 4.2

4.5. The regression analysis in Example 4.18 (page 97) produced the estimated regression equation $\hat{y} = 0.923307 - 2.24991x + 1.46865x^2 - 0.173206x^3$. Use equation (4.13) to find the sums of squares for β_1, β_2 and β_3 (that is, for testing that each equals 0). Verify that these equal the "adjusted sums of squares" for x, x^2 and x^3 in that example (listed in Table 4.3 under SS (adj)). (You will need to create the regression matrix $\mathbf{X}$ and compute $(\mathbf{X}'\mathbf{X})^{-1}$.)

Section 4.3

4.6. Consider the lattice of subspaces W_i in the two-factor experiment, as illustrated in Fig. 4.2 and described on page 93. We want to rewrite them in terms of the subspaces U_1, U_2, and U_{12} defined in Sect. 2.2.

(i) Express the orthocomplements of $W_0, \ldots, W_3$ in terms of U_1, U_2, and U_{12}.
(ii) Express $W_1, \ldots, W_6$ as orthogonal sums of U_1, U_2, U_{12} and $\langle \mathbf{1} \rangle$.
(iii) Show that $W_1 + W_3 = W_5$ and $W_1 \cap W_3 = W_0$. (This is part of what is needed to verify that the subspaces W_i form a lattice.)

4.7. Prove Proposition 4.15. The proof of (a) and (b) should work for *any* linear transformation between *any* vector spaces. The proof of (c) should work for *any* function $\mathbf{X}$ between *any* two sets, W_1 and W_2 being subsets.

4.8. In Proposition 4.15:

(i) Show that if the inclusion in (a) is proper for *every* pair of distinct subspaces $W_1 \subset W_2$ then $\mathbf{X}$ is one-to-one.
(ii) Show that if the equality in (c) holds for *every* W_1 and W_2 then $\mathbf{X}$ is one-to-one.

Section 4.5

4.9. Let $\mathbf{X}$, assumed full rank, be the regression matrix for the three-predictor regression model or the design matrix for the $a \times b$ factorial model, and consider the corresponding lattices of subspaces in Fig. 4.2. In both models, show that

(i) $V_0 = \langle \mathbf{1} \rangle$, the span of the vector of ones.
(ii) the vector of fitted values for this simplest model is $\mathbf{Y}_0 = \bar{Y}\mathbf{1}$, where $\bar{Y}$ is the grand average of the data.
(iii) the total sum of squares is given by $SST = \sum_j (Y_j - \bar{Y}.)^2$ in the regression case, and $SST = \sum_i \sum_j \sum_k (Y_{ijk} - \bar{Y}_{...})^2$ in the factorial case.

4.10. Prove Theorem 4.22. Part (a) is a direct application of Theorem 4.1(a). The proof of parts (b) and (c) is similar to the proof of that theorem.

4.11. Prove equations (4.21) and (4.22). (Equation (A.16) gives $V = (V \cap V^{\perp}{}_j) \oplus V_j$. Intersect both sides with $V^{\perp}{}_{j-1}$ and apply the modular law (A.6).)

4.12. Prove Corollary 4.24. For regression, use the subspaces given in Example 4.21. For the $a \times b$ experiment, just consider the sequence $W_4 \supset W_1 \supset W_0$ for the subspaces illustrated in Fig. 4.2 and described on page 93. (Note that there are 6 possible sequences we could consider.)

4.13. Consider equation (4.18). Show that $SS(\boldsymbol{\beta} \in W_{j-1}|\boldsymbol{\beta} \in W_j) + \cdots + SS(\boldsymbol{\beta} \in W_0|\boldsymbol{\beta} \in W_1) = SS(\boldsymbol{\beta} \in W_0|\boldsymbol{\beta} \in W_j)$. That is, the sum of the last j sequential sums of squares is the sum of squares for testing $\boldsymbol{\beta} \in W_0$ in the constrained model $\boldsymbol{\beta} \in W_j$. It may be easiest to recast the above questions in terms of equation (4.15).

Section 4.5

4.14. Consider the data in Example 4.25.

(i) Plot the data. Does a model with only a quadratic term seem reasonable?
(ii) Perform a regression in which the terms are entered in the order x^2, x, x^3, using the sequential sum of squares. Does this alter the ANOVA table given in Example 4.25?

4.15. Rerun the ANOVA for the data in Example 4.26 with Variety fitted before Soil. Does the conclusion change (i.e., which factor is significant)?

4.16. Consider the 2×3 experiment in Example 4.26 with n_{ij} observations in cell (i, j). Let $\boldsymbol{\beta} \in W_1$ be the hypothesis "Only soil effect present" (see Eq. (2.5)) and $\boldsymbol{\beta} \in W_0$ be the hypothesis "No effects present". Use Theorem 4.28 and its corollary to show that the associated hypothesis for the sequential sum of squares for Soil, $SS(\boldsymbol{\beta} \in W_0|\boldsymbol{\beta} \in W_1)$, is

$$\frac{1}{n_{1\cdot}}(n_{11}\mu_{11} + n_{12}\mu_{12} + n_{13}\mu_{13}) - \frac{1}{n_{2\cdot}}(n_{21}\mu_{21} + n_{22}\mu_{22} + n_{23}\mu_{23}) = 0.$$

Assume the effects are in the same sequence as given there.

(Use the theorem to show that the sequential df is 1. Then by the corollary, the effect is defined by a single nonzero element of $N(\mathbf{P}^*\mathbf{T}')$. Letting $\mathbf{c}^*$ be the coefficient vector of the contrast given above, show that $\mathbf{c}^* \in N(\mathbf{P}^*\mathbf{T}')$. To do this, define the orthogonal projections $\mathbf{P}$, $\mathbf{P}_1$ and $\mathbf{P}_0$ as in Theorem 4.28, and show:

(i) $\mathbf{P}_0\mathbf{T}'\mathbf{c}^* = \mathbf{0}$. (You can use Proposition 4.1, or direct calculation.)
(ii) $\mathbf{P}_1\mathbf{T}'\mathbf{c}^* = \mathbf{T}'\mathbf{c}^*$. This is the main problem.
(iii) $\mathbf{P}\mathbf{T}'\mathbf{c}^* = \mathbf{T}'\mathbf{c}^*$. (This follows from the preceding step, or from the more general fact that $\mathbf{P}\mathbf{T}' = \mathbf{T}'$.))

Section 4.6

4.17. Let the $n \times n$ matrix $\mathbf{A}$ be positive definite and symmetric.

(i) Show that

$$\langle \mathbf{x}, \mathbf{y} \rangle = \mathbf{x}\mathbf{A}^{-1}\mathbf{y} \tag{4.90}$$

defines an inner product on $\mathbb{R}^n$. (Use Theorem A.106.)

(ii) Suppose $\mathbf{A}$ has columns $\mathbf{a}_1, \ldots, \mathbf{a}_n$, and let $\mathbf{x} = (x_1, \ldots, x_n)$. Show that

$$x_i = \langle \mathbf{x}, \mathbf{a}_i \rangle.$$

(This is known as the *reproducing property* of the inner product (4.90), since the inner product with the columns of $\mathbf{A}$ "reproduces" the components of $\mathbf{x}$. The matrix $\mathbf{A}$ is said to be the *reproducing kernel* of the inner product. Such kernels play an important role in Hilbert space theory and in the theory of second order stochastic processes.)

4.18. Prove Lemma 4.36 and Corollary 4.35. For the lemma, you will need Proposition 4.11. You may assume the first part of Exercise 4.17.

4.19. Let $\mathbf{M}$ be an invertible matrix. Show: If $\mathbf{M}$ is scalar resp. diagonal resp. block diagonal, then so is $\mathbf{M}^{-1}$.

4.20. Prove Theorem 4.41. You may assume the result of Exercise 4.19. To generalize Lemma 4.39 you need to partition the set of basis elements $\mathbf{e}_i$ correspondingly into sets $E_1, \ldots, E_k$.

4.21. Prove the equivalence of equations (4.44) and (4.45).

4.22. Prove Theorem 4.46. (Show that the desired orthogonality holds iff $v_1/n_{1\cdot} = \cdots = v_a/n_{a\cdot}$ and $w_1/n_{\cdot 1} = \cdots = w_b/n_{\cdot b}$.)

4.23. Write out the contrast vectors defining the parameters α_i and β_j in a 2×3 experiment with the weights given by Theorem 4.46. (See Sect. 2.5.2.)

Section 4.7

4.24. Prove Theorem 4.48. (Fix $\boldsymbol{\beta}_0$ as in Lemma 4.47, and put $\mathbf{Z} = \mathbf{Y} - \mathbf{X}\boldsymbol{\beta}_0$ and $\boldsymbol{\beta}^* = \boldsymbol{\beta} - \boldsymbol{\beta}_0$. Show that H_0 is now a linear hypothesis about $\boldsymbol{\beta}^*$, find the Wald statistic for testing it, and show that the statistic can be written in the form (4.52).)

Section 4.8.1

4.25. (i) Prove the Boole inequality (4.56). (Apply induction, using the fact that $\mathrm{P}(A \cup B) = \mathrm{P}(A) + \mathrm{P}(B) - \mathrm{P}(A \cap B)$.)

(ii) Prove inequality (4.57). The sets R_i and Θ_{0i} are arbitrary.

(iii) Prove inequality (4.59). (This comes directly from the Boole inequality.) The sets S_i are arbitrary.

4.26. Write down formulas for simultaneous 95% confidence intervals for β_0, β_1 and σ^2 based on the model $\mathbf{Y} \sim N(\mathbf{X}\boldsymbol{\beta}, \sigma^2\mathbf{I})$ where $\mathbf{Y}$ is $N \times 1$. (Use t-intervals for β_i and a χ^2-interval for σ^2.)

4.27. (ii) Let I be an uncountable set, and assume $0 < \alpha_r \leq 1$ for each $r \in I$. Show that the set

$$\left\{ \sum_{r \in J} \alpha_r, \; J \text{ finite} \right\}$$

is unbounded. (Show that there exists an n such that $[1/n, 1]$ contains α_r for infinitely many r.)

(ii) Show that a "connect-the-dots" approach in Example 4.49 yields confidence bands for which the Bonferroni inequality gives a confidence level of zero.

Section 4.8.2

4.28. Prove Proposition 4.51. (Let $\mathbf{b} = \mathbf{C}'\hat{\boldsymbol{\beta}}$. Show that for each $\mathbf{c} \in U$ there is a unique $\mathbf{z} \in \mathbb{R}^d$ such that $\mathbf{c} = \mathbf{C}\mathbf{z}$. Apply the Maximization Lemma A.116 with this choice of $\mathbf{b}$ and $\mathbf{z}$ and the appropriate matrix $\mathbf{A}$. Make sure you verify the assumptions of the lemma.)

4.29. Verify that $\hat{\mathbf{c}}$ has the value given in Example 4.52 (up to scalar multiple), and that the sum of squares for $\hat{\mathbf{c}}'\boldsymbol{\beta}$ equals the sum of squares for Compaction. (You will need to form a matrix $\mathbf{C}$ for Eq. (4.66). Explain why you can replace $\mathbf{X}'\mathbf{X}$ by the identity matrix in that equation and in (4.13) in this example.)

4.30. Suppose we use (3.28) to create a confidence band for a simple linear regression. That is, suppose the upper boundary is the set of upper endpoints of the t-intervals, plotted as a function of x, and similarly for the lower boundary. Calculate the familywise confidence level of this procedure if $N = 29$ and if the individual intervals have confidence level 0.95. (Hint: Compare with the corresponding Scheffé formula.)

Section 4.9

4.31. Complete the proof of Theorem 4.55 (Eqs. (4.79) and (4.81)–(4.84)).

4.32. Suppose $\hat{\sigma}_\tau^2$ is given by (4.85). Letting $p = 4$ and $n = 5$, show that $\mathrm{P}(\hat{\sigma}_\tau^2 < 0) \doteq 0.58$ when $\sigma_\tau^2 = 0$. Find the probability when $\sigma_\tau^2/\sigma_e^2 = 1/2$; when $\sigma_\tau^2/\sigma_e^2 = 2$. Show that in general (for arbitrary, fixed n and p) this probability is a decreasing function of σ_τ^2/σ_e^2.

4.33. In Table 4.7, verify the formulas for

(i) $\mathrm{E}(MSE)$. (Write $\mathbf{I}_{bn} = \mathbf{I}_b \otimes \mathbf{I}_n$, and use the mixed-product formula with three terms in computing $(\mathbf{I} - \mathbf{P})\boldsymbol{\mu}$ and $(\mathbf{I} - \mathbf{P})\boldsymbol{\Sigma}$.)

(ii) $\mathrm{E}(MSB)$. (Imitate the derivation of $\mathrm{E}(MSA)$.)

Chapter 5
Multifactor Designs

Abstract We study two important decompositions of the parameter space of a factorial model with arbitrarily many factors. The first is the standard breakdown into main effects and interactions, the basis for the analysis of variance. The second, in classical symmetric factorial models, is a finer decomposition into main effects and components of interaction. In both cases we have some algebraic tools to generate effects from other effects. For the former there is a method given by multilinear algebra (the Kirkjian-Zelen construction), while for the latter we have a much more complete theory using the arithmetic of finite fields. A goal is to control confounding with blocks, and both cases rest upon some general results on blocking (partitioning of the set of treatment combinations).

The modern field of experimental design was created by Ronald A. Fisher while working at the Rothamsted Experimental Station in England. Sir John Russell was the director of the Station in 1919 when he hired Fisher as the Station's first statistician. In 1926 Russell wrote, "The chief requirement [in experiments] is simplicity; only one question should be asked at a time" [117, page 989]. Fisher was

> convinced that this view is wholly mistaken. Nature ... will best respond to a logical and carefully thought out questionnaire; indeed, if we ask her a single question, she will often refuse to answer until some other topic has been discussed. [56, page 511.]

(Joan Fisher Box gives an extensive discussion of the development of Fisher's thinking concerning experimental design in [26].)

Following a decade of research, general expositions of the subject appeared in 1935: Fisher's book *Design of Experiments* [57] and an extended paper [153] that his colleague Frank Yates read to the Royal Statistical Society. The following year a paper [10] appeared that had a pronounced effect on the direction of research in design. The author, Mildred M. Barnard, was a young Australian who had gone to the Galton Laboratory at University College, London, to work with Fisher as a doctoral student, and who moved to Rothamsted a year later to continue her work under Yates.

Barnard introduced the idea of a *generalized interaction* when dealing with the *problem of confounding* (see Sects. 5.5 and 5.6). She recognized that the contrast

J. H. Beder, *Linear Models and Design*,
https://doi.org/10.1007/978-3-031-08176-7_5

vectors in a 2^k design have "an internal symmetry" that she exploited to design confounding schemes. This symmetry turned out to be that of a group under componentwise multiplication. (The reader can already see this group structure in the 2^3 design if a column of ones is added to Table 2.1.) While some combinatorial methods had already been applied—for example, the use of Latin and Graeco-Latin squares—her paper launched decades of investigation into the application of algebra in problems of design.

A review of Barnard's scientific and personal life up to 1988 can be found in [53]. Barnard died in 2000.

This chapter is devoted to the study of factorial experiments with k factors, each factor being observed at some number of discrete levels. We will begin by studying partitions (blockings) of the set of treatment combinations, and the contrasts that result from a given partition. Section 5.3 will apply this to the general definition of main effects and interactions, and their mutual orthogonality, as ultimately expressed by Theorem 5.18. Section 5.4 introduces an important algebraic feature of multifactor experiments, brought to light by Kurkjian and Zelen, and expressed by Theorem 5.30 and its corollaries. Finally, we study the problem of confounding with blocks in Sect. 5.5, particularly in certain symmetric factorial designs. For such designs, Theorem 5.53 introduces the idea of components of interaction, a finer breakdown of "degrees of freedom" than Theorem 5.18, and Theorem 5.58 shows how to find "generalized interactions" of such components. The familiar naming convention and group theory for these components is introduced in Sect. 5.6.4.

5.1 Vectors and Functions: Notation

We denote the cardinality of a set E by $|E|$.

We have just mentioned the use of componentwise multiplication, an unusual operation on vectors[1] but one that is familiar to every calculus student when framed as the pointwise product of two functions. Similarly, it is unusual to refer to vectors that are "constant on rows" (as in Sect. 2.2), but not at all uncommon to consider functions that are constant on certain sets. Finally, we will typically need to deal with multi-indexed components of vectors (e.g., μ_{ijk}), which are rather cumbersome.

These and other issues motivate us to make use of the fact that a vector $\mathbf{v} = (v_1, \ldots, v_n)$ may be viewed as a function v on the set $\{1, \ldots, n\}$ defined by $v(i) = v_i$. Thus when we deal with vectors that typically have multi-indexed components (e.g., μ_{ijk}) *we will treat them as functions of several variables* (e.g., $\mu(i, j, k)$). In such cases the index set T is a Cartesian product, and is the domain of the corresponding function. Note that this approach avoids having to fix an order of the elements of T, which would be necessary in forming a vector $\mathbf{v}$.

The set of real-valued functions on a set T is denoted $\mathbb{R}^T$. It is a vector space over $\mathbb{R}$, where addition is the pointwise addition of functions and scalar multiplication

[1] The componentwise product of matrices is known by various names, such as the *Hadamard product*.

is the multiplication of a function by a constant. Pointwise multiplication makes it an *algebra* over $\mathbb{R}$: the function $w = uv$ is defined by $w(t) = u(t)v(t)$. This product is commutative and associative, and has a multiplicative identity, namely 1, the function that is constantly 1. The *Euclidean inner product* in $\mathbb{R}^T$ is

$$(u, v) = \sum_{t \in T} u(t)v(t). \tag{5.1}$$

If we need to view these functions as p-tuples, $p = |T|$, we need to fix an order of the elements of T and then represent the function v as a vector with component $v(t)$ in the tth position. When we do this, the inner product (5.1) is just the ordinary dot product in $\mathbb{R}^p$, the sum and scalar product are the usual ones for vectors in $\mathbb{R}^p$, and the pointwise product is the componentwise product mentioned above.

We have denoted by 1 the constant function taking the value 1:

$$1(t) \equiv 1 \text{ for all } t \in T.$$

Similarly, we write 1_C for the *indicator* or *characteristic* function of the set $C \subset T$:

$$1_C(t) = \begin{cases} 1 \text{ if } t \in C, \\ 0 \text{ if } t \notin C. \end{cases}$$

Thus 1 is 1_T. We record a few elementary observations:

Lemma 5.1

a. $1_C 1_D = 1_{C \cap D}$ *(pointwise product).*
b. *If* $D_1, \ldots, D_k$ *are pairwise disjoint, then* $\sum_i 1_{D_i} = 1_D$ *iff* $D = \cup_i D_i$.
c. *We have*

$$(1_C, 1_D) = |C \cap D|. \tag{5.2}$$

A *contrast function* $c \in \mathbb{R}^T$ is a function such that $\sum_{t \in T} c(t) = 0$. Equivalently, it is a function that is orthogonal to 1. A contrast in μ is therefore an expression $\sum_{t \in T} c(t)\mu(t)$ where c is a contrast function.

5.2 The General Theory of Block Effects

Let T be a finite set. For a given partition[2] $\mathcal{C}$ of T, we define

$$U_{\mathcal{C}} = \{c \in \mathbb{R}^T : c \text{ is a contrast function that is constant on each block of } \mathcal{C}\}.$$

[2] For a general review of partitions, see Sect. A.2.2.

When T is a set of treatments (or treatment combinations), we call $U_{\mathcal{C}}$ the *block effect* of $\mathcal{C}$. Since the "rows" of an $a \times b$ design are a partition of the ab cells, a row effect is a block effect, and similarly so is a column effect. These are of course the main effects in such a design, as we have seen in Sect. 2.2. Block effects will be used in defining main effects as well as interactions in a general factorial design. They are also central to the idea of confounding.

A convenient alternate way to define $U_{\mathcal{C}}$ is to introduce the *incidence space* of $\mathcal{C}$ to be the vector space

$$M_{\mathcal{C}} = \{u \in \mathbb{R}^T : u \text{ is constant on each block of } \mathcal{C}\}.$$

When $\mathcal{C}$ is the *trivial partition* $\{T\}$, $M_{\mathcal{C}}$ = the subspace of constant functions = $\langle 1 \rangle$, the subspace spanned by the function 1.

Lemma 5.2 *Let $\mathcal{C}$ be a partition of T. The indicators 1_C, $C \in \mathcal{C}$, form an orthogonal basis of $M_{\mathcal{C}}$, and $1 \in M_{\mathcal{C}}$. If $\mathcal{C}$ is non-trivial, then $U_{\mathcal{C}} = M_{\mathcal{C}} \ominus \langle 1 \rangle$ and*

$$\dim U_{\mathcal{C}} = |\mathcal{C}| - 1. \tag{5.3}$$

We leave the proof of the lemma as an easy exercise. By Theorem A.70(a) we also have

$$M_{\mathcal{C}} = U_{\mathcal{C}} \oplus \langle 1 \rangle \text{ (orthogonal sum)}.$$

Remark 5.3 If we fix an order of the elements of T, the basis vectors $\mathbf{1}_C$ may be viewed as columns of a matrix $\mathbf{A}$ known as the *incidence matrix* of $\mathcal{C}$; the term "incidence space" naturally suggests itself for the column space of $\mathbf{A}$.

We denote by Part(T) the set of partitions of T. We will rely heavily on the fact that Part(T) a lattice, the *partition lattice* of T (see Sect. A.2.2). In particular, we partially order partitions so that $\mathcal{B} \leq \mathcal{C}$ iff $\mathcal{C}$ is a *refinement* of $\mathcal{B}$. That is, we put "fine" above "coarse", for reasons that will become clear shortly.[3] We will naturally write $\mathcal{B} < \mathcal{C}$ if $\mathcal{B} \leq \mathcal{C}$ and $\mathcal{B} \neq \mathcal{C}$. We leave it as an exercise to show that $\mathcal{B} \leq \mathcal{C}$ iff every block of $\mathcal{C}$ is contained in a block of $\mathcal{B}$ (Lemma A.6). This is often a simpler condition to verify.

The join or supremum of partitions $\mathcal{C}$ and $\mathcal{D}$ is given by

$$\mathcal{C} \vee \mathcal{D} = \{C \cap D : C \in \mathcal{C}, D \in \mathcal{D}\}.$$

Their meet or infimum, $\mathcal{C} \wedge \mathcal{D}$, is defined by declaring that x and y are in the same block of $\mathcal{C} \wedge \mathcal{D}$ if there is a sequence $x = x_1, x_2, \ldots, x_n = y$ in T such that x_i

[3] Caution: Our ordering of partitions is the opposite of that used by many authors.

and x_{i+1} are in the same block of either $\mathcal{C}$ or $\mathcal{D}$. See Sect. A.2.2 for more detail, especially Theorem A.7.

Example 5.4 Let $T = \{1, \ldots, 8\}$, and consider the partitions

$$\mathcal{A} = \{\{1, 2\}, \{3, 4\}, \{5, 6, 7\}, \{8\}\} \text{ and}$$
$$\mathcal{B} = \{\{1\}, \{2, 3\}, \{4\}, \{5\}, \{6, 7, 8\}\}.$$

The reader can verify that

$$\mathcal{A} \vee \mathcal{B} = \{\{1\}, \{2\}, \{3\}, \{4\}, \{5\}, \{6, 7\}, \{8\}\} \text{ and}$$
$$\mathcal{A} \wedge \mathcal{B} = \{\{1, 2, 3, 4\}, \{5, 6, 7, 8\}\}.$$

For an arbitrary set T, consider the map

$$\tau : \text{Part}(T) \to \{\text{subspaces of } \mathbb{R}^T\}$$
$$\mathcal{C} \mapsto U_{\mathcal{C}}.$$

We know (Theorem A.21) that the subspaces of $\mathbb{R}^T$ form a lattice, where ordering is by inclusion, meet is intersection, and join is vector-space sum. The following facts were given by Tjur [141]:

Theorem 5.5 *The map τ is one-to-one and preserves order and infima. We have*

$$U_{\mathcal{C}\vee\mathcal{D}} \supseteq U_{\mathcal{C}} + U_{\mathcal{D}}. \tag{5.4}$$

We will refer to τ as the *Tjur map*. It is this proposition that makes our partial order on partitions natural. If we had defined $\leq$ so that "fine" were *below* "coarse", then the map τ would be order-*reversing* (as in Lemma 6.2 of [8]). See also Remark A.8.

Proof of Theorem 5.5 It is easy to see that $\mathcal{C} \leq \mathcal{D}$ implies that $U_{\mathcal{C}} \subseteq U_{\mathcal{D}}$, so that τ preserves order. In fact, the converse also holds. For let us assume that $U_{\mathcal{C}} \subseteq U_{\mathcal{D}}$, so that $M_{\mathcal{C}} \subseteq M_{\mathcal{D}}$. Let $C \in \mathcal{C}$; we claim that C is a union of blocks of $\mathcal{D}$. By assumption, $1_C \in M_{\mathcal{D}}$, so we have an orthogonal expansion

$$1_C = \sum_i a_i 1_{D_i},$$

and a quick computation using Lemma A.62 and Eq. (5.2) shows that this

$$= \sum_j 1_{D_{i_j}}$$

for some subfamily D_{i_j} of D_i. It follows from Lemma 5.1 that $C = \cup_j D_{i_j}$.

Thus in fact $U_{\mathcal{C}} \subseteq U_{\mathcal{D}}$ if *and only if* $\mathcal{C} \leq \mathcal{D}$. It follows in particular that τ is one-to-one. To show that τ preserves infima, we must show that

$$U_{\mathcal{C}\wedge\mathcal{D}} = U_{\mathcal{C}} \cap U_{\mathcal{D}}.$$

To show the inclusion $\supseteq$, let $u \in U_{\mathcal{C}} \cap U_{\mathcal{D}}$. Then u is a contrast function and is constant on the blocks of $\mathcal{C}$ and the blocks of $\mathcal{D}$. We must show that it is constant on the blocks of $\mathcal{C} \wedge \mathcal{D}$. To this end, let $E \in \mathcal{C} \wedge \mathcal{D}$, and let $x, y \in E$. Then there is a sequence $x = x_1, \ldots, x_k = y$ such that, for each i, x_i and x_{i+1} are in the same block of $\mathcal{C}$ or of $\mathcal{D}$. In either case, $u(x_i) = u(x_{i+1})$ for all i, so $u(x) = u(y)$. Thus u is constant on E.

The proofs of the reverse inclusion and of (5.4) are left as an exercise. □

Equality in display (5.4) would have asserted that τ also preserves suprema, but that is not true. In fact, this leads us to the following:

Definition 5.6 The *generalized interaction* of the effects $U_{\mathcal{C}}$ and $U_{\mathcal{D}}$ is the orthogonal difference $U_{\mathcal{C}\vee\mathcal{D}} \ominus (U_{\mathcal{C}} + U_{\mathcal{D}})$.

We will see (Remark 5.62) that this is the most general form of Barnard's generalized interaction.

To characterize the orthogonality of block effect subspaces, we let π be the uniform probability measure (normalized counting measure) on T:

$$\pi(E) = |E|/|T|. \tag{5.5}$$

We will say that two partitions $\mathcal{C}$ and $\mathcal{D}$ are *independent* (with respect to π)[4] if

$$\pi(C \cap D) = \pi(C)\pi(D) \tag{5.6}$$

for every $C \in \mathcal{C}$ and $D \in \mathcal{D}$. Our characterization is this [11]:

Lemma 5.7 *$U_{\mathcal{C}} \perp U_{\mathcal{D}}$ iff $\mathcal{C}$ and $\mathcal{D}$ are independent.*

Proof For any $B \subset T$ the function $u_B = 1_B - \pi(B)1$ is orthogonal to 1, and so for any blocking $\mathcal{C}$ the set $\{u_C : C \in \mathcal{C}\}$ spans $U_{\mathcal{C}}$. The lemma now follows by taking the inner products of u_C with u_D for all $C \in \mathcal{C}$ and $D \in \mathcal{D}$. □

Independence is a combinatorial condition, as (5.6) may be written

$$|C \cap D||T| = |C||D|. \tag{5.7}$$

[4] Some authors (see, e.g., [8]) use the term *orthogonal* rather than *independent* when referring to partitions. There are reasons to prefer a term like independent; see the paragraph before Example 5.8.

This is implicit in Tjur [141], and is mentioned by Loyer [94] in certain symmetric factorial designs. Bailey [8, Corollary 6.5] states condition (5.7) explicitly, while Bose gives an equivalent condition for pairwise independence [22, page 109].

More generally, independence of k partitions is defined in the obvious way as independence of all choices of 2, 3, ..., k sets taken one from each partition. Thus independence is actually a stronger condition than orthogonality of the corresponding vector spaces, which is only a pairwise relation. The reader may show, for example, that if $\mathcal{C}$, $\mathcal{D}$ and $\mathcal{E}$ are independent partitions then so are $\mathcal{C} \vee \mathcal{D}$ and $\mathcal{E}$ (see Exercise 5.5).

Example 5.8 A *Latin square of order n* is an $n \times n$ array filled with n symbols, each symbol occurring once in each row and once in each column. Here are two Latin squares of order 3:

0	1	2
1	2	0
2	0	1

0	2	1
1	0	2
2	1	0

If we label the rows and columns of the Latin squares above by 0, 1 and 2, then the first square partitions the 9 cells into {00, 12, 21}, {01, 10, 22}, and {02, 11, 20}. (The first block contains those cells having a 0.)

Similarly, a Latin square of order n partitions an $n \times n$ array into n blocks of equal size.

Lemma 5.9 *Let T be the cells of an $n \times n$ array, and let $\mathcal{A}$ and $\mathcal{B}$ be the partitions of T given by the rows and columns, respectively.*

If $\mathcal{L}$ is a Latin square of order n, and $\mathcal{C}$ is the partition of T determined by $\mathcal{L}$, then $\mathcal{C}$ is independent of $\mathcal{A}$ and $\mathcal{B}$.

Conversely, let $\mathcal{C}$ be a partition of T into n blocks of equal size, say $C_1, \ldots, C_n$. Let $c_1, \ldots, c_n$ be distinct symbols, and put c_i into each cell of C_i. If $\mathcal{C}$ is independent of $\mathcal{A}$ and $\mathcal{B}$, then the array is a Latin square.

Proof The latinity of $\mathcal{L}$ implies that if $A \in \mathcal{A}$ and $C \in \mathcal{C}$ then $|A \cap C| = 1$. Since $|A| = n$ and $|C| = n$, it follows that $|A \cap C||T| = |A||C|$, so that $\mathcal{A}$ and $\mathcal{C}$ are independent, by Eq. (5.7). The proof for $\mathcal{B}$ and $\mathcal{C}$ is the same.

Conversely, the same equation shows that if a partition $\mathcal{C}$ is independent of rows and columns, then the size of each block must be multiple of n. If we consider partitions in n blocks of size n, then the same equation shows that each block has one cell from each row and one from each column—in other words, it defines a Latin square. □

If in Example 5.8 we view the rows and columns as representing the levels of two factors, then $U_{\mathcal{A}}$ and $U_{\mathcal{B}}$ are what we have called U_1 and U_2, the main effects for the two factors. Since $U_{\mathcal{C}}$ is orthogonal to these, it must be a subspace of U_{12}, the interaction effect. In Sect. 5.6 we will call $U_{\mathcal{C}}$ a *component of interaction*.

We note another feature about the two Latin squares in this example: If we superimpose the one on the other, each of the nine possible ordered pairs of values occurs in exactly one cell. (For example, the pair (2, 1) occurs in row 1, column 3, and only there.) Two Latin squares of order n are said to be *orthogonal* if, when they are superimposed, every pair of symbols occurs exactly once. The following result provides a justification for using the term "orthogonal" with Latin squares:

Proposition 5.10 *Let $\mathcal{C}$ and $\mathcal{D}$ be the partitions formed by two Latin squares of order n. The following are equivalent:*

(a) The squares are orthogonal.
(b) $\mathcal{C}$ and $\mathcal{D}$ are independent partitions.
(c) $U_\mathcal{C}$ and $U_\mathcal{D}$ are orthogonal.

If there is a set of r mutually orthogonal Latin squares of order n then $r \leq n - 1$.

When $n = 3$, the maximum number $r = 2$ can be attained, as Example 5.8 shows. This is as special case of a more general result that we will meet later in this chapter. We leave the proof of Proposition 5.10 as an exercise.

Example 5.11 Condition (5.7) can give us a lot of information about what is possible in a given factorial experiment. Consider a 4×4 experiment with factors A (rows) and B (columns), let T be the set of 16 treatment combinations, and let $\mathcal{A}$ and $\mathcal{B}$ be the row- and column-partitions of T. Suppose we seek a partition $\mathcal{C}$ that is independent of both $\mathcal{A}$ and $\mathcal{B}$, so that the effect $U_\mathcal{C}$ is a component of interaction.

According to Eq. (5.7), each block C of $\mathcal{C}$ must satisfy $|A_i||C| = |A_i \cap C||T|$, or $4|C| = |A_i \cap C|16$, where A_i is the ith row. Then

$$|C| = 4|A_i \cap C|, \tag{5.8}$$

so $|C|$ must be a multiple of 4. Setting aside the trivial partition (where $C = T$), this means that $|C| = 4$ or 8.

If $|C| = 4$, then (5.8) says that $|A_i \cap C| = 1$, meaning that C has one cell in each row. Similarly, C must have one cell per column. If all the blocks of $\mathcal{C}$ have size 4, then $\mathcal{C}$ defines a Latin square of order 4. In Sect. 5.6 we will see how to construct three independent partitions of this type (you are asked to carry this out in Exercise 5.23). Since each of these has 4 blocks, each defines a block effect of dimension 3. But there are 9 degrees of freedom for interaction, so this will give an orthogonal decomposition of interaction into three components.

In Sect. 5.7 we will consider methods to construct a decomposition of interaction using nine partitions with blocksize 8.

Example 5.12 Lemma 5.7 already allows us to conclude orthogonality of many effects. Consider, for example, an $a \times b \times c$ design (see Sect. 2.3) with factors A, B and C. Let $\mathcal{A}$, $\mathcal{B}$ and $\mathcal{C}$ be the partitions determined by the levels of each factor, and let $A' \in \mathcal{A}$, $B' \in \mathcal{B}$, and $C' \in \mathcal{C}$ be blocks ("slices"). Then

$$\pi(A') = bc/abc = 1/a, \quad \pi(B') = 1/b, \quad \pi(C') = 1/c,$$
$$\pi(A' \cap B') = c/abc = 1/ab, \quad \pi(A' \cap C') = 1/ac, \quad \pi(B' \cap C') = 1/bc,$$
$$\pi(A' \cap B' \cap C') = 1/abc,$$

from which we see that A', B' and C' are independent. Thus we see that $U_{\mathcal{A}}, U_{\mathcal{B}}$, and $U_{\mathcal{C}}$ are mutually orthogonal. Of course, these are nothing but U_1, U_2 and U_3 defined earlier. From Lemma 5.2 we can see moreover that $\dim U_1 = a - 1, \dim U_2 = b - 1$, and $\dim U_3 = c - 1$.

We can say yet more. In terms of the present chapter, the subspace of A-by-B interactions defined in Sect. 2.3 is, in our present terminology,

$$U_{12} = U_{\mathcal{A} \vee \mathcal{B}} \ominus (U_{\mathcal{A}} + U_{\mathcal{B}}). \tag{5.9}$$

The blocks of $\mathcal{A} \vee \mathcal{B}$ are the "tubes" determined by the combined levels of factors A and B (see Fig. 2.2). Since $\mathcal{A} \vee \mathcal{B}$ and $\mathcal{C}$ are independent, we see that $U_{\mathcal{A} \vee \mathcal{B}} \perp U_{\mathcal{C}}$. But $U_{12} \subset U_{\mathcal{A} \vee \mathcal{B}}$, so $U_{12} \perp U_3$. Similarly $U_{13} \perp U_2$ and $U_{23} \perp U_1$. Moreover, from Lemma 5.2, Corollary A.71 and the orthogonality of U_i and U_j we see that

$$\begin{aligned}\dim U_{12} &= \dim U_{\mathcal{A}_1 \vee \mathcal{A}_2} - (\dim U_1 + \dim U_2) \\ &= (ab - 1) - (a - 1) - (b - 1) = (a - 1)(b - 1)\end{aligned}$$

and similarly $\dim U_{13} = (a - 1)(c - 1)$ and $\dim U_{23} = (b - 1)(c - 1)$.

Lemma 5.7 is not enough to prove that $U_{12} \perp U_{23}$, however. The difficulty is that $\mathcal{A} \vee \mathcal{B}$ and $\mathcal{B} \vee \mathcal{C}$ "overlap" at $\mathcal{B}$. For this we need more machinery.

One option is to strengthen the lemma. To accomplish this, we will work not with subspaces like (5.9), but rather with larger subspaces of the form $U_{\mathcal{A} \vee \mathcal{B}} \ominus U_{\mathcal{B}}$.

Consider partitions $\mathcal{C}$, $\mathcal{D}$ and $\mathcal{E}$ of the finite set T. Note that $U_{\mathcal{D}}$ is contained in both $U_{\mathcal{C} \vee \mathcal{D}}$ and $U_{\mathcal{D} \vee \mathcal{E}}$ (τ preserves order). We seek necessary and sufficient conditions on the partitions such that

$$U_{\mathcal{C} \vee \mathcal{D}} \ominus U_{\mathcal{D}} \perp U_{\mathcal{D} \vee \mathcal{E}} \ominus U_{\mathcal{D}}. \tag{5.10}$$

Let us denote intersections as "products" for simplicity ($C \cap D = CD$). The events C and E are *conditionally independent*[5] given D if

$$\pi(CE|D) = \pi(C|D)\pi(E|D). \tag{5.11}$$

[5] With respect to π.

Like independence, this is a combinatorial condition, namely

$$|CDE||D| = |CD||DE|.$$

We say that the partitions $\mathcal{C}$ and $\mathcal{E}$ are *conditionally independent* given $\mathcal{D}$ if (5.11) holds for all $C \in \mathcal{C}$, $D \in \mathcal{D}$, and $E \in \mathcal{E}$. The characterization we seek is the following:

Theorem 5.13 *Let $\mathcal{C}$, $\mathcal{D}$ and $\mathcal{E}$ be partitions of a finite set T. Then (5.10) holds if and only if $\mathcal{C}$ and $\mathcal{E}$ are conditionally independent, given $\mathcal{D}$.*

In particular, if $\mathcal{C}$, $\mathcal{D}$ and $\mathcal{E}$ are independent, then (5.10) holds.

Lemma 5.7 is a corollary of this theorem. For let $\mathcal{D}$ be the smallest element in Part(T): $\mathcal{D} = \{T\}$. Then conditional independence given $\mathcal{D}$ is ordinary independence, $U_{\mathcal{D}} = (0)$, $\mathcal{C} \vee \mathcal{D} = \mathcal{C}$, and $\mathcal{E} \vee \mathcal{D} = \mathcal{E}$. That is, $U_{\mathcal{C}} \perp U_{\mathcal{E}}$ iff $\mathcal{C}$ and $\mathcal{E}$ are independent.

Example 5.14 (Example 5.12 Continued) The orthogonality of U_{12} and U_{23} in an $a \times b \times c$ design follows from Theorem 5.13, as the independence of $\mathcal{A}$, $\mathcal{B}$ and $\mathcal{C}$ implies that $U_{\mathcal{A}\vee\mathcal{B}} \ominus U_{\mathcal{B}} \perp U_{\mathcal{B}\vee\mathcal{C}} \ominus U_{\mathcal{B}}$. But $U_{12} = U_{\mathcal{A}\vee\mathcal{B}} \ominus (U_{\mathcal{A}} + U_{\mathcal{B}}) \subset U_{\mathcal{A}\vee\mathcal{B}} \ominus U_{\mathcal{B}}$, and similarly $U_{23} \subset U_{\mathcal{B}\vee\mathcal{C}} \ominus U_{\mathcal{B}}$, so $U_{12} \perp U_{23}$.

Since U_{123} is defined as the subspace of contrasts orthogonal to all six of the subspaces $U_1, \ldots, U_{23}$, this verifies the orthogonality in the decomposition (2.16) of $\mathbb{R}^{abc}$. Because of orthogonality, a count of dimensions and a little algebra shows that $\dim U_{123} = (a-1)(b-1)(c-1)$.

Proof of Theorem 5.13 It is easy to see that (5.10) holds iff

$$M_{\mathcal{C}\vee\mathcal{D}} \ominus M_{\mathcal{D}} \perp M_{\mathcal{D}\vee\mathcal{E}} \ominus M_{\mathcal{D}}, \tag{5.12}$$

where $M_{\mathcal{F}}$ is the incidence space of the partition $\mathcal{F}$. □

Let $P =$ the orthogonal projection of $\mathbb{R}^T$ on $M_{\mathcal{D}}$. The functions 1_{CD}, $C \in \mathcal{C}$, $D \in \mathcal{D}$, form a basis of $M_{\mathcal{C}\vee\mathcal{D}}$, and since $I - P$ maps $M_{\mathcal{C}\vee\mathcal{D}}$ onto $M_{\mathcal{C}\vee\mathcal{D}} \ominus M_{\mathcal{D}}$ (Corollary A.93(A.93)), the images $(I - P)1_{CD}$ span $M_{\mathcal{C}\vee\mathcal{D}} \ominus M_{\mathcal{D}}$. A similar statement holds for $M_{\mathcal{D}\vee\mathcal{E}} \ominus M_{\mathcal{D}}$. Therefore, (5.12) holds iff

$$(I - P)1_{CD} \perp (I - P)1_{D'E} \quad \text{for all} \quad C \in \mathcal{C},\ D, D' \in \mathcal{D}, E \in \mathcal{E}. \tag{5.13}$$

We thus need to set $((I - P)1_{CD}, (I - P)1_{D'E}) = 0$. To do this we will need the following fact, whose proof we leave as an exercise:

Lemma 5.15 *Let $\mathcal{D}$ and P be as above. Then for all $C \subseteq T$ and $D \in \mathcal{D}$ we have $P1_{CD} = \pi(C|D)1_D$.*

Using Lemma 5.15 and the standard properties of the projection $I - P$, we find:

$$
\begin{aligned}
((I-P)1_{CD}, (I-P)1_{D'E}) &= ((I-P)1_{CD}, 1_{D'E}) \\
&= (1_{CD} - \pi(C|D)1_D, 1_{D'E}) \\
&= |CDD'E| - \pi(C|D)|DD'E| \\
&= \begin{cases} |CDE| - \pi(C|D)|DE| & \text{if } D = D', \\ 0 & \text{if } D \neq D'. \end{cases}
\end{aligned}
$$

When $D = D'$, this = 0 if and only if

$$|CDE| = \pi(C|D)|DE|. \tag{5.14}$$

Dividing by $|D|$, (5.14) becomes (5.11), that is, C and E are conditionally independent given D. Thus if (5.13) holds, then (5.11) must hold for all $C \in \mathcal{C}$, $D \in \mathcal{D}$, $E \in \mathcal{E}$, and conversely, as claimed.

The final statement of the theorem results from the fact that if $\mathcal{C}$, $\mathcal{D}$ and $\mathcal{E}$ are independent then $\mathcal{C}$ and $\mathcal{E}$ are conditionally independent given $\mathcal{D}$. □

5.3 The Multifactor Design: Reprise

In an influential expository paper [22, page 110] R. C. Bose gave the following definitions:

> A contrast (or the degree of freedom possessed by it) may be said to belong to the *main effect* F_i,[6] if the coefficients in the linear function constituting the contrast are independent of the levels of factors other than F_i (in other words the coefficients of all treatments in which F_i occurs at a given level are the same).
>
> A contrast (or the degree of freedom possessed by it) may be said to belong to the *first order interaction* $F_i F_j$ between the factors F_i and F_j if (i) the coefficients in the linear function constituting the contrast are independent of the levels of the factors other than F_i and F_j, [and] (ii) the contrast is orthogonal to any contrast belonging to the main effect of F_i or F_j.
>
> The above definitions may now be extended by induction. After defining when a contrast belongs to the $(k-1)$-th order interaction of any k factors, for $k = 2, 3, \ldots, r-1$, we can proceed to the following definition. A contrast belongs to the r-th order interaction of the factors $F_{i_1}, F_{i_2}, \ldots, F_{i_{r+1}}$ if (i) [the coefficients of the contrast are independent of the levels of the factors other than $F_{i_1}, F_{i_2}, \ldots, F_{i_{r+1}}$, and (ii)] the contrast is orthogonal to all contrasts belonging to the main effects of $F_{i_1}, F_{i_2}, \ldots, F_{i_{r+1}}$, as well as to all contrasts belonging to the $(k-1)$-th order interaction of any k of the above factors for $k = 2, 3, \ldots, r$. The $(k-1)$-th order interaction between $F_{i_1}, F_{i_2}, \ldots, F_{i_k}$ is called the k-factor interaction $F_{i_1} F_{i_2} \cdots F_{i_k}$.[7]

---

[6] Bose used F_i rather than A_i to denote the ith factor.

[7] The bracketed passage should have appeared in the original but was evidently dropped accidentally. Other minor typographic errors have been corrected as well.

In line with our discussion in Sect. 1.7, the hypothesis of "no F_2 effect" is the statement that all the contrasts belonging to the main effect of F_2 equal zero. The statement that there is no F_1F_3 interaction is the statement that all contrasts belonging to this interaction equal zero.

Bose's description extends to k-factor designs the spaces of contrasts that we developed for two- and three-factor designs in Sects. 2.2 and 2.3. In this section we rewrite his description in terms of such spaces. That is, for each $I \subset \{1, \ldots, k\}$ (that is, for each subset of factors) we define a set U_I of contrast vectors, namely those belonging to that interaction. We verify the mutual orthogonality of these subspaces (and count dimensions) using the results of the previous section.

As in Sect. 1.5, let $T = A_1 \times \cdots \times A_k$ be the set of treatment combinations in an $s_1 \times \cdots \times s_k$ factorial, where A_i indexes the levels of factor i and $s_i = |A_i|$. We begin by describing various partitions of T.

The most basic partitions are those defined by the levels of one factor. In the two-factor case these are "rows" and "columns", and in the three-factor case they are "slices", as described in Sects. 2.2 and 2.3. In the general case, the blocks of the partition defined by the ith factor are the sets

$$A_1 \times \cdots \times A_{i-1} \times \{r\} \times A_{i+1} \times \cdots \times A_k \tag{5.15}$$

where r ranges over A_i. These form a partition $\mathcal{A}_i$ consisting of s_i blocks of equal size.

For $i \neq j$ the blocks of $\mathcal{A}_i \vee \mathcal{A}_j$ are intersections of sets (5.15), and thus (for $i < j$) are of the form

$$A_1 \times \cdots \times A_{i-1} \times \{r\} \times A_{i+1} \times \cdots \times A_{j-1} \times \{s\} \times A_{j+1} \times \cdots \times A_k$$

where $r \in A_i$ and $s \in A_j$.

In general, for any nonempty subset $I \subset \{1, \ldots, k\}$ the factors $i \in I$ determine the partition $\vee_{i \in I} \mathcal{A}_i$ of T, where we use the shorthand

$$\vee_{i \in I} \mathcal{A}_i = \mathcal{A}_{i_1} \vee \cdots \vee \mathcal{A}_{i_d}$$

if $I = \{i_1, \ldots, i_d\}$. The blocks of $\vee_{i \in I} \mathcal{A}_i$ are formed by taking intersections of blocks, one from each $\mathcal{A}_i$, $i \in I$, and are subsets of T of the form $B_1 \times \cdots \times B_k$, where for fixed elements $r_i \in A_i$ we have

$$B_i = \begin{cases} \{r_i\} \text{ if } i \in I, \\ A_i \text{ if } i \notin I. \end{cases} \tag{5.16}$$

Example 5.16 Figure 2.2 (page 37) illustrated these partitions in a 3-factor design. We may rewrite that figure in the present notation, using $\mathcal{A}$, $\mathcal{B}$ and $\mathcal{C}$ for the partitions defined by factors A, B and C, respectively:

$$\mathcal{A} \vee \mathcal{B} \vee \mathcal{C}$$

$$\mathcal{A} \vee \mathcal{B} \qquad \mathcal{A} \vee \mathcal{C} \qquad \mathcal{B} \vee \mathcal{C}$$

$$\mathcal{A} \qquad\qquad \mathcal{B} \qquad\qquad \mathcal{C}$$

$$\{T\}$$

Note that the partitions increase in refinement from bottom to top, so that $\mathcal{A} \vee \mathcal{B}$ refines both $\mathcal{A}$ and $\mathcal{B}$, and so on.

We have introduced these partitions for the following reason: if $\mathcal{C} = \vee_{i \in I} \mathcal{A}_i$, the block effect $U_{\mathcal{C}}$ *is precisely the set of contrast functions* $c(t_1, \ldots, t_k)$ *that are independent of the values of* t_j *for* $j \notin I$ *– that is, which depend only on the levels of the factors indicated by* I.

We pause to record some simple observations that will be needed below. As before, independence is with respect to π, the uniform probability measure on T. For the remainder of this section it will be useful to use the notation

$$\mathcal{C}_I = \vee_{i \in I} \mathcal{A}_i. \tag{5.17}$$

Lemma 5.17 ([16])

a. $|\mathcal{C}_I| = \prod_{i \in I} s_i$, *and* $\pi(B) = \dfrac{1}{\prod_{i \in I} s_i}$ *for every block* $B \in \mathcal{C}_I$.
b. $\mathcal{C}_I \vee \mathcal{C}_J = \mathcal{C}_{I \cup J}$.
c. $\mathcal{C}_I$ *and* $\mathcal{C}_J$ *are independent iff* $I \cap J = \emptyset$.

Proof To prove (b), let $B' \in \mathcal{C}_I$ and $B'' \in \mathcal{C}_J$. Then $B' = B'_1 \times \cdots \times B'_k$ and $B'' = B''_1 \times \cdots \times B''_k$ where B'_i is of form (5.16) and B''_i is of the same form with I replaced by J (and possibly different elements r_i). We must show that either $B' \cap B''$ is also of this form, $I \cup J$ replacing I, or $B' \cap B'' = \emptyset$. But the first case occurs if B'_i and B''_i agree for all $i \in I \cap J$ (trivially if $I \cap J = \emptyset$), while the second occurs if they disagree. Thus $\mathcal{C}_I \vee \mathcal{C}_J \subset \mathcal{C}_{I \cup J}$.

Conversely, if $B \in \mathcal{C}_{I \cup J}$ then B is of form (5.16) with $I \cup J$ replacing I. Using the given values of r_i, $i \in I \cup J$, define

$$B'_i = \begin{cases} \{r_i\} & \text{if } i \in I, \\ A_i & \text{if } i \notin I. \end{cases}$$

and

$$B_i'' = \begin{cases} \{r_i\} & \text{if } i \in J, \\ A_i & \text{if } i \notin J \end{cases}$$

and put $B' = B_1' \times \cdots \times B_k'$ and $B'' = B_1'' \times \cdots \times B_k''$. Note that B' and B'' automatically agree on $I \cap J$, and that $B' \in \mathcal{C}_I$ and $B'' \in \mathcal{C}_J$. Then $B = B' \cap B'' \in \mathcal{C}_I \vee \mathcal{C}_J$, and so $\mathcal{C}_{I \cup J} \subset \mathcal{C}_I \vee \mathcal{C}_J$, proving (b).

The proofs of (a) and (c) are left as exercises. □

We now describe the contrasts belonging to main effects and to various interactions in the factorial experiment. First, the contrasts between the blocks of $\mathcal{A}_i$ define the main effect of factor i. The set of such contrast functions is then

$$U_i = U_{\mathcal{A}_i}.$$

The contrast functions belonging to the ij-interaction are defined to be

$$U_{ij} = \{c \in U_{\mathcal{A}_i \vee \mathcal{A}_j} : c \perp U_i \text{ and } U_j\}.$$

In general, for $\emptyset \neq I \subset \{1, \ldots, k\}$ we define the subspaces U_I inductively[8] as

$$U_I = \{c \in U_{\mathcal{C}_I} : c \perp U_J \text{ for all } J \subsetneq I\}. \tag{5.18}$$

When $|I| \geq 2$, U_I is the set of contrast functions belonging to the interaction between the factors listed in the set I. This is a slightly modernized version of the definition given by Bose quoted above.

We say that U_{ij} is a *first-order* interaction, and in general that the interaction U_I has *order* $|I| - 1$. Main effects may be said to be interactions of *order zero*.

The next result summarizes the basic facts underlying the analysis of variance. It generalizes Theorem 2.7. Again, $\mathcal{C}_I$ is given by (5.17).

Theorem 5.18

a. If $I \neq J$ then $U_I \perp U_J$.

b. We have the orthogonal decomposition

$$U_{\mathcal{C}_I} = \oplus_{J \subseteq I} U_J, \tag{5.19}$$

[8] In this induction, we assume that U_J has been defined for all $J \subsetneq I$. With a slight abuse of notation, we are writing U_{ij} for U_I where $I = \{i, j\}$.

summing over the nonempty subsets of I. In particular

$$\mathbb{R}^T = \langle 1 \rangle \oplus_I U_I, \tag{5.20}$$

the sum running over all nonempty subsets I of $\{1, \ldots, k\}$.

c. $\dim U_I = \prod_{i \in I} (s_i - 1)$ *for each nonempty subset I of $\{1, \ldots, k\}$.*

The subspace $\langle 1 \rangle$ represents the *effect of the grand mean* $\bar{\mu} = (1/|T|) \sum_{t \in T} \mu(t)$, in the sense that $\bar{\mu} = 0$ if and only if $\mu \perp 1$. Thus Eq. (5.20) separates all linear functions of cell means into the grand mean effect and the sets of contrasts corresponding to main effects and interactions. Equations (2.14) and (2.16) are special cases for $k = 2$ and 3. Item (c) gives the usual formula for the degrees of freedom for each main effect and interaction. It would be natural to let

$$U_\emptyset = \langle 1 \rangle,$$

so that (5.20) could be expressed as an orthogonal sum over *all* subsets of $\{1, \ldots, k\}$. That point of view will be useful when we study aliasing in Chap. 6. It should be noted, though, that $U_\emptyset$ consists of the constant functions rather than contrast functions.

Proof of Theorem 5.18 From (5.18) we see that $U_I \perp U_J$ if $J \subsetneq I$, so we consider U_I and U_J where neither I nor J contains the other.

If $I \cap J = \emptyset$ then $\mathcal{C} = \vee_{i \in I} \mathcal{A}_i$ and $\mathcal{E} = \vee_{i \in J} \mathcal{A}_i$ are independent (Lemmas 5.17), so that $U_\mathcal{C} \perp U_\mathcal{E}$ (Lemma 5.7). Since $U_I \subset U_\mathcal{C}$ and $U_J \subset U_\mathcal{E}$, we again have $U_I \perp U_J$.

If $I \cap J \neq \emptyset$, put

$$\mathcal{C} = \bigvee_{i \in I \setminus J} \mathcal{A}_i, \quad \mathcal{D} = \bigvee_{i \in I \cap J} \mathcal{A}_i, \quad \mathcal{E} = \bigvee_{i \in J \setminus I} \mathcal{A}_i.$$

Then $\mathcal{C}$, $\mathcal{D}$ and $\mathcal{E}$ are independent, so $U_{\mathcal{C} \vee \mathcal{D}} \ominus U_\mathcal{D} \perp U_{\mathcal{D} \vee \mathcal{E}} \ominus U_\mathcal{D}$ by Theorem 5.13. But $\mathcal{C} \vee \mathcal{D} = \vee_{i \in I} \mathcal{A}_i$ and $\mathcal{D} \vee \mathcal{E} = \vee_{i \in J} \mathcal{A}_i$, so $U_I \subset U_{\mathcal{C} \vee \mathcal{D}} \ominus U_\mathcal{D}$ and $U_J \subset U_{\mathcal{D} \vee \mathcal{E}} \ominus U_\mathcal{D}$, and so once again we have $U_I \perp U_J$. This proves (a).

The proofs of parts (b) and (c) are left as exercises. □

Theorem 5.18 is the result that allowed us to conclude the independence of order (Corollary 4.42) in equireplicate factorial designs. It is for this reason that the orthogonality of hypotheses is so important. Together with Corollary 4.5 (page 84), Theorem 5.18 also allows us to extend earlier results (Corollaries 4.24 and 4.16) to multifactor experiments:

Corollary 5.19 *Given the notation of Theorem 5.18, if all cells are filled in a factorial experiment then the sequential and adjusted degrees of freedom for testing $\boldsymbol{\beta} \perp U_I$ are equal, and are given by $\prod_{i \in I} (s_i - 1)$.*

The proof is left as an easy exercise.

Example 5.20 The following table contains simulated data (Y) from a $2 \times 3 \times 4$ experiment with 2 observations per treatment combination. The factors are labeled A, B and C; the levels of C are labeled 1, 2, 3 and 4, those of A and B similarly.

cell	Y	cell	Y	cell	Y	cell	Y
111	2.7, 2.7	123	6.1, 7.5	211	1.9, 2.8	223	7.8, 8.5
112	2.4, 2.1	124	10.1, 10.8	212	3.3, 4.8	224	12.8, 10.4
113	4.1, 5.2	131	3.8, 4.4	213	4.8, 5.0	231	5.3, 3.7
114	4.0, 6.3	132	6.8, 7.2	214	4.3, 6.2	232	6.8, 7.3
121	2.3, 3.3	133	10.4, 8.5	221	3.3, 4.0	233	11.4, 10.3
122	4.6, 5.7	134	14.2, 12.9	222	7.4, 4.8	234	14.3, 14.6

Below is the analysis of variance table for this data set. Since the design is balanced and the various effects are orthogonal (according to Theorem 5.18), the corresponding sequential and adjusted sums of squares are the same, and are additive. The degrees of freedom are given by (c) of the theorem, or by Corollary 5.19. For example, the $B \times C$ interaction has $(3-1)(4-1) = 6$ df.

Source	*SS*	df	*MS*	*F*	p-value
A	6.435	1	6.435	7.32	0.012
B	199.297	2	99.648	113.35	0.000
C	300.665	3	100.222	114.00	0.000
$A \times B$	0.812	2	0.406	0.46	0.636
$A \times C$	0.872	3	0.291	0.33	0.803
$B \times C$	56.794	6	9.466	10.77	0.000
$A \times B \times C$	2.840	6	0.473	0.54	0.774
Error	21.099	24	0.879		
Total	588.814	47			

5.4 The Kurkjian-Zelen Construction

Table 2.1 contains the contrast columns for the main effects and interactions in a 2^3 factorial design. In Example 2.10 we saw how to derive the interaction columns of this table from those for A, B and C by orthogonalization. It turns out that they can be generated very easily by componentwise multiplication: The column for AB is the product of those for A and B, and so on, as the reader can check. This observation, applying to 2^k designs in general, seems to have originated with Barnard [10, page 197]. (She saw more than this pattern, and we will take this up in Sect. 5.5.)

We can see something similar in other designs.

Example 5.21 Example 1.32 gave the contrasts for main effects and interactions in a 2×3 design, which we summarize here:

Cell	A	B		AB	
11	1	1	0	1	1
12	1	−1	1	−1	0
13	1	0	−1	0	−1
21	−1	1	0	−1	−1
22	−1	−1	1	1	0
23	−1	0	−1	0	1

If we multiply column A componentwise by the first B column, we do indeed get the first AB column. However, multiplying A by the second B column gives $(0, 1, -1, 0, -1, 1)'$. While this is not the second AB column, it is indeed a contrast vector for interaction (it represents additivity between columns 2 and 3).

What is true, as we shall see, is that the componentwise product of *any* column of U_1 and *any* column of U_2 will belong to U_{12}. Moreover, the product of a basis of U_1 and a basis of U_2 will give us a basis of U_{12}. This will apply to any two-factor design, and in fact holds in a natural way in arbitrary factorial designs, as indicated in Corollaries 5.32 and 5.33. *This is the key application of this section.*

A key to understanding this may be seen in another aspect of our 2×3 example.

Example 5.22 (Continuation of Example 5.21) Consider the vectors $\mathbf{v} = (1, -1)'$, $\mathbf{w}_1 = (1, -1, 0)'$, $\mathbf{w}_2 = (1, 0, -1)'$, and the vectors $\mathbf{1}_2$ and $\mathbf{1}_3$ of lengths 2 and 3. The reader can easily verify that the *Kronecker product* $\mathbf{v} \otimes \mathbf{1}_3$ is precisely the A column and that $\mathbf{1}_2 \otimes \mathbf{w}_1$ and $\mathbf{1}_2 \otimes \mathbf{w}_2$ are the columns for B.

Note that the vector $\mathbf{v}$ encodes the contrast between the two levels of factor A, while $\mathbf{w}_1$ and $\mathbf{w}_2$ encode contrasts between level 1 and either level 2 or level 3 of B.

Something similar happens with more than two factors, for which we need to consider Kronecker products with more than two factors, an approach that has its origin in the work of Kurkjian and Zelen [82]. One can see that with three or more factors the ordering of cells starts to become a significant issue. We avoid this by abandoning the need to write vectors as n-tuples and writing them instead as functions, as suggested in Sect. 5.1. For example, the Kronecker product $\mathbf{v} \otimes \mathbf{w}$ is a vector whose components are the products $v_i w_j$ listed in lexicographic order (Lemma A.118). We may write this in function form $v(i)w(j)$ if we understand the Kronecker product in a different way, which we now explore.

Hardin and Kurkjian [70] gave an extensive review of the literature stemming from [82] as of 1989.

5.4.1 Multilinear Algebra

The material in this subsection and the first part of the next is somewhat technical, and is only used in order to establish Corollaries 5.32 and 5.33.

Let $T = A \times B$, A and B arbitrary sets, and consider the three vector spaces $\mathbb{R}^A$, $\mathbb{R}^B$, and $\mathbb{R}^T$. For $v \in \mathbb{R}^A$ and $w \in \mathbb{R}^B$, the function $v \otimes w$ on T defined by

$$v \otimes w(r, s) = v(r)w(s), \ \ (r, s) \in T, \tag{5.21}$$

is an element of $\mathbb{R}^T$. Such functions are called *decomposable*. For example, if A and B are sets of numbers, then $g(r, s) = 2^{r+s}$ is decomposable, but $h(r, s) = r + s$ is not.

From their definition we see that decomposable functions obey some simple algebraic rules. In particular, it is easy to see that $v \otimes w$ is *linear in* v, that is,

$$(a_1 v_1 + a_2 v_2) \otimes w = a_1(v_1 \otimes w) + a_2(v_2 \otimes w),$$

and similarly in w. Thus a constant multiple of a decomposable function is decomposable, since

$$a(v \otimes w) = (av) \otimes w;$$

we refer to this as *absorbing a constant*. Finally, the pointwise product of two decomposable functions is computed by "factorwise" multiplication:

$$(v_1 \otimes w_1)(v_2 \otimes w_2) = v_1 v_2 \otimes w_1 w_2.$$

For example, if $v_1(r) = 2^r$, $v_2(r) = \sin r$, $w_1(s) = 2^s$, and $w_2(s) = \cos s$, this says that $(2^{r+s})(\sin r \cos s) = (2^r \sin r)(2^s \cos s)$.

Let $V \subset \mathbb{R}^A$ and $W \subset \mathbb{R}^B$ be vector subspaces. Define[9]

$$V \otimes W = \langle \{v \otimes w : v \in V, w \in W\} \rangle.$$

That is, $V \otimes W$ is the vector space of functions on T which are sums $\sum_i v_i \otimes w_i$ of decomposable functions (initially, linear combinations, but one may absorb the scalar coefficients, as observed above). In particular we denote $V \otimes \langle 1 \rangle$ by $V \otimes 1$, and similarly for $1 \otimes V$. This is not really an abuse of notation, as $\sum_i v_i \otimes a_i 1 = (\sum_i a_i v_i) \otimes 1$.

[9] The reader who is becoming concerned about unauthorized use of $\otimes$ is invited to look ahead to Remark 5.39.

Lemma 5.23 *If $f \in V \otimes W$ and $t \in B$, then the function f_t defined by*

$$f_t(\cdot) = f(\cdot, t)$$

belongs to V.

Proof If $f = \sum_i v_i \otimes w_i$, then $f(\cdot, t) = \sum_i v_i(\cdot)w_i(t)$, which is a linear combination of functions $v_i \in V$. □

The next result is useful in constructing spanning sets and bases of $V \otimes W$ from those of V and W.

Proposition 5.24 *Let $T = A \times B$.*

a. *If $\{v_i\}$ is linearly independent in $\mathbb{R}^A$ and $\{w_j\}$ is linearly independent in $\mathbb{R}^B$, then $\{v_i \otimes w_j\}$ is linearly independent in $\mathbb{R}^T$.*
b. *Assume V and W are finite-dimensional. If $\{v_i\}$ and $\{w_j\}$ are spanning sets of V and W, then $\{v_i \otimes w_j\}$ spans $V \otimes W$.*
c. *Assume V and W are finite-dimensional. If $\{v_i\}$ and $\{w_j\}$ are bases of V and W, then $\{v_i \otimes w_j\}$ is a basis of $V \otimes W$, and* $\dim(V \otimes W) = (\dim V)(\dim W)$.
d. *If A and B are finite, then $\mathbb{R}^T = \mathbb{R}^A \otimes \mathbb{R}^B$.*

Proof (b) Let $f \in V \otimes W$. We must find coefficients b_{ij}, only finitely many non-zero, such that

$$f = \sum_i \sum_j b_{ij} v_i \otimes w_j, \tag{5.22}$$

that is, such that for every $s \in A$ and $t \in B$ we have

$$f(s, t) = \sum_i \sum_j b_{ij} v_i(s) w_j(t).$$

Since V and W are finite-dimensional, we may assume without loss of generality that $\{v_i\}$ and $\{w_j\}$ are finite, so that sums of the type (5.22) are always finite.

As we remarked above, for each $t \in B$ the function f_t belongs to V, and so there exists a set of coefficients *depending on t*, say $a_i(t)$, such that

$$f_t = \sum_i a_i(t) v_i.$$

But as a function of t, $a_i \in W$ for each i, so

$$a_i = \sum_j b_{ij} w_j.$$

Therefore

$$f_t = \sum_i \left(\sum_j b_{ij} w_j(t) \right) v_i$$

for every $t \in B$. But then

$$f(s,t) = f_t(s) = \sum_i \sum_j b_{ij} v_i(s) w_j(t)$$

for every $s \in A$ and $t \in B$, as desired.

The proofs of parts (a), (c) and (d) are left as an exercise. □

Remark 5.25 Since A and B are arbitrary in (a), the indices i and j run over index sets which may not be finite or even countable. The finiteness condition in (b) and (c) holds in particular when A and B are finite sets.

One can show that Proposition 5.24 (b) holds if *at most one* factor is infinite-dimensional. This finiteness assumption appears to be necessary in the absence of other structure on T (compare [101, Proposition 6.6]). The difficulty is in insuring that in any linear combination only finitely many coefficients are nonzero.

We continue assuming that $T = A \times B$. If f_1 and f_2 are in $\mathbb{R}^T$, then their inner product is

$$(f_1, f_2) = \sum_{t \in T} f_1(t) f_2(t) = \sum_{(r,s) \in A \times B} f_1(r,s) f_2(r,s).$$

Since f_1 and f_2 are sums of decomposable functions, computing this reduces to computing inner products of decomposable functions. The latter can be expressed in terms of the inner products in $\mathbb{R}^A$ and $\mathbb{R}^B$ in a simple way:

Lemma 5.26 *For $v_1, v_2 \in \mathbb{R}^A$ and $w_1, w_2 \in \mathbb{R}^B$ we have*

$$(v_1 \otimes w_1, v_2 \otimes w_2) = (v_1, v_2)(w_1, w_2). \tag{5.23}$$

In particular, $v_1 \otimes w_1 \perp v_2 \otimes w_2$ iff either $v_1 \perp v_2$ or $w_1 \perp w_2$.

Proof We have

$$\begin{aligned}
(v_1 \otimes w_1, v_2 \otimes w_2) &= \sum_{(r,s) \in A \times B} v_1 \otimes w_1(r,s)\; v_2 \otimes w_2(r,s) \\
&= \sum_{(r,s) \in A \times B} v_1(r) w_1(s) v_2(r) w_2(s) \\
&= \sum_{r \in A} v_1(r) v_2(r) \sum_{s \in B} w_1(s) w_2(s) \;=\; (v_1, v_2)(w_1, w_2).
\end{aligned}$$

□

For vectors in Euclidean spaces (n-tuples), Eq. (5.23) must be restated in terms of the Kronecker product, as in this example.

Example 5.27 Suppose that in vector notation $\mathbf{v} = (1, 2)'$ and $\mathbf{w} = (2, -1, -1)'$. Then $(\mathbf{v} \otimes \mathbf{1}_3, \mathbf{1}_2 \otimes \mathbf{w}) = (\mathbf{v}, \mathbf{1})(\mathbf{1}, \mathbf{w}) = 0$. One could also verify this by writing out $\mathbf{v} \otimes \mathbf{1}_3 = (1, 1, 1, 2, 2, 2)'$ and $\mathbf{1}_2 \otimes \mathbf{w} = (2, -1, -1, 2, -1, -1)'$ and taking the dot product.

The results above extend without any surprises to products of more than two factors. Thus if $T = A_1 \times \cdots \times A_k$, the functions $f \in \mathbb{R}^T$ are functions of k variables. The function $v_1 \otimes \cdots \otimes v_k \in \mathbb{R}^T$ is defined by

$$v_1 \otimes \cdots \otimes v_k(t_1, \ldots, t_k) = v_1(t_1) \cdots v_k(t_k) \tag{5.24}$$

($v_i \in \mathbb{R}^{A_i}$). As before, $v_1 \otimes \cdots \otimes v_k$ is *multilinear*, that is, linear in each "factor" v_i, and the pointwise product of two decomposable functions is computed by multiplying "factorwise":

$$(v_1 \otimes \cdots \otimes v_k)(w_1 \otimes \cdots \otimes w_k) = v_1 w_1 \otimes \cdots \otimes v_k w_k. \tag{5.25}$$

Finally, given subspaces $V_i \subset \mathbb{R}^{A_i}$, we define

$$V_1 \otimes \cdots \otimes V_k = \langle \{v_1 \otimes \cdots \otimes v_k : v_i \in V_i\} \rangle.$$

That is, $V_1 \otimes \cdots \otimes V_k$ is the span in $\mathbb{R}^T$ of the decomposable functions $v_1 \otimes \cdots \otimes v_k$.

Lemma 5.23 and inner-product equation (5.23) have natural extensions to more than two factors:

Lemma 5.28 *For $f \in V_1 \otimes \cdots \otimes V_k$, define f_i by fixing all arguments of f except the ith. Then $f_i \in V_i$.*

For $v_i, w_i \in V_i$ we have

$$(v_1 \otimes \cdots \otimes v_k,\ w_1 \otimes \cdots \otimes w_k) = (v_1, w_1) \cdots (v_k, w_k). \tag{5.26}$$

In order to state Proposition 5.24 conveniently with k factors, we let S_i denote a set of vectors. More precisely:

Proposition 5.29 *Let $T = A_1 \times \cdots \times A_k$, and let $S_i \subset \mathbb{R}^{A_i}$.*

a. *If S_i is a linearly independent set in $\mathbb{R}^{A_i}$, then $\{v_1 \otimes \cdots \otimes v_k : v_i \in S_i\}$ is a linearly independent set in $\mathbb{R}^T$.*
b. *Let $V_i \subset \mathbb{R}^{A_i}$ be a finite-dimensional subspace. If S_i spans V_i, then $\{v_1 \otimes \cdots \otimes v_k : v_i \in S_i\}$ spans $V_1 \otimes \cdots \otimes V_k$.*
c. *If S_i is a basis of V_i then $\{v_1 \otimes \cdots \otimes v_k : v_i \in S_i\}$ is a basis of $V_1 \otimes \cdots \otimes V_k$, and* $\dim V_1 \otimes \cdots \otimes V_k = (\dim V_1) \cdots (\dim V_k)$.
d. *If A_i are finite sets, then $\mathbb{R}^T = \mathbb{R}^{A_1} \otimes \cdots \otimes \mathbb{R}^{A_k}$.*

The proofs of Lemma 5.28 and Proposition 5.29 are left as exercises.

5.4.2 Application to Factorial Designs

We now begin to connect the preceding with the spaces U_I that we defined in Sect. 5.3.

Given a subspace $V \subset \mathbb{R}^A$ we let

$$V^\alpha = \begin{cases} V, & \alpha = 1, \\ \langle 1_A \rangle, & \alpha = 0, \end{cases} \tag{5.27}$$

where 1_A is the function in $\mathbb{R}^A$ that is constantly 1.[10] Adapting a notation of [82], if V_i is a subspace of $\mathbb{R}^{A_i}$, then each *binary vector* $(\alpha_1, \dots, \alpha_k) \in \{0, 1\}^k$ defines a space

$$V = V_1^{\alpha_1} \otimes \cdots \otimes V_k^{\alpha_k}. \tag{5.28}$$

In particular, if $I \subset \{1, \dots, k\}$ and if $\boldsymbol{\alpha}_I$ is the binary vector such that

$$\begin{aligned} \alpha_i &= 1 \text{ if } i \in I, \\ &= 0 \text{ if } i \notin I, \end{aligned}$$

then V is the set of functions that are sums of functions of the form $v = v_1 \otimes \cdots \otimes v_k$ where

$$\begin{aligned} v_i &\in V_i \quad \text{if } i \in I, \\ v_i &= 1_{A_i} \text{ if } i \notin I. \end{aligned}$$

(Initially, v_i is a multiple of 1_{A_i} if $i \notin I$, but we may write $v_i = 1_{A_i}$ by absorbing constants into other factors.) Note that if $v \in V$ then the value of $v(t_1, \dots, t_k)$ is independent of t_j, $j \notin I$. In other words, $v \in U_{\mathcal{C}}$ where $\mathcal{C} = \vee_{i \in I} \mathcal{A}_i$.

We specialize the construction (5.28) to certain subspaces. Namely, let

$$U_{A_i} = 1_{A_i}^{\perp},$$

the set of contrast functions in $\mathbb{R}^{A_i}$. The next theorem gives us a new way to construct the subspaces U_I.

Theorem 5.30 *For every $I \subset \{1, \dots, k\}$ and for $\boldsymbol{\alpha}_I = (\alpha_1, \dots, \alpha_k)$,*

$$U_I = U_{A_1}^{\alpha_1} \otimes \cdots \otimes U_{A_k}^{\alpha_k}. \tag{5.29}$$

---

[10] The function 1_A would correspond to the vector $\mathbf{1}_s$ of length $s = |A|$.

To establish this we will need the following lemma, whose proof we leave as an exercise.

Lemma 5.31 *Let $\dot{U}_I$ be the subspace of $\mathbb{R}^T$ on the right-hand side of (5.29). If $I \neq J$ then $\dot{U}_I \perp \dot{U}_J$.*

Proof of Theorem 5.30 We need to show that $U_I = \dot{U}_I$ for all I. We first note that this is true for $I = \emptyset$, since clearly $\dot{U}_\emptyset = \langle 1_{A_1} \otimes \cdots \otimes 1_{A_k} \rangle = \langle 1 \rangle = U_\emptyset$.

Proceeding inductively, we fix $I \subset \{1, \ldots, k\}$, and assume that $\dot{U}_J = U_J$ for all $J \subsetneq I$. We need to show that $\dot{U}_I$ satisfies the definition (5.18) of U_I. Now $\dot{U}_I \subset U_{\mathcal{C}}$ where $\mathcal{C} = \vee_{i \in I} \mathcal{A}_i$, as we remarked above. We claim that $\dot{U}_I \perp U_J$ for $J \subsetneq I$. By the induction hypothesis this is equivalent to showing that $\dot{U}_I \perp \dot{U}_J$. But this is true by Lemma 5.31.

This shows that $\dot{U}_I \subseteq U_I$ for each I. Assuming this, equality will follow if we just show that $\dim \dot{U}_I = \dim U_I$. But if $s_i = |A_i|$ then U_{A_i} has a basis of $s_i - 1$ elements, and so Proposition 5.29(c) implies that $\dim \dot{U}_I = \prod_{i \in I}(s_i - 1)$, which is $\dim U_I$. □

We can now explain the examples with which we opened this section.

Corollary 5.32 *Suppose I and J are disjoint subsets of $\{1, \ldots, k\}$. If $v \in U_I$ and $w \in U_J$, then $vw \in U_{I \cup J}$, where vw is the pointwise product of the functions v and w.*

Proof of Corollary 5.32 First consider decomposable functions $v = v_1 \otimes \cdots \otimes v_k \in U_I$ and $w = w_1 \otimes \cdots \otimes w_k \in U_J$. Here

$$\begin{cases} v_i \in U_{A_i} & \text{if } i \in I \\ v_i = 1_{A_i} & \text{if } i \notin I \end{cases} \quad \text{and} \quad \begin{cases} w_j \in U_{A_j} & \text{if } j \in J \\ w_j = 1_{A_j} & \text{if } j \notin J. \end{cases}$$

Now by (5.25),

$$vw = v_1 w_1 \otimes \cdots \otimes v_k w_k.$$

Clearly $v_i w_i = 1_{A_i}$ if $i \notin I \cup J$. On the other hand, since $I \cap J = \emptyset$ it follows that $v_i w_i \in U_{A_i}$ if $i \in I$ or $i \in J$. Thus $vw \in U_{I \cup J}$.

The proof for general functions v and w follows easily when we view them as sums of decomposable functions. □

We can make a more precise statement about the product of decomposables:

Corollary 5.33 *If I and J are subsets of $\{1, \ldots, k\}$, not necessarily disjoint, if $v \in U_I$ and $w \in U_J$ are decomposable, and if $K = \{i : v_i w_i \neq 1\}$, then $K \subseteq I \cup J$ and $vw \in U_K$.*

Note that it is possible to have $K = \emptyset$, in which case $vw = 1$. The proof of Corollary 5.33 is left as an exercise.

Combining Corollary 5.32 with Proposition 5.29(c), *we are able to create a basis of contrast vectors for each main effect and interaction in a factorial design, once we are given a basis for each main effect.* Examples 5.21 and 5.22 showed how to do this in the case of a 2×3 design. We also see why the contrast vectors of the 2^3 design in Example 2.10 can be constructed by componentwise multiplications, as we noted at the beginning of this section.

The 2^3 example also explains the need for disjointness of I and J in Corollary 5.32: Multiplying the columns for AB and BC does not give us the column for ABC. In fact, the product of AB and BC turns out to be the column AC, which is consistent with Corollary 5.33.

Let us take a moment to construct the contrast vectors for two more designs.

Example 5.34 (The 3×3 *Design)* Here there are two factors, each at 3 levels. Let us index the levels of both factors by 0, 1 and 2, so that $T = A \times B$ where $A = B = \{0, 1, 2\}$. As a basis of $\mathbb{R}^A$ or of $\mathbb{R}^B$ we may take the vectors $\mathbf{u}_1 = (1, -1, 0)'$ and $\mathbf{u}_2 = (1, 0, -1)$. Then a basis for U_1 is $\{\mathbf{u}_1 \otimes \mathbf{1}_3, \mathbf{u}_2 \otimes \mathbf{1}_3\}$, while a basis for U_2 is $\{\mathbf{1}_3 \otimes \mathbf{u}_1, \mathbf{1}_3 \otimes \mathbf{u}_2\}$. We enter these vectors in the respective columns for A and B in the table below, and then complete the table by multiplying each vector for A with each vector for B:

Cell	A		B		Interaction			
00	1	1	1	1	1	1	1	1
01	1	1	−1	0	−1	0	−1	0
02	1	1	0	−1	0	−1	0	−1
20	−1	0	1	1	−1	−1	0	0
22	−1	0	−1	0	1	0	0	0
21	−1	0	0	−1	0	1	0	0
20	0	−1	1	1	0	0	−1	−1
21	0	−1	−1	0	0	0	1	0
22	0	−1	0	−1	0	0	0	1

Example 5.35 (The 2^4 *Design)* Each of the four factors has 2 levels, which may be indexed by 0 and 1. Thus $T = A \times B \times C \times D$ where $A = B = C = D = \{0, 1\}$. A basis for $\mathbb{R}^A$ is the vector $\mathbf{u} = (1, -1)'$, and similarly for $\mathbb{R}^B$, $\mathbb{R}^C$ and $\mathbb{R}^D$. The column for A is thus $\mathbf{u} \otimes \mathbf{1}_2 \otimes \mathbf{1}_2 \otimes \mathbf{1}_2$, for B, $\mathbf{1}_2 \otimes \mathbf{u} \otimes \mathbf{1}_2 \otimes \mathbf{1}_2$, and similarly for C and D. The other columns are products of these. Note that we can compute the column for ABC several ways—$(A)(B)(C)$, $(A)(BC)$, and so on, and similarly for the other columns. The result is Table 5.1.

As with the 2^3 example, we see that the product of two "overlapping" interactions is only a *subset* of their "union"—for example, multiplying columns ABC and ABD results in the column CD, not $ABCD$, consistent with Corollary 5.33. In Sect. 5.6.4 we will find a simple way to predict the result of this multiplication for 2^k factorials, and indeed for s^k factorials when s is a prime or a power of a prime.

Table 5.1 Contrast vectors in a 2^4 experiment (Example 5.35)

Cell	A	B	C	D	AB	AC	AD	BC	BD	CD	ABC	ABD	ACD	BCD	$ABCD$
0000	1	1	1	1	1	1	1	1	1	1	1	1	1	1	1
0001	1	1	1	−1	1	1	−1	1	−1	−1	1	−1	−1	−1	−1
0010	1	1	−1	1	1	−1	1	−1	1	−1	−1	1	−1	−1	−1
0011	1	1	−1	−1	1	−1	−1	−1	−1	1	−1	−1	1	1	1
0100	1	−1	1	1	−1	1	1	−1	−1	1	−1	−1	1	−1	−1
0101	1	−1	1	−1	−1	1	−1	−1	1	−1	−1	1	−1	1	1
0110	1	−1	−1	1	−1	−1	1	1	−1	−1	1	−1	−1	1	1
0111	1	−1	−1	−1	−1	−1	−1	1	1	1	1	1	1	−1	−1
1000	−1	1	1	1	−1	−1	−1	1	1	1	−1	−1	−1	1	−1
1001	−1	1	1	−1	−1	−1	1	1	−1	−1	−1	1	1	−1	1
1010	−1	1	−1	1	−1	1	−1	−1	1	−1	1	−1	1	−1	1
1011	−1	1	−1	−1	−1	1	1	−1	−1	1	1	1	−1	1	−1
1100	−1	−1	1	1	1	−1	−1	−1	−1	1	1	1	−1	−1	1
1101	−1	−1	1	−1	1	−1	1	−1	1	−1	1	−1	1	1	−1
1110	−1	−1	−1	1	1	1	−1	1	−1	−1	−1	1	1	1	−1
1111	−1	−1	−1	−1	1	1	1	1	1	1	−1	−1	−1	−1	1

Example 5.36 (Quantitative Factors) As we've seen in Sect. 2.4, when factor levels are quantitative we can define contrasts representing various polynomial effects—linear, quadratic and so on. We defined these only in the one-factor case, but indicated that they extend to the multifactor case with appropriate repetition of components. We now see how to do this. For example, suppose quantitative factors A and B have a and b levels, respectively; if the contrast vector $\mathbf{c}$ represents the quadratic effect of A in a one-factor design, then $\mathbf{c} \otimes \mathbf{1}$ represents that effect in the $a \times b$ design. Similarly, if $\mathbf{d}$ represents the quadratic effect of B in a one-factor design, then $\mathbf{1} \otimes \mathbf{d}$ represents that effect in the $a \times b$ design. Moreover, $\mathbf{c} \otimes \mathbf{d}$ is a contrast vector belonging to interaction and represents the quadratic-by-quadratic effect of A and B.

We end with an alternate characterization of the subspaces U_I, whose proof is left as an exercise.

Corollary 5.37 *A contrast function $c \in \mathbb{R}^T$ belongs to U_I if and only if (a) its value $c(t_1, \ldots, t_k)$ depends only on the arguments t_i, $i \in I$, and (b) for each $i \in I$ and for any fixed values of t_j, $j \neq i$, we have $\sum_{t_i \in A_i} c(\ldots, t_i, \ldots) = 0$.*

This characterization of the spaces U_I is sometimes given as a definition [98, 130]. It is straightforward to prove once we have Theorem 5.30 in hand.

Remark 5.38 The reader may have noticed that the three facts listed in Theorem 5.18 are fairly easy to show for the subspaces $\dot{U}_I$ defined in Lemma 5.31. These are all spaces of contrasts, and the issue is to show that they are the same as the subspaces U_I that we started with.

As pointed out in [137], the orthogonal decomposition $\mathbb{R}^T = \oplus_I \dot{U}_I$ holds more generally if we consider just arbitrary subspaces U_i of $\mathbb{R}^{A_i}$ and their orthocomplements (instead of 1 and $1^\perp$).

Remark 5.39 The $\otimes$ operation we have referred to above is of course the usual tensor product.

The tensor product of two vector spaces V and W (not just spaces of functions) is constructed as the vector space of formal linear combinations of ordered pairs $[v, w] \in V \times W$ modulo certain relations. The equivalence class of $[v, w]$ is denoted $v \otimes w$. This turns out to be our definition when V and W are spaces of functions.

The reader familiar with Hilbert space theory will recognize Eq. (5.23) as the definition of an inner product in the tensor product of two (pre-)Hilbert spaces [101]. (One extends this definition to arbitrary elements by linearity and completeness.) Thus this definition coincides with the given inner product on $\mathbb{R}^{A \times B}$.

5.5 Confounding with Blocks

Suppose there are too many treatment combinations in an experiment for us to be able to observe all of them simultaneously. For example, one may be preparing samples in an oven that has limited capacity, so that samples must be treated in batches. These batches are then called *incomplete blocks*. In this usage, an *incomplete block* is a (nonempty) proper subset of the set T of treatment combinations. The overall problem is that our experiment may be introducing a new and unknown *block effect*, which we need to account for. The usual assumption is that block effects are *additive*—that is, that each block adds an unknown constant (possibly zero) to the mean responses in that block.

Certain designs may allow overlapping blocks. Suitably restricted, these include *balanced (BIB)* and *partially balanced incomplete block (PBIB)* designs. We will be concerned instead with designs in which the batches form a partition of T. These are often referred to as *confounded designs*. (For BIB and PBIB designs the reader is referred to texts such as [81, 151] or, for a more abstract treatment, [8, 108] or [136].)

5.5.1 Generalities

A simple, classic example is that of a 2×2 experiment in which we can only observe two of the four treatment combinations at once. The unblocked experiment was described in Example 2.8 (page 21), where the cells and the contrasts for A, B, and interaction were given as follows:

Cell	A	B	AB
00	1	1	1
01	1	−1	−1
10	−1	1	−1
11	−1	−1	1

How should we partition the four cells? If we put 00 and 01 in one block and the others in the second block, then the block effect will be identical with the main effect of A. Thus, for example, if we detect a significant effect of factor A, we will not be able to say whether it is due to A or to a difference between blocks. We say that the main effect of A is *confounded with blocks*.

The same thing will happen if we put cells 00 and 10 in one block and the others in the second block, except that now the effect of B will be confounded with blocks. There is one further choice, of course, and that is to partition the cells into $\{00, 11\}$ and $\{01, 10\}$. This confounds the AB interaction with blocks, but we may be willing to live with this, especially because we are still able to make inferences about the main effects of A and B. Why is that?

Suppose that block $\{00, 11\}$ adds a constant d_1 to the means μ_{00} and μ_{11}, and block $\{01, 10\}$ adds a constant d_2. The contrast for A is unchanged, since

$$\mu_{00} + d_1 + \mu_{01} + d_2 - (\mu_{10} + d_2) - (\mu_{11} + d_1) = \mu_{00} + \mu_{01} - \mu_{10} - \mu_{11},$$

and similarly for the contrast for B. We say that A and B are *unconfounded with blocks*. Clearly this unconfoundedness is due to the fact that the contrasts for A and B are orthogonal to the contrast for blocks (and to the vector $\mathbf{1}$). We are thus led to the following definition.

Definition 5.40 Let T be the set of treatment combinations of an experiment, and let $U_{\mathcal{B}}$ be a block effect for some partition $\mathcal{B}$ of T. An effect[11] U is

- *confounded with blocks* if $U \subset U_{\mathcal{B}}$;
- *unconfounded with blocks* if $U \perp U_{\mathcal{B}}$.

We will call an effect *partly confounded with blocks* if it is neither confounded nor unconfounded.

The term "partly confounded" is not often found in the literature, although it is there implicitly. It is not to be confused with the more common term *partially confounded*. In an experiment that is *replicated* several times, an effect is *partially confounded* if a different blocking is used in each replication and if the effect is unconfounded in at least one. This is discussed briefly in Example 5.65 of Sect. 5.6.

Example 5.41 Suppose we need to run a symmetric $n \times n$ experiment in n equal blocks. How may we do this without confounding either main effect with blocks?

[11] A set of contrast functions; see page 39.

Think of the treatment combinations as the cells defined by n rows and n columns. If $\mathcal{A}$ and $\mathcal{B}$ denote the partitions by rows and by columns, respectively, then $U_{\mathcal{A}} = U_1$ and $U_{\mathcal{B}} = U_2$, the two main effects. We saw in Example 5.8 that a Latin square of order n defines a partition $\mathcal{C}$ of the n^2 cells in n equal blocks such that $U_{\mathcal{C}}$ is orthogonal to both U_1 and U_2. Thus main effects are unconfounded with the blocks of $\mathcal{C}$. Note that this is always possible to implement, as there are Latin squares of every order.

At the other extreme, in an $a \times b$ experiment, if a and b are relatively prime then every blocking must confound a main effect, at least partly. We leave this as an exercise.

A problem arises when we use two partitions simultaneously. To illustrate, consider the $2 \times 2 \times 2$ (or 2^3) experiment described in Table 2.1 (page 38), and suppose we need to run our experiment in four blocks of two. We might choose to confound both ABC and AB by superimposing the two corresponding blockings. The partition that confounds ABC would assign cells to one of two blocks depending on the sign of the ABC contrast vector, and similarly for AB. We would thus end up with the following partition:

		ABC	
		+	−
AB	+	000 110	001 111
	−	011 101	010 100

The general contrast between these four blocks is an expression of the form

$$a\mu_{000} + a\mu_{110} + b\mu_{001} + b\mu_{111} + c\mu_{011} + c\mu_{101} + d\mu_{010} + d\mu_{100}$$

where $a + b + c + d = 0$. This of course includes the contrasts for AB and ABC. The problem is that it also includes the contrast for C ($a = d = 1, b = c = -1$), so that this partition confounds the main effect of C with blocks.

We should not be surprised that this partition confounds more than just the "generating" contrasts AB and ABC. After all, there are four blocks, and so the set of block contrasts has dimension 3.

This was understood before Barnard's paper [10] appeared. What she did was to recognize a simple algorithm for determining this extra confounded effect. Namely, we may multiply the contrast vectors for AB and ABC componentwise to get that for C, as the reader can easily verify in Table 2.1. Here is how she says it, regarding a 2^k experiment:

> It will be seen that the interaction between any two main effects is represented by the set of signs obtained by multiplying together the corresponding signs of the pair of main effects considered, and that the same is true of any two treatment comparisons which have no treatment factor in common. This rule can be extended to include the generalized interaction

> of any two lines,[12] provided that if the comparisons represented by these two lines have a factor, or factors, in common (such as AB and BC), these factors do not appear in the resultant generalized interaction (AC, in the example chosen). [10, page 197. The "example chosen" is in the original.]
>
> ...the treatment comparisons represented by the first two lines and by the interaction between them, which represent the three possible comparisons which can be made between the blocks of this replication, are confounded [with blocks]. [10, page 198]

Barnard has introduced several ideas here:

(a) Ordinary interactions be computed by multiplying contrast vectors componentwise (something that Kurkjian and Zelen generalized two decades later, as in Corollary 5.33).
(b) The componentwise product of *any* two contrast vectors yields another one representing another effect. She thus calls the latter the *generalized interaction* of the first two.
(c) There is a simple algebraic way to determine the generalized interaction: Multiply letters, and omit any letter that is squared.
(d) If two effects are confounded with blocks, so will their generalized interaction be.

The algebra that Barnard introduced here is group theory, although she doesn't identify it as such. In any case, her paper opened an entire area of research with the goal of extending her ideas to more general factorial experiments. More specifically, one would like to find a way to predict, and thereby to control, the confounding with blocks. *It is not at all clear, at first glance, just how to go about doing this.* For example, in the 3×3 experiment in Example 5.34, multiplying the first A column by the first interaction column does not produce a contrast vector belonging to either a main effect or interaction.

The most successful results concern those symmetric or s^k experiments in which s is a prime or a power of a prime. We will call these *classical* symmetric factorial experiments. These results were obtained during the decade following Barnard's paper, by Bose and Kishen [23] and by Fisher [58, 59], the former using geometric approach, the latter a group-theoretic one.

Basic to both approaches is the use of finite fields. We will not need any deep results concerning such fields, but the reader will need to be reasonably comfortable with their arithmetic. We will denote the finite field with s elements by $GF(s)$ (for Galois field). Such a field exists if, and only if, s is a prime or a prime power. See Appendix A.3 for a brief introduction.

[12] Barnard writes the contrast vectors as rows, or "lines".

5.6 Confounding in Classical Symmetric Factorial Designs

In a symmetric factorial experiment with k factors, the set of treatment combinations may be taken to be $T = A^k$, where the same set A is used to index the levels of each factor. In a *classical* symmetric factorial experiment (i.e., where $s = |A|$ is a prime or prime power), we may take A to be the field $GF(s)$. With this choice,

$$T = (GF(s))^k$$

becomes a vector space over $GF(s)$ of dimension k. We will consider a special set of partitions of T, whose blocks are solution sets of systems of linear equations of the form

$$a_1t_1 + \cdots + a_kt_k = b, \tag{5.30}$$

where the variables t_i, the coefficients a_i, and the quantity b are in $GF(s)$. For each partition $\mathcal{B}$ we have the block effect $U_{\mathcal{B}}$, and these effects will be main effects and "components of interaction". Our first goal is to study these partitions.

Notation We will denote elements of $(GF(s))^k$ by boldface letters in order to think of them as vectors. These elements play two different roles, and will be distinguished by different letters: $\mathbf{t} = (t_1, \ldots, t_k)'$ is a treatment combination, while $\mathbf{a} = (a_1, \ldots, a_k)'$ is the vector of coefficients in an equation such as (5.30). Similarly,

$$T = (GF(s))^k = \text{the set of treatment combinations } \mathbf{t}\text{, and}$$

$$V = (GF(s))^k = \text{the set of coefficient vectors } \mathbf{a}.$$

We will also use the notation $(GF(s))^*$, T^* and V^* for the set of nonzero elements of $GF(s)$ of T and of V, respectively. The zero element of $(GF(s))^k$ is the k-tuple $\mathbf{0} = (0, \ldots, 0)'$.

5.6.1 Special Blockings and Block Effects

For each $\mathbf{a} = (a_1, \ldots, a_k) \in V^*$, we define the linear functional[13] $L_{\mathbf{a}} : T \to GF(s)$ by

$$L_{\mathbf{a}}(\mathbf{t}) = a_1t_1 + \cdots + a_kt_k, \tag{5.31}$$

[13] See Remark 5.49 below.

where $\mathbf{t} = (t_1, \ldots, t_k)$. For each $b \in GF(s)$, we define $B(L_\mathbf{a}, b)$ to be the solution set of $L_\mathbf{a}(\mathbf{t}) = b$; that is,

$$B(L_\mathbf{a}, b) = \{\mathbf{t} \in T\text{:}a_1 t_1 + \cdots + a_k t_k = b\} \tag{5.32}$$

Note that $B(L_\mathbf{a}, 0)$ is a subspace, and $B(L_\mathbf{a}, b)$ is a flat, of the vector space T (Theorem A.39). More generally, if $\mathbf{a}_1, \ldots, \mathbf{a}_j \in V^*$, then $B(L_{\mathbf{a}_1}, b_1) \cap \cdots \cap B(L_{\mathbf{a}_j}, b_j)$ is the solution set to the system

$$\begin{aligned} a_{11}t_1 + \cdots + a_{1k}t_k &= b_1 \\ \vdots \qquad\quad \vdots \quad &\quad \vdots \\ a_{j1}t_1 + \cdots + a_{jk}t_k &= b_j, \end{aligned} \tag{5.33}$$

where $\mathbf{a}_i = (a_{i1}, \ldots, a_{ik})'$. This set also has a simple geometric description:

Lemma 5.42 *If the vectors $\mathbf{a}_i$ are linearly independent, then the solution set of (6.5) is a $(k - j)$-flat. That is, it is of the form $U + \mathbf{t}_0$ where U is a subspace of T of dimension $k - j$ and $\mathbf{t}_0$ is a particular solution.*

The sets $B(L_\mathbf{a}, b)$ and their intersections will be the blocks of treatment combinations in what follows.

Lemma 5.43 *With the above notation:*

a. *$B(L_\mathbf{0}, 0) = T$, and $B(L_\mathbf{0}, b) = \emptyset$ if $b \neq 0$.*
b. *For distinct $b, b' \in GF(s)$, $B(L_\mathbf{a}, b) \cap B(L_\mathbf{a}, b') = \emptyset$.*
c. *For every $\mathbf{a} \in V^*$ and $b \in GF(s)$, $|B(L_\mathbf{a}, b)| = s^{k-1}$.*
d. *If $\mathbf{a}_1, \ldots, \mathbf{a}_j \in V^*$ are linearly independent over $GF(s)$, then for any $b_1, \ldots, b_j \in GF(s)$ (not necessarily distinct), $|B(L_{\mathbf{a}_1}, b_1) \cap \cdots \cap B(L_{\mathbf{a}_j}, b_j)| = s^{k-j}$.*

The proofs of the previous two lemmas are left as exercises.

For any $L = L_\mathbf{a}$ let us write

$$\mathcal{B}(L) = \{B(L, b) : b \in GF(s)\}. \tag{5.34}$$

That is, $\mathcal{B}(L)$ is the family of solution sets (5.32) as b varies over $GF(s)$. It is a blocking of the set of treatment combinations:

Proposition 5.44 *For each $\mathbf{a} \in V^*$, $\mathcal{B}(L_\mathbf{a})$ is a partition of T into s blocks of equal size, while $\mathcal{B}(L_\mathbf{0}) = \{T\}$, the trivial partition. If $\mathbf{a}_1, \ldots, \mathbf{a}_j$ are linearly independent, then $\mathcal{B}(L_{\mathbf{a}_1}) \vee \cdots \vee \mathcal{B}(L_{\mathbf{a}_j})$ consists of s^j blocks of equal size, and $\mathcal{B}(L_{\mathbf{a}_1}), \ldots, \mathcal{B}(L_{\mathbf{a}_j})$ are independent. If $\mathbf{a}_1$ and $\mathbf{a}_2$ are linearly dependent, then $\mathcal{B}(L_{\mathbf{a}_1}) = \mathcal{B}(L_{\mathbf{a}_2})$.*

Proof The first two statements follow immediately from the lemma. In particular, independence comes from the fact that $\pi(B_1 \cap \cdots \cap B_r) = 1/s^r$ for any $r \geq 1$, where $B_i \in \mathcal{B}(L_{\mathbf{a}_i})$. For the last, the linear dependence of $\mathbf{a}_1$ and $\mathbf{a}_2$ means that $\mathbf{a}_2 = c\mathbf{a}_1$ for some $c \in (GF(s))^*$. But then the equation $L_{\mathbf{a}_1}(\mathbf{t}) = b$ is equivalent to the equation $L_{\mathbf{a}_2}(\mathbf{t}) = cb$, and so each block of $\mathcal{B}(L_{\mathbf{a}_1})$ is a block of $\mathcal{B}(L_{\mathbf{a}_2})$, and vice versa. □

We may define an equivalence relation $\sim$ on V by saying that

$$\mathbf{a}_1 \sim \mathbf{a}_2 \quad \text{iff} \quad \mathbf{a}_2 = c\mathbf{a}_1 \quad \text{for some } c \in (GF(s))^*. \tag{5.35}$$

Note that $\mathbf{0}$ is its own equivalence class, and so we may regard $\sim$ as a relation on V^*. Clearly $\mathbf{a}_1 \sim \mathbf{a}_2$ iff $\mathbf{a}_1$ and $\mathbf{a}_2$ are linearly dependent. Proposition 5.44 asserts that if $\mathbf{a}_1 \sim \mathbf{a}_2$ then $\mathcal{B}(L_{\mathbf{a}_1}) = \mathcal{B}(L_{\mathbf{a}_2})$. The block $B(L_{\mathbf{a}}, 0)$ is called the *principal block* of $\mathcal{B}(L_{\mathbf{a}})$. It is a subspace of T. Note that equivalent vectors define the same principal block, since $L_{c\mathbf{a}}(\mathbf{t}) = 0$ iff $L_{\mathbf{a}}(\mathbf{t}) = 0$.

We may record a couple of important observations about $\sim$-equivalence.

Proposition 5.45 *Every (nonzero) equivalence class of the relation (5.35) contains a unique vector* $\mathbf{a}$ *with "leading component" 1, that is, having 1 as its first nonzero component. There are* $(s^k - 1)/(s - 1)$ *equivalence classes.*

Proof If the first nonzero component of $\mathbf{a}$ is a, then the first nonzero component of $a^{-1}\mathbf{a}$ is 1. Uniqueness follows because if both $\mathbf{a}$ and $\mathbf{b}$ have this property and $\mathbf{b} = c\mathbf{a}$ for some $c \in (GF(s))^*$, then $c = 1$.

For the second statement, the equivalence class of $\mathbf{a}$ is the set of vectors $c\mathbf{a}$ as c ranges over $(GF(s))^*$, so the equivalence class has $|(GF(s))^*| = s - 1$ vectors. Since $|V^*| = s^k - 1$, there are $(s^k - 1)/(s - 1)$ equivalence classes. □

It is customary to represent each equivalence class by the vector with leading component 1. By analogy with polynomials, let us agree to call such vectors *monic*. Thus each equivalence class of vectors in V^* contains a unique monic representative. In 2^k factorials all vectors in V^* are monic as the only nonzero element of $\mathbb{Z}/2$ is 1, and each equivalence class contains only one vector, so this complication doesn't arise.

Now consider the effects $U_{\mathcal{B}(L_{\mathbf{a}})}$ defined by the blockings $\mathcal{B}(L_{\mathbf{a}})$; for simplicity, let us write $U_{\mathcal{B}_{\mathbf{a}}}$. These are subspaces of $\mathbb{R}^T$, and from the preceding we see the following:

- $U_{\mathcal{B}_{\mathbf{a}_1}} = U_{\mathcal{B}_{\mathbf{a}_2}}$ iff $\mathbf{a}_1 \sim \mathbf{a}_2$;
- $U_{\mathcal{B}_{\mathbf{a}_1}} \perp U_{\mathcal{B}_{\mathbf{a}_2}}$ iff $\mathbf{a}_1 \not\sim \mathbf{a}_2$;
- $U_{\mathcal{B}_{\mathbf{0}}} = \langle 1 \rangle$, the space of constant functions;
- $\dim(U_{\mathcal{B}_{\mathbf{a}}}) = s - 1$ for $\mathbf{a} \neq 0$;
- There are $(s^k - 1)/(s - 1)$ distinct subspaces $U_{\mathcal{B}_{\mathbf{a}}}$ for $\mathbf{a} \neq \mathbf{0}$.

By considering dimensions, we immediately have the following:

Theorem 5.46 *In a symmetric* s^k *design, s a prime or prime power, we have*

$$\mathbb{R}^T = \langle 1 \rangle \oplus_{\mathbf{a}} U_{\mathcal{B}_{\mathbf{a}}}, \tag{5.36}$$

where $\mathcal{B}_{\mathbf{a}} = \mathcal{B}(L_{\mathbf{a}})$ and where the (orthogonal) sum is taken over representatives of the nonzero equivalence classes in V. In particular, the sum may be taken over the monic vectors in V.

If the design is equireplicate, then the sequential sums of squares for main effects and components of interaction are independent of the order of nesting. A sequential sum of squares for testing a main effect or component interaction is equal to its adjusted sum of squares.

For 2^k designs, the decomposition (5.36) is the same as Eq. (5.20) of Theorem 5.18, while for classical s^k designs with $s > 2$ it is similar to (5.20) but with more terms. In the latter case we will see (Sect. 5.6.2) that it is actually a refinement of (5.20). The second part of the present theorem extends Corollary 4.42.

Example 5.47 Consider the 2^3 experiment with factors A, B and C. Here $T = V = (\mathbb{Z}/2)^3$, so $|V| = 8$ and $|V^*| = 7$. We have

$$V^* = \{1, 0, 0), (0, 1, 0), (0, 0, 1), (1, 1, 0), (1, 0, 1), (0, 1, 1), (1, 1, 1)\}.$$

The vector $\mathbf{a} = (1, 0, 0)$ determines the function $L_{(1,0,0)}(t_1, t_2, t_3) = t_1$, and so the blocks of $\mathcal{B}(L_{\mathbf{a}})$ are simply the solution sets of the equations $t_1 = 0$ and $t_1 = 1$. But these are the blocks determined by factor A, and the block contrasts are the scalar multiples of the contrast in column A of Table 2.1. The blockings for factors B and C arise similarly.

The vector $\mathbf{a} = (1, 1, 0)$ determines the function $L_{(1,1,0)}(\mathbf{t}) = t_1 + t_2$, and so the blocks of $\mathcal{B}(L_{\mathbf{a}})$ are the following solution sets (for simplicity we write ijk for cell (i, j, k)):

$t_1 + t_2 = 0$	$t_1 + t_2 = 1 \pmod 2$
000	010
001	011
110	100
111	101

Every contrast between these blocks is a scalar multiple of the AB contrast in Table 2.1. The other interaction contrasts in the table arise in the same way.

Example 5.48 Consider the 3×3 experiment of Example 5.34, where $\mathbb{Z}/3$ (= $GF(3)$) indexes the levels of each factor. Here $T = V = \mathbb{Z}/3 \times \mathbb{Z}/3$, and so $|V^*| = 8$. There are $(3^2 - 1)/(3 - 1) = 4$ equivalence classes in V^*, represented by the monic vectors $(1, 0)$, $(0, 1)$, $(1, 1)$ and $(1, 2)$. Each of the other four vectors of V^* is equivalent to one of these. For example, $(2, 1) \sim (1, 2)$ since $(2, 1) = 2(1, 2)$ (mod 3), using relation (5.35).

The corresponding linear functionals are

$$L_{(1,0)}(\mathbf{t}) = t_1, \ L_{(0,1)}(\mathbf{t}) = t_2, \ L_{(1,1)}(\mathbf{t}) = t_1 + t_2, \text{ and } L_{(1,2)}(\mathbf{t}) = t_1 + 2t_2.$$

If we calculate the value of each of these at each cell $\mathbf{t} \in T$, we get the four columns after "cell" in Table 5.2. Entering each of those columns in a 3×3 array allows us to visualize the four resulting partitions:

00	01	02
10	11	12
20	21	22

cells

$L =$

0	0	0
1	1	1
2	2	2

t_1

0	1	2
0	1	2
0	1	2

t_2

0	1	2
1	2	0
2	0	1

$t_1 + t_2$

0	2	1
1	0	2
2	1	0

$t_1 + 2t_2$

Note that the last two of these are the Latin squares in Example 5.8.

To illustrate the breakdown of interaction into components, we reanalyze an earlier data set in a 3×3 experiment (see Table 4.6). Note that the source of non-additivity has been isolated in the AB component.

Source	SS	df	MS	F	p-value
A	25.794	2	12.897	11.75	0.003
B	68.951	2	34.476	31.42	0.000
AB	26.855	2	13.428	12.24	0.003
AB^2	2.628	2	1.314	1.20	0.346
Error	9.876	9	1.097		
Total	134.104	17			

We conclude this example by bringing out several features to be explored in more detail later in this section:

Components of interaction. Let the four blockings be denoted $\mathcal{B}_1$ through $\mathcal{B}_4$. Since $\mathcal{B}_1$ is the set of rows and $\mathcal{B}_2$ is the set of columns of the array, $U_{\mathcal{B}_1}$ and $U_{\mathcal{B}_2}$ are the main effects of the two factors. The independence of the partitions $\mathcal{B}_i$ implies the mutual orthogonality of $U_{\mathcal{B}_1}, U_{\mathcal{B}_2}, U_{\mathcal{B}_3}$ and $U_{\mathcal{B}_4}$. Thus, in our earlier notation, $U_{\mathcal{B}_1} = U_1$, $U_{\mathcal{B}_2} = U_2$, and $U_{\mathcal{B}_3} \oplus U_{\mathcal{B}_4} = U_{12}$. The subspaces $U_{\mathcal{B}_3}$ and $U_{\mathcal{B}_4}$ will be called *components of interaction*. We will discuss this more generally in Sect. 5.6.2.

Generalized interactions. A quick check shows that if we create a blocking $\mathcal{B}$ using, say, both $\mathcal{B}_1$ and $\mathcal{B}_4$ (i.e., $\mathcal{B} = \mathcal{B}_1 \vee \mathcal{B}_4$), then $\mathcal{B}$ will partition the cells into 9 blocks of size 1.[14] It follows that $U_{\mathcal{B}}$ will have dimension $9 - 1 = 8$. But $U_{\mathcal{B}}$ contains $U_{\mathcal{B}_1}$ and $U_{\mathcal{B}_4}$, and $\dim(U_{\mathcal{B}_1} + U_{\mathcal{B}_4}) = 2 + 2 = 4$, so evidently $U_{\mathcal{B}_2}$ and $U_{\mathcal{B}_3}$ account for the missing piece of $U_{\mathcal{B}}$. They are thus the *generalized interactions* of $U_{\mathcal{B}_1}$ and $U_{\mathcal{B}_4}$. While it is not necessary in this example, it is significant that we could have predicted this by the following calculations

[14] This would be the case with any two of the blockings, and illustrates Lemma 5.43(d) with $k = j = 2$.

Table 5.2 A 3×3 experiment. The first four columns after "cell" show four blocking functions along with their values modulo 3. The last four columns give contrast vectors for the corrersponding effects, including the two components of interaction. The notations AB and AB^2 are explained in Example 5.48. Compare the contrasts with those constructed in Example 5.34

Cell	t_1	t_2	t_1+t_2	t_1+2t_2	A		B		AB		AB^2	
00	0	0	0	0	1	1	1	1	1	1	1	1
01	0	1	1	2	1	1	−1	0	−1	0	0	−1
02	0	2	2	1	1	1	0	−1	0	−1	−1	0
10	1	0	1	1	−1	0	1	1	−1	0	−1	0
11	1	1	2	0	−1	0	−1	0	0	−1	1	1
12	1	2	0	2	−1	0	0	−1	1	1	0	−1
20	2	0	2	2	0	−1	1	1	0	−1	0	−1
21	2	1	0	1	0	−1	−1	0	1	1	−1	0
22	2	2	1	0	0	−1	0	−1	−1	0	1	1

modulo 3, where $\mathbf{a} = (a_1, a_2)$ corresponds to the function $L(\mathbf{t}) = a_1t_1 + a_2t_2$:

$$(1,0) + (1,2) = (2,2) \sim (1,1)$$
$$(1,0) + 2(1,2) = (0,1).$$

This is what extends Barnard's method of calculation to the 3×3 experiment. The general case is described in detail in Sect. 5.6.3.

Multiplicative notation. Being main effects, $U_{\mathcal{B}_1}$ and $U_{\mathcal{B}_2}$ are naturally labeled A and B in Table 5.2. The labels AB and AB^2 for $U_{\mathcal{B}_3}$ and $U_{\mathcal{B}_4}$ encode the corresponding blocking functions by letting the coefficients of t_1 and t_2 be exponents of A and B, respectively—for example, $t_1 + 2t_2 \leftrightarrow (1,2) \leftrightarrow A^1B^2$. This is a convenient notation that will be described more fully in Sect. 5.6.4.

Remark 5.49 The element $\mathbf{a} \in V$ defines a linear function $L_\mathbf{a}$ on T with values in the field of scalars, in this case $GF(s)$. Such functions are usually called *linear functionals*. The set $\mathcal{L}$ of linear functionals on a vector space V is what is known as the *dual space* of V. We will have more to say about $\mathcal{L}$ below (Proposition 5.66).

On several occasions we will make use of the following elementary observation:

Lemma 5.50 $L_{\mathbf{a}+\mathbf{b}} = L_\mathbf{a} + L_\mathbf{b}$, *and* $L_{c\mathbf{a}} = cL_\mathbf{a}$ *for* $c \in GF(s)$. *In general, if* $\mathbf{a} = \sum_i c_i\mathbf{a}_i$ *then* $L_\mathbf{a} = \sum_i c_i L_{\mathbf{a}_i}$.

5.6.2 Components of Interaction

We continue to use the notation T and V for $(GF(s))^k$, as explained above.

Recall that each main effect or interaction in a k-factor experiment is defined by a subspace $U_I \subset \mathbb{R}^T$ of contrast functions, where I is a subset of factors. For example, if the factors are $A, B, C, \ldots$, then the subspace U_3 contains the contrasts defining the main effect of C, and U_{124} similarly represents the $A \times B \times D$ interaction. (The exact definition of these subspaces was given in Sect. 5.3.) Our main goal here is to show that for each $I \subset \{1, \ldots, k\}$ the effect U_I is an orthogonal sum of block effects $U_{\mathcal{B}}$ defined in Sect. 5.6.1. This is the content of Theorem 5.53 below.

Our first step is to identify blockings $\mathcal{B} = \mathcal{B}(L_{\mathbf{a}})$ for which $U_{\mathcal{B}}$ can be a component of U_I. For any vector $\mathbf{a} = (a_1, \ldots, a_k) \in V$, we define the *support* of $\mathbf{a}$ to be the set

$$\text{supp}(\mathbf{a}) = \{i : a_i \neq 0\}.$$

Proposition 5.51 *Let* $\emptyset \neq I \subset \{1, \ldots, k\}$*, and let* $\mathbf{a} \in V$ *be such that* $\text{supp}(\mathbf{a}) = I$*. Let* $\mathcal{B} = \mathcal{B}(L_{\mathbf{a}})$*. Then* $U_{\mathcal{B}} \subset U_I$*. If* $I = \{i\}$*, then* $U_{\mathcal{B}} = U_i$*, the main effect of factor* i*.*

Thus, for example, in an experiment with factors $A, B, C, \ldots$, if the linear function $a_1t_1 + a_2t_t + a_4t_4$ (with nonzero coefficients) defines a blocking $\mathcal{B}$, then $U_{\mathcal{B}}$ is a potential component of the $A \times B \times D$ interaction.

Proof Let $c \in U_{\mathcal{B}}$. To show that $c \in U_I$, we need to show that it satisfies the two conditions of Corollary 5.37, namely (a) that the value of $c(t_1, \ldots, t_k)$ depends only on the arguments $t_i, i \in I$, and (b) that for $i \in I$ and for fixed values $t_j, j \neq i$, we have

$$\sum_{t \in GF(s)} c(\ldots, t_{i-1}, t, t_{i+1}, \ldots) = 0.$$

First, let B be a block of $\mathcal{B}$. That is, B is the solution set of an equation

$$a_1t_1 + \cdots + a_kt_k = b. \tag{5.37}$$

The truth of the statement $\mathbf{t} = (t_1, \ldots, t_k) \in B$, and thus the value of the indicator function $1_B(\mathbf{t})$, will be unaffected if the value of a variable $t_j, j \notin I$, is changed, since t_j doesn't actually appear in (5.37). Thus the value of the $1_B(\mathbf{t})$ depends only on the values of $t_i, i \in I$. This is therefore true for $1_{B_1}, \ldots, 1_{B_s}$, where $B_1, \ldots, B_s$ are the blocks of $\mathcal{B}$, and so is true for their span, the incidence space $M_{\mathcal{B}}$. Since $c \in U_{\mathcal{B}} \subset M_{\mathcal{B}}$, this is true for c. This verifies condition (a).

For (b), we note that c is constant on the blocks of $\mathcal{B}$, so that there are constants $c_1, \ldots, c_s$ such that

$$c(\mathbf{t}) = c_i \text{ if } \mathbf{t} \in B_i$$

where we continue to denote the blocks of $\mathcal{B}$ by $B_1, \ldots, B_s$. Since $|B_i| = s^{k-1}$, and since c is a contrast, we have

$$0 = \sum_{\mathbf{t}\in T} c(\mathbf{t}) = \sum_{i=1}^{s} \sum_{\mathbf{t}\in B_i} c(\mathbf{t}) = s^{k-1} \sum_{i=1}^{s} c_i,$$

so

$$\sum_{i=1}^{s} c_i = 0.$$

Now let $i \in I$ and fix t_j for all $j \neq i$; as t varies over $GF(s)$, the function

$$L_{\mathbf{a}}(\mathbf{t}) = a_1 t_1 + \cdots + a_{i-1} t_{i-1} + \ a_i t \ + a_{i+1} t_{i+1} + \cdots + a_k t_k$$

must take on s distinct values, so that for each $t \in GF(s)$, $\mathbf{t} = (t_1, \ldots, t_{i-1}, t, t_{i+1}, \ldots, t_k)$ solves an Eq. (5.37) for a different b. That is, the k-tuple $\mathbf{t}$ falls in each block of $\mathcal{B}$ exactly once. But then $c(\mathbf{t})$ takes each value $c_1, \ldots, c_s$ exactly once, and so $\sum_{t\in GF(s)} c(\ldots, t_{i-1}, t, t_{i+1}, \ldots) = \sum_i c_i = 0$. That is, c satisfies condition (b).

When $I = \{i\}$, $\mathcal{B}$ has s blocks, so $\dim U_{\mathcal{B}} = s - 1 = \dim U_i$, and so $U_{\mathcal{B}} = U_i$. □

For a fixed nonempty subset I of $\{1, \ldots, k\}$, define

$$V_I = \{\mathbf{a} \in V\colon \operatorname{supp}(\mathbf{a}) = I\} = \{(a_1, \ldots, a_k) \in V\colon a_i \neq 0 \text{ iff } i \in I\}.$$

For example, $\mathbf{a} \in V_{\{1,2\}}$ if $a_1 \neq 0$, $a_2 \neq 0$, and $a_3 = \cdots = a_k = 0$; the proposition asserts that if $\mathcal{B} = \mathcal{B}(L_{\mathbf{a}})$, then we have $U_{\mathcal{B}} \subset U_{12}$. While there are $(s-1)^{|I|}$ vectors in V_I, some of them are equivalent under the relation $\sim$ given by (5.35), so the blockings they determine are not all distinct.

Lemma 5.52 *The number of* distinct *blockings* $\mathcal{B}(L_{\mathbf{a}})$, $\mathbf{a} \in V_I$, *is* $(s-1)^{|I|-1}$.

Proof First we observe that V_I is closed under multiplication by $c \in (GF(s))^*$, since this doesn't change the positions of the nonzero entries of a vector, so if $\mathbf{a} \in V_I$ and $\mathbf{b} \sim \mathbf{a}$, then $\mathbf{b} \in V_I$. Thus V_I is a union of $\sim$-equivalence classes. Choose the monic representative of each class. It has the general form

$$(0, \cdots, 0, 1, *, \cdots *),$$

where there are precisely $|I| - 1$ nonzero entries among the $*$'s, in positions fixed by I. Every choice of these nonzero entries represents a different equivalence class and therefore a distinct blocking, and each entry can be any element of $(GF(s))^*$, so there are $(s-1)^{|I|-1}$ such vectors, and therefore that many distinct blockings $\mathcal{B}(L_{\mathbf{a}})$, $\mathbf{a} \in V_I$. □

Theorem 5.53 *Let* $\emptyset \neq I \subset \{1, \ldots, k\}$. *Then*

$$U_I = \oplus_{\mathbf{a}} U_{\mathcal{B}_{\mathbf{a}}}, \tag{5.38}$$

where $\mathcal{B}_{\mathbf{a}} = \mathcal{B}(L_{\mathbf{a}})$ *and where the sum is taken over representatives of the equivalence classes in* V_I. *In particular, the sum may be taken over the monic vectors in* V_I.

Proof The representatives $\mathbf{a}$ are inequivalent and therefore pairwise linearly independent, so by Proposition 5.44 the partitions $\mathcal{B}_{\mathbf{a}}$ are pairwise independent. But then Lemma 5.7 implies that the subspaces $U_{\mathcal{B}}$ are mutually orthogonal. Since each is contained in U_I (Proposition 5.51), so is their orthogonal sum. By counting dimensions, we will show that U_I equals this sum, as claimed.

From Proposition 5.44 we know that $\mathcal{B}_{\mathbf{a}}$ has s blocks, so that $\dim U_{\mathbf{a}} = s - 1$ for each $\mathbf{a}$. But by Lemma 5.52 there are $(s-1)^{|I|-1}$ distinct blockings, and thus that many summands $U_{\mathbf{a}}$ in (5.38). Thus the right-hand side of (5.38) has dimension $(s-1)^{|I|}$. On the other hand, Theorem 5.18(c) implies that $\dim U_I = (s-1)^{|I|}$ as well. This proves our claim. □

Because of Eq. (5.38), the summands $U_{\mathcal{B}_{\mathbf{a}}}$ are called the *components of the interaction* U_I.

Theorem 5.53 decomposes each interaction U_I into a sum of components of dimension $s-1$. But we know from Theorem 5.18 that $\mathbb{R}^T$ itself may be decomposed into a sum of effects U_I. Combining these theorems gives us another proof of the decomposition (5.36) of Theorem 5.46. It also confirms that the latter decomposition is a refinement of that in Theorem 5.18, as we mentioned earlier.

Example 5.54 Since each interaction in a 2^k experiment has 1 degree of freedom, the only components of interaction are the interactions themselves. Each interaction is given by a linear functional over $\mathbb{Z}/2$, and these are easy to see. For example, in a 2^4 experiment with factors A, B, C and D, the BCD interaction is given by $L_{(0,1,1,1)}(\mathbf{t}) = t_2 + t_3 + t_4$. Setting this $= 0$ or $= 1 \pmod 2$ gives two blocks, and the BCD interaction will be the corresponding block effect. The reader can verify that a contrast for this effect is the column for BCD in Table 5.1. The span of this column vector is the subspace U_I representing the BCD interaction, where $I = \{2, 3, 4\}$.

For 2^k experiments, Theorem 5.53 adds nothing new, since each interaction contains only one component. But for factors with $s > 2$ levels, the analysis of variance can be expanded.

Example 5.55 Consider a 3^3 experiment with factors A, B and C. We index the levels of each factor by $\mathbb{Z}/3$. Let $I = \{1, 2\}$. There are four vectors $\mathbf{a} \in V_I$, namely

$$\begin{matrix} (1,1,0) & (1,2,0) \\ (2,2,0) & (2,1,0) \end{matrix}$$

and their monic representatives are $(1, 1, 0)$ and $(1, 2, 0)$. The first determines the blocking $\mathcal{B}_1$ of T given by equations of the form $t_1 + t_2 = b \pmod 3$, the second the blocking $\mathcal{B}_2$ given by $t_1 + 2t_2 = b \pmod 3$. Each blocking has 3 blocks, and so gives rise to a space of contrast functions of dimension 2. Theorem 5.53 tells us that $U_{12} = U_{\mathcal{B}_1} \oplus U_{\mathcal{B}_2}$. That is, the $A \times B$ interaction has two components, given by $\mathbf{a} = (1, 1, 0)$ and $(1, 2, 0)$. Similarly, the $B \times C$ interaction will have two components, given by $\mathbf{a} = (0, 1, 1)$ and $(0, 1, 2)$.

Table 5.3 gives the $(3^3 - 1)/(3 - 1) = 13$ blockings that define the components of interaction in this experiment, each indicated by the blocking function at the top of the corresponding column. The values 0, 1 and 2 in each column separate the 27 cells into 3 blocks of 9. The blocking $\mathcal{B}$ defined by a given column specifies one of the effects $U_{\mathcal{B}}$ appearing in Eq. (5.36). Note that each two-factor interaction has two components of interaction, while the three-factor interaction has four components, as predicted by Lemma 5.52.

We make a couple of further observations in this table:

- The columns for t_1, t_2 and t_3 together give the cells.
- The rest of the columns are computed from them componentwise, by arithmetic modulo 3.

Example 5.56 For two-factor experiments, the results of this section tell us something important about sets of mutually orthogonal Latin squares (or MOLS, as they are often referred to).

An $s \times s$ experiment has $(s - 1)^2$ degrees of freedom for interaction, and Theorem 5.53 tells us that this interaction is an orthogonal sum of $s - 1$ subspaces of the form $U_{\mathcal{B}_\mathbf{a}}$, where $\mathcal{B}_\mathbf{a}$ is the partition of the set T of treatment combinations whose s blocks are the solution sets to equations $L_\mathbf{a}(\mathbf{t}) = c$, $c \in GF(S)$. Each of these subspaces is orthogonal to the main effects subspaces U_1 and U_2, which are determined by the row- and column-partitions, so each partition $\mathcal{B}_\mathbf{a}$ is independent of rows and of columns (Lemma 5.7). But an easy application of Eq. (5.7) shows that each block of $\mathcal{B}_\mathbf{a}$ intersects each row and each column in just one cell—that is, $\mathcal{B}_\mathbf{a}$ defines a Latin square of order s. By Proposition 5.10 the orthogonality of the subspaces $U_{\mathcal{B}_\mathbf{a}}$ is equivalent to the orthogonality of these $s - 1$ Latin squares, the maximum possible number of MOLS of this order.[15]

That is, for there to be a set of $s - 1$ MOLS of order s, it is sufficient that s be a prime or prime power (in which case the method of this section gives a construction, as in Exercise 5.23). Whether this condition is necessary is unknown.

[15] To be clear, there can be a set of fewer than $s - 1$ MOLS that is maximal in the sense that it can't be extended by adding in another Latin square. There are even single Latin squares that don't have an "orthogonal mate." So $s - 1$ is the maximum size of a maximal set of MOLS.

Table 5.3 Components of interaction in a 3^3 experiment, discussed in Example 5.55. Column headings are functions of t_1, t_2 and t_3 written vertically to save space, and indicate a component of interaction. Columns contain the values of each function at each cell. Each column determines a partition of the cells into 3 blocks according to the values 0, 1 and 2, and thus a main effect or a component of interaction

cell	t_1	t_2	t_3	t_1+t_2	t_1+2t_2	t_1+t_3	t_1+2t_3	t_2+t_3	t_2+2t_3	$t_1+t_2+t_3$	$t_1+2t_2+t_3$	$t_1+t_2+2t_3$	$t_1+2t_2+2t_3$
000	0	0	0	0	0	0	0	0	0	0	0	0	0
001	0	0	1	0	0	1	2	1	2	1	1	2	2
002	0	0	2	0	0	2	1	2	1	2	2	1	1
010	0	1	0	1	2	0	0	1	1	1	2	1	2
011	0	1	1	1	2	1	2	2	0	2	0	0	1
012	0	1	2	1	2	2	1	0	2	0	1	2	0
020	0	2	0	2	1	0	0	2	2	2	1	2	1
021	0	2	1	2	1	1	2	0	1	0	2	1	0
022	0	2	2	2	1	2	1	1	0	1	0	0	2
100	1	0	0	1	1	1	1	0	0	1	1	1	1
101	1	0	1	1	1	2	0	1	2	2	2	0	0
102	1	0	2	1	1	0	2	2	1	0	0	2	2
110	1	1	0	2	0	1	1	1	1	2	0	2	0
111	1	1	1	2	0	2	0	2	0	0	1	1	2
112	1	1	2	2	0	0	2	0	2	1	2	0	1
120	1	2	0	0	2	1	1	2	2	0	2	0	2
121	1	2	1	0	2	2	0	0	1	1	0	2	1
122	1	2	2	0	2	0	2	1	0	2	1	1	0
200	2	0	0	2	2	2	2	0	0	2	2	2	2
201	2	0	1	2	2	0	1	1	2	0	0	1	1
202	2	0	2	2	2	1	0	2	1	1	1	0	0
210	2	1	0	0	1	2	2	1	1	0	1	0	1
211	2	1	1	0	1	0	1	2	0	1	2	2	0
212	2	1	2	0	1	1	0	0	2	2	0	1	2
220	2	2	0	1	0	2	2	2	2	1	0	1	0
221	2	2	1	1	0	0	1	0	1	2	1	0	2
222	2	2	2	1	0	1	0	1	0	0	2	2	1
	A	B	C	$A \times B$		$A \times C$		$B \times C$		$A \times B \times C$			

5.6.3 *Finding Generalized Interactions*

Given j linearly independent elements $\mathbf{a}_1, \ldots, \mathbf{a}_j$ of V^*, let $L_i = L_{\mathbf{a}_i}$ be the corresponding linear functionals. The partition $\mathcal{B} = \mathcal{B}(L_1) \vee \cdots \vee \mathcal{B}(L_j)$ has s^j blocks of blocksize s^{k-j}, each block being the solution set of a system of simultaneous equations

$$\begin{aligned} L_1(\mathbf{t}) &= b_1 \\ &\vdots \\ L_j(\mathbf{t}) &= b_j \end{aligned} \tag{5.39}$$

(written out, this is the system (5.33)). Now $\mathcal{B}(L_i) < \mathcal{B}$ implies that $U_i \subset U_{\mathcal{B}}$, where for the moment we put $U_i = U_{\mathcal{B}(L_i)}$, so each U_i is confounded with $\mathcal{B}$-blocks. But $\dim U_1 + \cdots + \dim U_j = j(s-1) < s^j - 1 = \dim U_{\mathcal{B}}$, so it is clear that more effects are confounded with $\mathcal{B}$-blocks. These are called *generalized interactions* of the effects U_i, and the question is how to find them. The answer involves the subspace $E \subset V$ spanned by $\mathbf{a}_1, \ldots, \mathbf{a}_j$. We first note the following.

Lemma 5.57 *Let E be a subspace of V of dimension j. Then E^* is the union of $(s^j-1)/(s-1)$ equivalence classes of V^*, equivalence given by (5.35). If $\mathbf{a}_1, \ldots, \mathbf{a}_j$ is a basis of E, then a set of representatives of the equivalence classes is given by the expressions $\sum_{i=1}^{j} c_i \mathbf{a}_i$ with $c_i \in GF(s)$ such that $(c_1, \ldots, c_j)$ is monic.*

Proof If $\mathbf{a} \in E$ then $c\mathbf{a} \in E$ for any $c \in (GF(s))^*$, so E contains the entire equivalence class of $\mathbf{a}$, and so E^* is the disjoint union of such classes, and each class has $s-1$ elements. If $\mathbf{a}_1, \ldots, \mathbf{a}_j$ is a basis of E, then every element of E has a unique representation $\sum_{i=1}^{j} c_i \mathbf{a}_i$. Each equivalence class in E^* contains a unique element for which $(c_1, \ldots, c_j)$ is monic, and there are $s^{j-1} + \cdots + s + 1 = (s^j - 1)/(s-1)$ such elements. □

Alternatively, E is isomorphic to $(GF(s))^j$, and so has s^j elements. Moreover, E^* corresponds to $(GF(s)^j)^*$ under this isomorphism, and the lemma now follows from Proposition 5.45.

With this result, we can answer our question.

Theorem 5.58 *Given the linearly independent vectors $\mathbf{a}_1, \ldots, \mathbf{a}_j \in V$, let $E = \langle \mathbf{a}_1, \ldots, \mathbf{a}_j \rangle$ be their span, and let $\mathcal{B} = \mathcal{B}(L_{\mathbf{a}_1}) \vee \cdots \vee \mathcal{B}(L_{\mathbf{a}_j})$. Define $\mathbf{a}_{j+1}, \ldots, \mathbf{a}_r$ so that $\mathbf{a}_1, \ldots, \mathbf{a}_r$ are representatives of the $r = (s^j-1)/(s-1)$ equivalence classes of E^*. Then $U_{\mathcal{B}}$ has the orthogonal decomposition*

$$U_{\mathcal{B}} = \oplus_{i=1}^{r} U_{\mathcal{B}(L_{\mathbf{a}_i})}. \tag{5.40}$$

The subspaces on the right-hand side of (5.40) are all confounded with $\mathcal{B}$-blocks, and the components numbered $j+1, \ldots, r$, are the *generalized interactions* of the first r components. Before proving Theorem 5.58, we give two examples.

Example 5.59 For 2^k experiments, the only linear combinations of vectors in $V = (GF(2))^k$ are sums, since the only scalars are 0 and 1. Consider the 2^3 example of Sect. 5.5.1. The linear functionals corresponding to AB and ABC are $L_{\mathbf{a}}(\mathbf{t})$ where $\mathbf{a} = (1, 1, 0)$ and $(1, 1, 1)$, respectively. Their sum modulo 2 is $(0, 0, 1)$, and the blocking given by $L_{(0,0,1)}(\mathbf{t})$ is precisely that defining the main effect of C. Thus C is the generalized interaction of ABC and AB. That is what we found earlier, though with more work.

Example 5.60 In Example 5.55 we saw that in a 3^3 experiment with factors A, B and C, the vector $\mathbf{a}_1 = (1, 1, 0)$ determined a component of the $A \times B$ interaction, and we noted that $\mathbf{a}_2 = (0, 1, 2)$ would determine a component of the $B \times C$ interaction. Therefore, blocking by the functional $L_{(1,1,0)}$ would confound (part of) the $A \times B$ interaction, and blocking by $L_{(0,1,2)}$ would confound (part of) the $B \times C$ interaction. Each of these creates 3 blocks of size 9, and confounds 2 degrees of freedom (df).

Suppose we simultaneously partition the 27 cells using both these functionals. That would create 9 blocks of size 3, accounting for 8 df confounded with blocks. These include the components of interaction determined by $\mathbf{a}_1$ and $\mathbf{a}_2$. Their generalized interactions should confound another 4 df. They are determined by taking linear combinations $c_1\mathbf{a}_1 + c_2\mathbf{a}_2$ where $c_i \in \mathbb{Z}/3$ and (c_1, c_2) is monic. Aside from $\mathbf{a}_1$ and $\mathbf{a}_2$ themselves, these are $\mathbf{a}_3 = \mathbf{a}_1 + \mathbf{a}_2$ and $\mathbf{a}_4 = \mathbf{a}_1 + 2\mathbf{a}_2$.

Thus the generalized interactions we seek are given by $\mathbf{a}_3 = (1, 2, 2)$ and $\mathbf{a}_4 = (1, 0, 1)$. According to Theorem 5.53, the first determines a component of the $A \times B \times C$ interaction, the second a component of the $A \times C$ interaction.

This method of calculating generalized interactions is effective but may seem a bit cumbersome. In Sect. 5.6.4 we will introduce a type of notation that makes these calculations much simpler.

The crux of Theorem 5.58 is the following observation, a particular case of which we observed in the 2^3 illustration near the beginning of Sect. 5.5. We leave the proof of this lemma as an exercise.

Lemma 5.61 *Let* $E = \langle \mathbf{a}_1, \ldots, \mathbf{a}_j \rangle$ *and* $\mathcal{B} = \mathcal{B}(L_{\mathbf{a}_1}) \vee \cdots \vee \mathcal{B}(L_{\mathbf{a}_j})$. *Then for every* $\mathbf{a} \in E^*$ *we have* $\mathcal{B}(L_{\mathbf{a}}) < \mathcal{B}$.

Proof of Theorem 5.58 From Lemma 5.61 we see that $U_{\mathcal{B}(L_{\mathbf{a}_i})} \subset U_{\mathcal{B}}$ for every i, and thus that

$$U_{\mathcal{B}(L_{\mathbf{a}_1})} + \cdots + U_{\mathcal{B}(L_{\mathbf{a}_r})} \subseteq U_{\mathcal{B}}. \tag{5.41}$$

Since the the vectors $\mathbf{a}_i$ are pairwise independent, the partitions $\mathcal{B}(L_{\mathbf{a}_i})$ are pairwise independent as well (Proposition 5.44), so that the sum in (5.41) is orthogonal. To show equality, we may show that the two sides of (5.41) have the same dimension. But the orthogonal sum has dimension $r(s-1) = s^j - 1$, by Lemma 5.57, and this is $\dim U_{\mathcal{B}}$ as $\mathcal{B}$ has s^j blocks. □

Remark 5.62 The notion of generalized interaction in s^k experiments, $s > 2$, is implicit in Fisher [58, 59], and is made explicit by Bose and Kishen [23].

Writing $\mathcal{C} = \mathcal{B}(L_{\mathbf{a}_1})$ and $\mathcal{D} = \mathcal{B}(L_{\mathbf{a}_2})$, we see from Eq. (5.40) with $j = 2$ that the generalized interaction of the block effects $U_{\mathcal{C}}$ and $U_{\mathcal{D}}$ is the orthogonal difference $U_{\mathcal{C}\vee\mathcal{D}} \ominus (U_{\mathcal{C}} + U_{\mathcal{D}})$, consistent with Definition 5.6.

Remark 5.63 As a vector space, $V = (GF(s))^k$ is an *affine geometry*, a kind of geometry that includes the usual Euclidean geometry (which also has concepts of length and angle). The notation often used for $(GF(s))^k$ is $EG(k, s)$ or $AG(k, s)$. Borrowing terminology from geometry, one also calls the partition $\mathcal{B}(L_{\mathbf{a}})$ defined by (5.34) a *pencil of parallel flats*. By extension, **a** itself may be referred to as a pencil.

The equivalence relation (5.35) has a geometric meaning: an equivalence class is either the set $\{\mathbf{0}\}$ or a line through $\mathbf{0}$ but with $\mathbf{0}$ removed, so that for nonzero points we have $\mathbf{a} \sim \mathbf{b}$ iff **a** and **b** lie on the same line through the origin. Moreover, the lines turn out to be the points of another finite geometry, namely the *projective geometry* of dimension $k - 1$ over $GF(s)$, often denoted $PG(k - 1, s)$. Finite geometries are developed in a number of texts, for example [108].

While we don't need the geometric properties of projective space, it is not uncommon to use the notation $\mathbf{a} \in PG(k-1, s)$ to mean that **a** is the representative of its equivalence class in V^*. In the literature the representative is always assumed to be a *monic* vector.

5.6.4 Multiplicative Notation: The Effects Group

As we noted above, Barnard described her method of computing generalized interactions by saying that "if the comparisons represented by ... two lines have a factor, or factors, in common (such as AB and BC), these factors do not appear in the resultant generalized interaction (AC, in the example chosen)". It was noticed early that this method of calculating could be given algebraically by multiplication:

$$AB \cdot BC = AC,$$

which works provided that $B^2 = I$, an identity element. We now provide the basis for this kind of computation.

Continuing to write $V = (GF(s))^k$, we define the *effects group*

$$G = \{A_1^{a_1} \cdots A_k^{a_k} \colon (a_1, \ldots, a_k) \in V\}$$

with multiplication given as follows: For F_1 and $F_2 \in G$ given by

$$F_1 = A_1^{a_1} \cdots A_k^{a_k} \text{ and } F_2 = A_1^{b_1} \cdots A_k^{b_k},$$

the product $F_1 F_2$ is

$$F_1 F_2 = A_1^{a_1+b_1} \cdots A_k^{a_k+b_k}.$$

In effect, the elements A_i are permitted to commute with each other. Note that the identity element of G is

$$I = A_1^0 \cdots A_k^0,$$

and the inverse of F_1 above is

$$F_1^{-1} = A_1^{-a_1} \cdots A_k^{-a_k}.$$

Moreover, since $GF(s)$ is of *characteristic* p ($pa = 0$ for all $a \in GF(s)$) where s is a power of the prime p, every element of G is of *order* p:

$$F^p = I \text{ for all } F \in G.$$

Note how all of these properties are inherited from those of the vector space V. Finally, scalar multiplication in V becomes becomes the action of $GF(s)$ on G via exponentiation:

$$\left(A_1^{a_1} \cdots A_k^{a_k}\right)^b = A_1^{a_1 b} \cdots A_k^{a_k b} \text{ for } b \in GF(s).$$

With this, we have defined G to be an abelian group, with *generators* $A_1, \ldots, A_k$. The elements of G are referred to as *words* in the letters A_i. When k, the number of effects, is small, we usually use $A, B, C, \ldots$ in place of $A_1, A_2, A_3, \ldots$.

Linear independence in V becomes the following condition in G: the elements $F_1, \ldots, F_r$ are *independent* in G if

$$F_1^{c_1} \cdots F_r^{c_r} = I \quad \text{implies} \quad c_1 = \cdots = c_r = 0. \tag{5.42}$$

There doesn't seem to be an accepted term for this condition, so we will simply refer to it as "independence".

The equivalence relation (5.35) on V^* defines an equivalence relation on G^*, the non-identity elements of G:

$$F_1 \sim F_2 \quad \text{iff} \quad F_2 = F_1^c \quad \text{for some } c \in (GF(s))^*. \tag{5.43}$$

The equivalence class of the element $F \in G$ is thus the set

$$\{F^c\colon\ c \in (GF(s))^*\}. \tag{5.44}$$

A given class can be represented by a word whose first nonzero exponent is 1. It is natural for us to refer to such elements of G as *monic words.*[16] One can always convert a word F to an equivalent monic word by raising it to an appropriate exponent.

If $\mathbf{a} = (a_1, \ldots, a_k)$, **the convention is to name the effect $U_{\mathcal{B}(L_\mathbf{a})}$ by the word $A_1^{a_1} \cdots A_k^{a_k}$**. In particular, we use the *monic* word representing the effect.

Example 5.64 For 2^k experiments the method is especially simple. Here every generator (and in fact every element) has order 2. Thus, for example, the generalized interaction of AB and BC (Barnard's example) is

$$AB \cdot BC = AB^2C = AC,$$

since $B^2 = I$. Similarly, the generalized interaction of AB and ABC is

$$AB \cdot ABC = A^2B^2C = C.$$

Note how this encodes the computation $(1, 1, 0) + (1, 1, 1) = (0, 0, 1) \pmod 2$ of Example 5.59.

Example 5.65 In a 3^3 experiment the effects group G has three generators, A, B and C, each of order 3. If we use the functional $L_{(1,1,0)}$ to partition the 27 cells, the component of interaction confounded with blocks will be AB; if we use $L_{(0,1,2)}$, then BC^2 will be confounded. If we use both functionals simultaneously to create 9 blocks of size 3, both of these will be confounded, along with their generalized interactions, which we compute to be

$$AB \cdot BC^2 = AB^2C^2, \text{ and}$$

$$AB \cdot (BC^2)^2 = AB \cdot B^2C^4 = AC,$$

as $B^3 = I$ and $C^4 = C$. This mirrors the computation we did in Example 5.60. If we blocked this experiment to confound AB, AC, BC^2 and AB^2C^2, the ANOVA table with N observations would have this analysis:

Source	A	B	C	AB^2	AC^2	BC	ABC	AB^2C	ABC^2	Blocks	Error	Total
df	2	2	2	2	2	2	2	2	2	8	$N - 26$	$N - 1$

If the design is equireplicate with r observations per treatment combination, then $N = 27r$. With $r = 4$, though, another possibility opens: We may choose to confound each of AB, AC, BC^2 and AB^2C^2 in a different replicate. These four effects are then only *partially confounded*. To analyze this, one introduces a new

[16] The group identity element I is not considered a monic word.

factor called Replicate, and the Block factor is nested within Replicate. Designs like this are said to be *resolvable*. The reader can find more information about resolvable designs in [108] and [136] and in applied texts such as [81].

A slightly different computation with the same four effects illustrates a further point. The generalized interactions of AB and AC are

$$AB \cdot AC = A^2BC \sim (A^2BC)^2 = AB^2C^2, \text{ and}$$
$$AB \cdot (AC)^2 = AB \cdot A^2C^2 = BC^2.$$

The computation of BC^2 is similar to earlier ones. In the computation of AB^2C^2, we make use of the equivalence relation (5.43), specifically

$$F^2 \sim F,$$

in order to find the monic representative of the component of interaction.

Finally, note that we may work backwards to determine the blocking functionals needed to confound given components of interaction. For example, $AB = A^1B^1C^0$ corresponds to $\mathbf{a} = (1, 1, 0)$, and so is confounded with the blocks defined by $L_{(1,1,0)}$ (mod 3). Similarly, BC is confounded by the blocks of $L_{(0,1,1)}$.

The last point in Example 5.65 is important. It makes use of one of the following one-to-one correspondences:

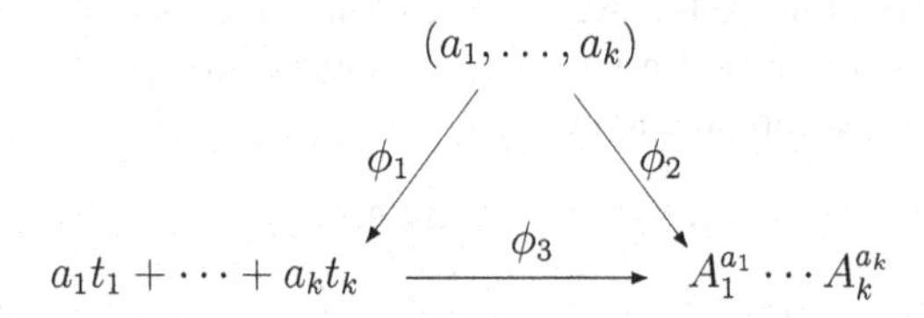

Under correspondence ϕ_3, the variables t_i are replaced by symbols A_i, sums by products, and (scalar) products by exponentiation. Thus, the blocking functional at left determines the component of interaction that will be confounded, at right. Conversely, given a component of interaction, one may determine the blocking functional $L_{\mathbf{a}}$ that will confound it.

As in Remark 5.49, we let $\mathcal{L}$ be the set of linear functionals $L_{\mathbf{a}}$. The maps ϕ_i are correspondences between three sets:

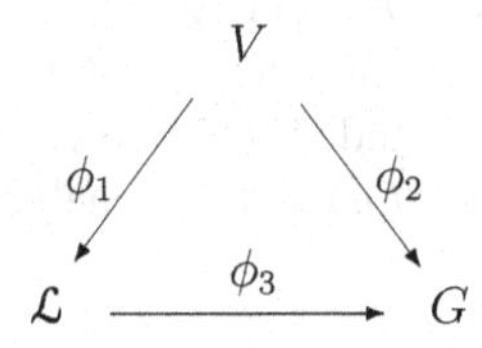

We note also that not only the three sets but also the operations within them correspond naturally. For example, $2(a_1, \ldots, a_k)$ corresponds to $2(a_1t_1+\cdots+a_kt_k)$. We state this formally as follows:

Proposition 5.66 *The set $\mathcal{L}$ is a vector space over $GF(s)$, and the map ϕ_1 is a vector space isomorphism. The maps ϕ_2 and ϕ_3 are isomorphisms that take sums to products and scalar multiplication to exponentiation.*

Proof The statements about $\mathcal{L}$ and ϕ_1 are immediate from Lemma 5.50. The claim about ϕ_2 is valid due to the way we defined G. The statement about ϕ_3 holds because $\phi_3 = \phi_2 \circ \phi_1{}^{-1}$. □

The map we have denoted by ϕ_3 is really the important one. It allows us to "read off" the function $L(t_1, t_2, \ldots) = t_1 + 2t_2 + t_3$ from the effect that it defines, which we have denoted by AB^2C, and vice versa.

Remark 5.67 A technical point about G: When the exponent b is actually an integer, exponentiation F^b has its usual meaning (e.g., $F^3 = FFF$). However, when exponents come from $GF(s)$ but not its subfield $\mathbb{Z}/p$, exponentiation F^b must be interpreted as the *operation* on G by the element $b \in GF(s)$. This is not of practical importance, as the usual rules of exponents still work. For the definition of a *group with operators*, see [143, Section 43] or [25, Chapter 2]. The map ϕ_2 must be understood as an isomorphism between groups with operators, where a vector space is viewed as an additive group whose operators are given by scalar multiplication.

The equivalence classes of G are called *orbits*. The set (5.44) is the orbit of F under the action of $(GF(s))^*$.

The designation of G as the effects group is traditional (see, e.g., [103, page 180]), although somewhat inaccurate. It is not the elements of G that are confounded by various blockings but rather the orbits of G^*.

Remark 5.68 Just as we encode the element $\mathbf{a} = (a_1, \ldots, a_k) \in V^*$ by an expression of the form $A_1^{a_1} \cdots A_k^{a_k}$ when representing a linear functional $L_{\mathbf{a}}(\mathbf{t})$, so may we also encode the treatment combination $\mathbf{t} = (t_1, \ldots, t_k) \in T$. The custom here is to use lower-case letters, omitting any letter to the 0th power. Since we allow $\mathbf{t} = \mathbf{0}$, we usually represent it by (1). With this new representation, the treatment combinations form an abelian group G', say, on k generators. As with effects, when k is small we usually use the letters $a, b, \ldots$. Thus, for example, the treatment combinations of a 2^3 experiment are

$$(1), a, b, c, ab, ac, bc, abc.$$

In addition, we do not impose a similarity relation on treatment combinations. Thus the cells of a 3^2 experiment are written

$$(1), a, a^2, b, ab, a^2b, b^2, ab^2, a^2b^2,$$

corresponding to

$$00, 10, 20, 01, 11, 21, 02, 12, 22.$$

With this new representation, the treatment combinations form a group on the generators $a, b, \ldots$, or $a_1, \ldots, a_k$.

We observed earlier that the principal block is a subspace of the vector space T. In this new notation, it is a subgroup of G', known as the *intrablock subgroup* [58].

5.6.5 Complex Contrasts

Barnard [10] made her discovery by studying the componentwise multiplication of contrast vectors in a two-level (2^k) factorial design. It is natural to ask whether there isn't a similar way of working directly with contrast vectors in more general s^k designs.

In fact there is, at least when s is prime.

Consider the columns in Table 5.1 (page 175), the contrast vectors in a 2^4 factorial design. Augmenting these by a column of 1's that we label I, we note the following:

1. The column labels are the 16 elements of the effects group G.
2. The columns themselves form a group isomorphic to G under componentwise multiplication. In fact, this *is* G if we think of the labels $A, B, \ldots$ not as abstract symbols but as simply the names of the columns.
3. The values ± 1 in each column indicate the partition of the 16 cells that defines that effect.
4. The rows of columns A, B, C, D indicate the treatment combinations of the experiment.
5. Each column gives the coefficients c of a contrast $\sum c_{ijk\ell}\, \mu_{ijk\ell}$ in cell means.

We cannot satisfy all of these conditions when $s \neq 2$, but we can achieve all but the last when $s = p$, a prime.

Example 5.69 Let us revisit the 3×3 experiment discussed in Example 5.48, and extract from Table 5.2 the following:

cell	t_1	t_2	$t_1 + t_2$	$t_1 + 2t_2$
00	0	0	0	0
01	0	1	1	2
02	0	2	2	1
10	1	0	1	1
11	1	1	2	0
12	1	2	0	2
20	2	0	2	2
21	2	1	0	1
22	2	2	1	0

Note that each cell is exactly the value of (t_1, t_2). Also, the last two columns can be computed from those for t_1 and t_2 by componentwise computation modulo 3. Finally, the values 0, 1 and 2 define four partitions of the cells corresponding to the factors A and B and the interaction components AB and AB^2.

Apart from row and column headings, the table above consists of a 9×4 matrix whose entries are integers—in fact, elements of $\mathbb{Z}/3$. Now let $\omega = e^{2\pi i/3} = (-1 + i\sqrt{3})/2$, a primitive cube root of unity,[17] and replace each entry j by ω^j. Relabeling the columns, this would give the following table:

cell	A	B	AB	AB^2
00	1	1	1	1
01	1	ω	ω	ω^2
02	1	ω^2	ω^2	ω
10	ω	1	ω	ω
11	ω	ω	ω^2	1
12	ω	ω^2	1	ω^2
20	ω^2	1	ω^2	ω^2
21	ω^2	ω	1	ω
22	ω^2	ω^2	ω	1

The new labels give the same information as before. The key point is that *arithmetic modulo 3 has been replaced by multiplication*, taking into account that $\omega^3 = 1$. That is, $AB = A \cdot B$ and $AB^2 = A \cdot B^2$, where multiplication and squaring are componentwise. Multiplication of columns has the convenience of conforming to multiplication in the effects group. Let's follow this further.

The generalized interaction of A and AB^2, say, should be AB, because

$$A \cdot AB^2 = A^2B^2 \sim AB.$$

[17] Roots of unity are discussed in the Appendix.

Table 5.4 Complex contrast vectors in a 3^2 factorial experiment

cell	I	A	B	A^2	B^2	AB	A^2B^2	AB^2	A^2B
00	1	1	1	1	1	1	1	1	1
01	1	1	ω	1	ω^2	ω	ω^2	ω^2	ω
02	1	1	ω^2	1	ω	ω^2	ω	ω	ω^2
10	1	ω	1	ω^2	1	ω	ω^2	ω	ω^2
11	1	ω	ω	ω^2	ω^2	ω^2	ω	1	1
12	1	ω	ω^2	ω^2	ω	1	1	ω^2	ω
20	1	ω^2	1	ω	1	ω^2	ω	ω^2	ω
21	1	ω^2	ω	ω	ω^2	1	1	ω	ω^2
22	1	ω^2	ω^2	ω	ω	ω	ω^2	1	1

However, componentwise multiplication simply gives us A^2B^2, as the reader can check. Of course, this gives the same blocking as AB, where we simply interchange ω and ω^2. In fact, the table above is missing five columns, corresponding to five more elements of the effects group. The additional columns give us Table 5.4.

Table 5.4 has four of the properties mentioned above:

1. The column labels are the 9 elements of the effects group G.
2. The columns themselves form a group isomorphic to G under componentwise multiplication. The product of two columns is indicated by the product of the column headings.
3. The values $1, \omega, \omega^2$ in each column indicate the partition of the 9 cells that defines that effect.
4. The rows of columns A and B indicate the treatment combinations of the experiment.

We also note the following:

5. Each column is a *complex contrast vector*, i.e., its components sum to zero. That is because each symbol occurs the same number of times, and because $1 + \omega + \omega^2 = (1 - \omega^3)/(1 - \omega) = 0$.
6. The columns are mutually orthogonal with respect to the *complex (or Hermitian) inner product*

$$\mathbf{u} \cdot \mathbf{v} = \sum_i u_i \bar{v}_i, \tag{5.45}$$

where $\bar{v}$ is the complex conjugate of v.

To generalize this, let us examine this table more closely. The lower right is a 9×9 array, the rows indexed by cell (that is, by $(\mathbb{Z}/3)^2$) and the columns by the elements of the effects group G. The cells and the elements of G are ordered differently, the columns following the order

$$(0, 0), (1, 0), (0, 1), (2, 0), (0, 2), (1, 1), (2, 2), (1, 2), (2, 1),$$

as is evident from the exponents on A and B. Finally, the 81 entries in the body of the table are of the form ω raised to the power $L_{\mathbf{a}_c}(\mathbf{t}_r)$, where $\mathbf{t}_r$ is a row value (a cell), $\mathbf{a}_c$ is a column value, and $L_{\mathbf{a}}(\mathbf{t})$ is defined by (5.31).

To describe the general form of such arrays, let us put $q = s^k$, s a prime power, so that $q = |(GF(s))^k| = |G|$, and let us fix an ordering $\mathbf{a}_0, \mathbf{a}_1, \ldots, \mathbf{a}_{q-1}$ of the elements of $V = (GF(s))^k$ such that $\mathbf{a}_0 = \mathbf{0}$. (We will choose a convenient order later.) Let us also fix an order $\mathbf{t}_0, \mathbf{t}_1, \ldots, \mathbf{t}_{q-1}$ of the cells of the experiment (also an ordering of the elements of $(GF(s))^k$, not necessarily the same as that of the vectors $\mathbf{a}_i$). Since

$$L_{\mathbf{a}}(\mathbf{t}) = \mathbf{t}'\mathbf{a},$$

it is convenient to write the entries of our table in the form $\mathbf{t}'\mathbf{a}$.

cell	$\mathbf{a}_0$	$\cdots$	$\mathbf{a}_i$	$\cdots$	$\mathbf{a}_{q-1}$
$\mathbf{t}_0$	$\mathbf{t}_0'\mathbf{a}_0$	$\cdots$	$\mathbf{t}_0'\mathbf{a}_i$	$\cdots$	$\mathbf{t}_0'\mathbf{a}_{q-1}$
$\mathbf{t}_1$	$\mathbf{t}_1'\mathbf{a}_0$	$\cdots$	$\mathbf{t}_1'\mathbf{a}_i$	$\cdots$	$\mathbf{t}_1'\mathbf{a}_{q-1}$
$\vdots$	$\vdots$		$\vdots$		$\vdots$
$\mathbf{t}_{q-1}$	$\mathbf{t}_{q-1}'\mathbf{a}_0$	$\cdots$	$\mathbf{t}_{q-1}'\mathbf{a}_i$	$\cdots$	$\mathbf{t}_{q-1}'\mathbf{a}_{q-1}$

Let $\mathbf{M}$ be the $q \times q$ array in the lower right of this table. The entries of $\mathbf{M}$ belong to $GF(s)$, the ijth element being $\mathbf{t}_i'\mathbf{a}_j$. Since $\mathbf{a}_0 = \mathbf{0}$, the entries in the first column are zeros. In addition, we have the following:

Theorem 5.70 *Let* $\mathbf{M}$ *be as above.*

a. *Each column of* $\mathbf{M}$ *except the first contains all the elements of* $GF(s)$ *repeated* s^{k-1} *times.*
b. *Let* $\mathcal{V}$ *be the set of columns of* $\mathbf{M}$*. Then* $\mathcal{V}$ *is a vector space over* $GF(s)$*.*
c. *The map* $\phi : V \to \mathcal{V}$ *given by*

$$\phi(\mathbf{a}) = \textit{column } \mathbf{a} \textit{ of } \mathbf{M}$$

is a vector space isomorphism.

Proof The jth column of $\mathbf{M}$ consists of the values of $L_{\mathbf{a}_j}(\mathbf{t})$ as $\mathbf{t}$ ranges over all the treatment combinations. Part (a) thus follows immediately from Lemma 5.43(c).

Since $\mathcal{V} \subset (GF(s))^q$ and since ϕ maps V onto $\mathcal{V}$, we see that (b) will follow as soon as we show that ϕ is linear (Theorem A.35). Since ϕ is obviously one-to-one, this will also show (c). Now, the linearity of ϕ means that

$$\phi(\text{col } \mathbf{a}_i + \text{col } \mathbf{a}_j) = \phi(\text{col } \mathbf{a}_i) + \phi(\text{col } \mathbf{a}_j) \quad \text{and} \quad \phi(c \text{ col } \mathbf{a}_i) = c\phi(\text{col } \mathbf{a}_i). \tag{5.46}$$

Table 5.5 Complex contrast vectors in a full p^k factorial experiment, p prime. Here $q = p^k$ and $\omega = e^{2\pi i/p}$. Columns are contrast vectors: If $\mathbf{a} = (a_1, \ldots, a_k)$, then the column heading $\mathbf{a}$ denotes the effect $A_1^{a_1} \cdots A_k^{a_k}$ (See Corollary 5.71)

cell	$\mathbf{a}_0$	$\cdots$	$\mathbf{a}_i$	$\cdots$	$\mathbf{a}_{q-1}$
$\mathbf{t}_0$	$\omega^{\mathbf{t}_0'\mathbf{a}_0}$	$\cdots$	$\omega^{\mathbf{t}_0'\mathbf{a}_i}$	$\cdots$	$\omega^{\mathbf{t}_0'\mathbf{a}_{q-1}}$
$\mathbf{t}_1$	$\omega^{\mathbf{t}_1'\mathbf{a}_0}$	$\cdots$	$\omega^{\mathbf{t}_1'\mathbf{a}_i}$	$\cdots$	$\omega^{\mathbf{t}_1'\mathbf{a}_{q-1}}$
$\vdots$	$\vdots$		$\vdots$		$\vdots$
$\mathbf{t}_{q-1}$	$\omega^{\mathbf{t}_{q-1}'\mathbf{a}_0}$	$\cdots$	$\omega^{\mathbf{t}_{q-1}'\mathbf{a}_i}$	$\cdots$	$\omega^{\mathbf{t}_{q-1}'\mathbf{a}_{q-1}}$

But the entries of column $\mathbf{a}_i$ are the quantities $\mathbf{t}'\mathbf{a}_i$ as $\mathbf{t}$ ranges over $\mathbf{t}_0, \ldots, \mathbf{t}_{q-1}$, and we have

$$\mathbf{t}'(\mathbf{a}_i + \mathbf{a}_j) = \mathbf{t}'\mathbf{a}_i + \mathbf{t}'\mathbf{a}_j \quad \text{and} \quad \mathbf{t}'(c\mathbf{a}_i) = c\mathbf{t}'\mathbf{a}_i$$

for each $\mathbf{t}$, which establishes (5.46). □

It is natural to adopt the following order of the elements of V for the columns: $\mathbf{a}_0 = \mathbf{0}$ (as above), then

$$\mathbf{a}_1 = (1, 0, \ldots, 0),\ \mathbf{a}_2 = (0, 1, 0, \ldots, 0), \ldots, \mathbf{a}_k = (0, \ldots, 0, 1),$$

with $\mathbf{a}_{k+1}, \ldots, \mathbf{a}_{q-1}$ enumerated in an arbitrary but fixed order. Thus $\mathbf{a}_1, \ldots, \mathbf{a}_k$ are the standard basis of $(GF(s))^k$ (elsewhere denoted $\mathbf{e}_1, \ldots, \mathbf{e}_k$), and the elements $\mathbf{a}_{k+1}, \ldots, \mathbf{a}_{q-1}$ are linear combinations of them. This means that the first k columns of N after column I are $A_1, \ldots, A_k$, and these generate the rest of the columns by (componentwise) multiplication, just as the elements $A_1, \ldots, A_k$ generate G. Table 5.4 illustrates this for the 3^2 factorial experiment.

Now suppose that $s = p$, a prime. Then entries of $\mathbf{M}$ belong to $\mathbb{Z}/p$, and $q = p^k$. Let $\omega = e^{2\pi i/p}$, a primitive pth root of unity. Create from $\mathbf{M}$ a new $q \times q$ matrix $\mathbf{N}$ in which the entry m_{ij} is replaced by $\omega^{m_{ij}}$. This means, in particular, that the first column is a vector of ones. The result is Table 5.5. In Sect. 6.8 we will make use of the following: If $\mathbf{c_a}$ is the column for $\mathbf{a}$, then the $\mathbf{t}$-th entry of that column may be written

$$c_{\mathbf{a}}(\mathbf{t}) = \prod_{i=1}^{k} \omega^{a_i t_i} \tag{5.47}$$

where $\mathbf{a} = (a_1, \ldots, a_k)'$ and $\mathbf{t} = (t_1, \ldots, t_k)'$.

The following corollary is an immediate consequence of Theorem 5.70; its proof is left as an exercise.

Corollary 5.71 *Let* $\mathbf{N}$ *be the* $q \times q$ *matrix in the lower right of Table 5.5, and let* $\mathbf{a}_0 = \mathbf{0}$.

a. *Except for the first column, the columns of* **N** *are complex contrast vectors, and all the columns are mutually orthogonal with respect to the complex inner product (5.45).*
b. *Under componentwise multiplication, the columns form a group G' isomorphic to the effects group G. The isomorphism is the map $\psi : G \to G'$ given by*

$$\psi(g) = \textit{column } g \textit{ of } \mathbf{N}.$$

In part (a) of this corollary we are using Proposition 5.66 to relabel the column headings of the table, replacing **a** by the corresponding element g of the effects group G. This is how we displayed Table 5.4.

Corollary 5.71 was our main goal. Note that *when $p = 2$, we recover Barnard's theory for 2^k factorial experiments*, since the square root of unity is -1. In that case, of course, the contrast vectors are all real. In this sense, perhaps, the corollary is the true generalization of Barnard's idea.

It should be noted that while the corollary applies only when s is a prime p, Theorem 5.70 only assumes that s is a prime or prime power. In fact, columns of the original matrix **M** may be viewed as contrast vectors but with values in $GF(s)$, since Theorem 5.70(a) implies that the sum of each column is zero (Exercise 5.25).

Complex contrasts were studied by Bailey [7], though for different reasons. We will make use of them in Sect. 6.8.

5.7 Confounding in Arbitrary Factorial Designs

Fisher introduced the concept of confounding in 1926 [56]. Over the next decade, various *ad hoc* combinatorial methods were devised to deal with confounding in a variety of experiments. The biggest breakthrough is probably Barnard's introduction of a group-theoretic algorithm to control confounding in 2^k factorial experiments.

Barnard's 1936 paper [10] initiated a search for similar approaches for more general experiments, the earliest and most successful of which is the theory we have described in Sect. 5.6. This gives a fairly complete framework to treat symmetric experiments in which all factors have a common number of levels, this number being a prime or prime power. Numerous ways to extend these results have been proposed, and while they often provide useful results for many practical problems, no overarching method has emerged that attains the theoretical power of that in the classical symmetric case. The purpose of this section is to provide a brief introduction to some of these approaches.

One way to emulate Barnard's approach is to consider multiplying ordinary (real) contrast vectors, but as we observed earlier, this doesn't produce generalized interactions, although it does produce higher-order interactions from lower-order ones (Corollaries 5.32 and 5.33). This was not understood until the 1960s, with the work of Kurkjian and Zelen [82].

The analysis of what we have called the classical symmetric factorial experiment was developed in the decade ending in 1945. The key here was not to multiply contrast vectors, but instead to analyze spaces of blocking functions $L_{\mathbf{a}}$, and more fundamentally of vectors $\mathbf{a} \in (GF(s))^k$. If this is obvious today, it is only so in retrospect.

5.7.1 A Survey of Methods of Confounding

In this section we will briefly survey various ways that have been suggested in order to move beyond the classical case.

Modular Arithmetic in s^k Designs, s Divisible by Two or More Primes The classical case works by indexing the set of levels of each factor by the finite field $GF(s)$, which makes the set of treatment combinations a vector space over that field. By far the most common path to generalizing this is to use some other algebraic object (typically a group or a ring) as the index set for a factor.

Example 5.72 The smallest symmetric case not handled by the classical approach is the 6×6 experiment. Suppose we index the levels of the factors (say A and B) by $\mathbb{Z}/6$, the ring of integers modulo 6, and form blocks by solving equations $a_1t_1 + a_2t_2 = r \pmod 6$ for $r = 0, 1, \ldots, 5$, where a_i and t_i are in $\mathbb{Z}/6$, a_i are fixed, and t_1 and t_2 are levels of A and B, respectively.

For example, suppose we consider the solution sets of $t_1 + 2t_2 = r$. We may display the results with a 6×6 array by putting the number r in cell (t_1, t_2) if that pair satisfies that equation:

		B					
		0	1	2	3	4	5
A	0	0	2	4	0	2	4
	1	1	3	5	1	3	5
	2	2	4	0	2	4	0
	3	3	5	1	3	5	1
	4	4	0	2	4	0	2
	5	5	1	3	5	1	3

The cells containing a 0 form the principal block, which we may denote by C_0. The rest of the cells separate similarly into blocks $C_1, \ldots, C_5$, so that this blocking—call it $\mathcal{C}$—has six equal blocks, analogous to what occurs in the classical case. But here the difference emerges. Letting A_i = row i and B_j = column j, we note that

$$C_0 \cup C_2 \cup C_4 = A_0 \cup A_2 \cup A_4, \text{ and}$$

$$C_1 \cup C_3 \cup C_5 = A_1 \cup A_3 \cup A_5,$$

which means that certain block contrasts (those between $C_0 \cup C_2 \cup C_4$ and $C_1 \cup C_3 \cup C_5$) are the same as those between the "even" and "odd" rows of the array. These account for 1 degree of freedom (d.f.) confounded with A. On the other hand,

$$|C_i \cap B_j| = 1$$

for all i and j, so that Eq. (5.7) is satisfied. Thus B is unconfounded with $\mathcal{C}$-blocks. Since $\mathcal{C}$ has 6 blocks, $\dim U_{\mathcal{C}} = 5$, and so the effect $U_{\mathcal{C}}$ is the orthogonal sum of two subspaces, one (of dimension 1) a subset of the main effect U_1, the other, of dimension 4, a subset of the interaction effect U_{12}. That is, the blocking $\mathcal{C}$ confounds 4 degrees of freedom of interaction. Both the main effect of A and the $A \times B$ interaction are partly confounded with blocks.

One could similarly analyze the blocking resulting from solving $t_1 + t_2 = r \pmod 6$. The 6×6 array that this produces is actually the addition table of $\mathbb{Z}/6$, which is easily seen to be a Latin square of order 6. The corresponding partition is independent of both rows and columns, and so leaves the main effects unconfounded with blocks, and confounds 5 degrees of freedom with interaction.

It is common to imitate the multiplicative notation of the classical case by referring to the first block effect above as A^1B^2 and the second as A^1B^1, the exponents being the coefficients in the corresponding blocking function.

A complete analysis of this example can be found in [144, Table 2].

We make two observations about Example 5.72, one paralleling the classical case, the other not:

- The set of treatment combinations in the example, namely $\mathbb{Z}/6 \times \mathbb{Z}/6$, is an abelian group under componentwise addition. Moreover, $\mathbb{Z}/6 \times \mathbb{Z}/6$ admits scalar multiplication by the elements of $\mathbb{Z}/6$, which makes it a *module* over $\mathbb{Z}/6$, a module being a generalization of a vector space in which the field of scalars is replaced by a ring. An expression $a_1t_1 + a_2t_2$ defines a linear functional from $\mathbb{Z}/6 \times \mathbb{Z}/6$ to $\mathbb{Z}/6$. Finally, the principal block defined by any linear functional is a sub-group (and in fact a sub-module) of $\mathbb{Z}/6 \times \mathbb{Z}/6$, and the other five blocks are its cosets. This observation can facilitate the determination of the confounding pattern created by each linear functional.
- The ring $\mathbb{Z}/6$ is not a field: 2, 3 and 4 lack a multiplicative inverse, and they are zero-divisors (for example, $(2)(3) = 0 \pmod 6$ even though $2 \neq 0$ and $3 \neq 0$ in $\mathbb{Z}/6$.) This means, among other things, that we cannot automatically put (a_1, a_2) in monic form $(1, *)$. For example, $(3, 1)$ can't be transformed to $(1, *)$ by scalar multiplication as 3 has no inverse in $\mathbb{Z}/6$. Therefore we must distinguish the main effect A^1 from the effects A^2, A^3 and A^4, and we can't write A^2B^1 as A^1B^c. Moreover, blockings may have 6, 3, or 2 blocks, depending on the coefficients a_i.

These consequences apply more generally to any s^k factorial design if we represent the set of treatment combinations as $(Z/s)^k$.

Modular Arithmetic in Asymmetric Designs: The Chinese Remainder Theorem If we try to extend the preceding approach to asymmetric factorial experiments, a new issue emerges. For example, consider an $a \times b$ experiment. If we try to use the method above, we would associate $\mathbb{Z}/a$ to the levels of factor A and $\mathbb{Z}/b$ to B. How, then, can we perform the arithmetic operations required in the equation $a_1 t_1 + a_2 t_2 = r$? How do we define addition between $\mathbb{Z}/a$ and $\mathbb{Z}/b$, and where should r live? Similar questions apply in experiments with more than two factors.

An early and influential paper [149] by White and Hultquist suggested a method for experiments of type $a^\ell b^m$, that is, where ℓ factors have a levels and m have b levels, but where a and b are primes. The idea is to embed the rings $\mathbb{Z}/a$ and $\mathbb{Z}/b$ in a larger ring, namely $\mathbb{Z}/ab$. One solves an equation $\sum_i a_i t_i = r$ with $a_i, t_i, r \in \mathbb{Z}/ab$ and then reinterprets t_i as an element of $\mathbb{Z}/a$ or $\mathbb{Z}/b$, depending on whether factor i has a or b levels. Their result was extended by Raktoe [109] to k primes, while Sihota and Banerjee [132] extended the result in a different direction, where all the factors have either a or b levels but where a and b are just relatively prime (as in a $5 \times 5 \times 6$ experiment). These are special cases of general method of embedding rings $\mathbb{Z}/s_i$ into a larger *residue ring*, that is, a ring of the form $\mathbb{Z}/n$, as follows. Suppose that among the numbers s_i there are exactly ℓ distinct values, say $s'_1, \ldots, s'_\ell$, and that these are pairwise relatively prime. Then we have a ring isomorphism

$$\prod_{i=1}^{\ell} \mathbb{Z}/s'_i \leftrightarrow \mathbb{Z}/n, \tag{5.48}$$

where $n = \prod_i s'_i$. The isomorphism (in particular, the surjectivity of the $\leftarrow$ map) is an application of the Chinese Remainder Theorem. Such a construction was carried out in [91] by P. Lin. (The isomorphism is proved in various texts, such as [86].)

General Factorial Designs: Cosets in Product Groups How might we go beyond the previous method in an arbitrary k-factor experiment? Certainly the left-hand side of (5.48) contains an image of each $\mathbb{Z}/s'_i$ as a subring (the element $x \in \mathbb{Z}/s'_i$ corresponding to the k-tuple $(0, \ldots, 0, x, 0, \ldots, 0)$), though in general we don't have an isomorphism (5.48) with some residue ring $\mathbb{Z}/n$. But if all we really need is a principal block that is a group, we can dispense with linear equations and simply choose any additive subgroup of $\prod_{i=1}^{k} \mathbb{Z}/s_i$ as our principal block, so that it and its cosets partition the treatment combinations.[18] A method for doing this, and for calculating the resulting confounding pattern, is given by John and Dean in [76] and [41].

General Factorial Designs: Bilinear Forms in Product Groups Bailey, Gilchrist and Patterson [9] give an alternative approach that, like the Chinese Remainder Theorem methods, requires solving certain equations modulo n where n =

[18] Voss and Dean [145] call these designs *generalized cyclic*.

$\text{lcm}(s_1, \ldots, s_k)$. Here we don't require the numbers s_i to be pairwise relatively prime. The equations are of the form $[\mathbf{z}, \mathbf{t}] = r \pmod{n}$, where $\mathbf{z}$ and $\mathbf{t}$ are elements of $\prod_i \mathbb{Z}/s_i$, $[\mathbf{z}, \mathbf{t}]$ is a bilinear form (i.e., linear in each argument), and $\mathbf{t}$ represents a treatment combination. For a given $\mathbf{z}$, the different values of $[\mathbf{z}, \mathbf{t}]$ define a partition of the set of treatment combinations. The principal block, which is the solution set of $[\mathbf{z}, \mathbf{t}] = 0$, is a subgroup of the additive group of the ring $\prod_i \mathbb{Z}/s_i$ and the other blocks are its cosets. Designs of this type are called *bilinear classical* in [145].

General Factorial Designs: Combining Sub-Designs Consider an $s_1 \times \cdots \times s_k$ experiment in which each s_i is prime, with at least two s_i distinct. The factors having the same values of s_i form a sub-design, in the sense that we may view the experiment as an equireplicate, classical s_i^ℓ design if we ignore the other factors. We take a blocking of each subdesign, and form a blocking from the intersections of their blocks—the join of these blockings. If the blocking in each subdesign leaves the corresponding main effects unconfounded, then the new blocking leaves all main effects in the experiment unconfounded. The reasoning is captured in the following result. We state it for just two distinct values of s_i, without requiring them to be prime.

Proposition 5.73 *In an $s_1 \times \cdots \times s_k$ experiment with factors $A_1, \ldots, A_k$, where $s_1 = \cdots = s_j$ and $s_{j+1} = \cdots = s_k$, let $\mathcal{C}$ and $\mathcal{D}$ be blockings such that $\mathcal{C}$ depends only on the levels of factors $A_1, \ldots, A_j$ and $\mathcal{D}$ the same for factors $A_{j+1}, \ldots, A_k$. If $\mathcal{C}$ and $\mathcal{D}$ leave main effects unconfounded, then so does $\mathcal{C} \vee \mathcal{D}$.*

In order to leave main effects unconfounded, a blocking has to be independent[19] of the blockings $\mathcal{A}_i$ defined by each factor (whose blocks were described in display (5.15)). Note that $\mathcal{C} \vee \mathcal{D}$ is a refinement of both $\mathcal{C}$ and $\mathcal{D}$. Normally, refinement can destroy independence (see Problem 5.4) but in this case it doesn't!

Proof We have assumed that $\mathcal{C} < \vee_{i=1}^{j} \mathcal{A}_i$ and $\mathcal{D} < \vee_{i=j+1}^{k} \mathcal{A}_i$, in the notation of Sect. 5.3, and we know that $\vee_{i=1}^{j} \mathcal{A}_i$ and $\vee_{i=j+1}^{k} \mathcal{A}_i$ are independent. In addition, we are assuming that $\mathcal{A}_i$ and $\mathcal{C}$ are independent for all i, and similarly $\mathcal{A}_i$ and $\mathcal{D}$. To show that $\mathcal{A}_i$ is independent of $\mathcal{C} \vee \mathcal{D}$, let $A \in \mathcal{A}_i$ and let $C \cap D \in \mathcal{C} \vee \mathcal{D}$ where $C \in \mathcal{C}$ and $D \in \mathcal{D}$. If $i \leq j$, then $A \in \vee_{i=1}^{j} \mathcal{A}_i$, and thus $A \cap C \in \vee_{i=1}^{j} \mathcal{A}_i$ as well. Thus $\pi(A \cap (C \cap D)) = \pi((A \cap C) \cap D) = \pi(A \cap C)\pi(D) = \pi(A)\pi(C)\pi(D) = \pi(A)\pi(C \cap D)$. A similar argument holds if $i > j$. □

When the values of the numbers s_i are prime (or even prime powers), we may apply the classical theory to each subdesign in order to obtain a blocking that leaves main effects unconfounded, as in the following example.

Example 5.74 Consider a $3 \times 2 \times 2$ experiment with factors A, B and C. First we apply Eq. (5.7) to determine the blocksize that we would need in order to avoid

[19] Recall that independence of partitions is defined with reference to the uniform probability measure π on the set of treatment combinations.

confounding the main effects. Let D be the block of such a partition of the 12 cells. If we re-use the letter A to denote a block (a "slab", as in Fig. 2.2) determined by one level of factor A, then A and D are independent iff $|A||D| = |A \cap D||T|$, or in other words $4|D| = 12|A \cap D|$, so that $|D|$ is a multiple of 3. Similarly, if B denotes a block determined by a level of factor B, then $|B| = 6$, and so a similar computation shows that $|D|$ is even. Thus $|D|$ is a multiple of 6, and the only non-trivial blocking of this type has two blocks of size 6. We now find such a blocking.

Consider the "sub-experiment" with factors B and C—that is, the 2×2 experiment that results from ignoring A. Here the only blocking that doesn't confound the main effects of B or C is the one that confounds BC. Its blocks are $\{00, 11\}$ and $\{01, 10\}$, or $\{x00, x11, x = 0, 1, 2\}$ and $\{x01, x10, x = 0, 1, 2\}$ in the original experiment. Written out, they are:

Block 1	Block 2
000	001
011	010
100	101
111	110
200	201
211	210

There are various ways to show that this blocking doesn't confound the main effect of A—for example, it carries one degree of freedom, as does the BC interaction, so that it can *only* confound the BC interaction.

Kempthorne [79, Section 18.4.1] gives three other blockings of this experiment that he credits to Yates, claiming that they are the only ones that leave main effects unconfounded. This is not quite right. Kempthorne's three blockings indeed leave main effects unconfounded, but they are to be run in three separate replications of the experiment, in each of which the BC interaction is partly confounded. (To investigate what else is confounded with blocks, the reader is invited to try Exercise 5.29.) Each of Kempthorne's replications gives some information about the BC interaction—what we call *partial confounding*. Our blocking, on the other hand, completely confounds the BC interaction, and only that.

Example 5.75 Consider a $2^2 3^2$ experiment with factors A, B, C and D, where A and B are at 2 levels and C and D at 3, and suppose we wish to construct a blocking that leaves main effects unconfounded. As in the previous example, an easy application of Eq. (5.7) shows that the blocksizes must be multiples of 6. Let us find a blocking consisting of 6 blocks of size 6.

We may write treatment combinations as (t_1, t_2, t_3, t_4). Viewing factors A and B as constituting a 2×2 subexperiment, and C and D a 3×3 subexperiment, we will take $t_1, t_2 \in \mathbb{Z}/2$ and $t_3, t_4 \in \mathbb{Z}/3$. As in Example 14.4.1 of [43], let us choose a blocking $\mathcal{E}$ that confounds the AB and CD^2 interactions. The equations $t_1 + t_2 = 0, 1 \pmod 2$ define a blocking $\mathcal{E}_1$ consisting two blocks of size 18, while $t_3 + 2t_4 = 0, 1, 2 \pmod 3$ give us a blocking $\mathcal{E}_2$ containing 3 blocks of size 12.

Since $\mathcal{E}_1$ and $\mathcal{E}_2$ are independent (why?), we have $|E \cap F| = 6$ for all $E \in \mathcal{E}_1$, $F \in \mathcal{E}_2$, and so $\mathcal{E} = \mathcal{E}_1 \vee \mathcal{E}_2$ works.

Now $\mathcal{E}$ has 6 blocks, so it confounds 5 degrees of freedom, of which the AB interaction accounts for 1 and the CD^2 for 2. The remaining 2 degrees of freedom belong to the generalized interaction of these two (see Definition 5.6), and the notation $ABCD^2$ suggests itself for this effect.[20] A direct application of Corollary 5.32 tells us that it belongs to the $A \times B \times C \times D$ interaction. A basis for it could be given by vw_i, $i = 1, 2$, where v and w_i are functions of (t_1, t_2, t_3, t_4), v is a contrast function for AB, and w_i are independent contrast functions for CD^2.

General Factorial Designs: Pseudofactors Another approach, one that makes direct use of the analysis of classical symmetric designs, is that of *pseudofactors*. This venerable technique was described as far back as 1937 by Yates [154, Example 14b].

Example 5.76 Yates sets out the problem of designing a 4×4 experiment in blocks of 8 and blocks of 4, confounding only interactions. He starts by declaring that "[a] 4×4 design is the equivalent of a 2^4 design." In what sense does he mean this?

Let the two factors be A and B, each having levels $0, 1, \alpha, \beta$, the four elements of $GF(4)$. (Yates does not use this.) Introduce the pseudofactors A_1, A_2, B_1 and B_2, each having levels labeled 0 and 1, and make the following correspondence:

$GF(4)$	$\mathbb{Z}/2 \times \mathbb{Z}/2$
0	$(0, 0)$
1	$(0, 1)$
α	$(1, 0)$
β	$(1, 1)$

This correspondence preserves addition, if addition in $\mathbb{Z}/2 \times \mathbb{Z}/2$ is componentwise.[21] Then the treatment combination (α, β), for example, would be represented by $((1, 0), (1, 1))$, or more simply by $(1, 0, 1, 1)$, an element of $(\mathbb{Z}/2)^4$. In terms of the four pseudofactors, this 4-tuple satisfies $x_1 + x_3 = 0$, as do 7 other cells in the 4×4 experiment. The reader can check that these 8 cells are those labeled 0 in the following:

	0	1	α	β
0	0	0	1	1
1	0	0	1	1
α	1	1	0	0
β	1	1	0	0

(5.49)

[20] In [43] the confounded effect is denoted by the pair $(ABCD^2, ABC^2D)$. This notation indicates that there are 2 degrees of freedom. It doesn't describe a specific basis for the effect.

[21] The correspondence does not preserve multiplication!

Moreover, this partition corresponds to a contrast for interaction, since it is independent of rows and columns, by Eq. (5.7).

There are 14 other nonzero linear functionals $a_1x_1 + a_2x_2 + a_3x_3 + a_4x_4$ with $a_i, x_i \in \mathbb{Z}/2$. Like $x_1 + x_3$, each defines a partition of the 16 cells into two (equal) blocks, and therefore defines an effect having 1 d.f. Moreover, regarding the 16 treatment combinations as the elements of $(\mathbb{Z}/2)^4$, the classical symmetric theory implies that the partitions are pairwise independent. Thus the 15 partitions define 15 mutually orthogonal effects.

In particular, the functionals x_1, x_2 and $x_1 + x_2$ define partitions belonging to the main effect of A. This can be seen by writing down three tables like (5.49), or by noting, for example, that $a_1x_1 + a_2x_2$ takes values independent of x_3 and x_4, and therefore depends only on the levels of A. Since the main effect of A has 3 d.f., these three functionals therefore give an orthogonal decomposition of this main effect. The three functionals x_3, x_4 and $x_3 + x_4$ likewise define three partitions belonging to B and give an orthogonal decomposition of its main effect. The remaining nine functionals define nine partitions, whose effects must belong to interaction. This gives the decomposition of interaction promised in Example 5.11. But we can say a bit more.

The classical theory (using $GF(4)$) already decomposes interaction into three effects, AB, AB^α and AB^β, each having 3 degrees of freedom. The construction of the corresponding partitions of the 16 treatment combinations, carried out in Exercise 5.23, results in a set of 3 mutually orthogonal Latin squares of order 4. Consider, for example, the partition for AB. It is defined by the equations $t_1 + t_2 = r$ as r ranges over $GF(4)$, and its Latin square is simply the addition table for $GF(4)$ (see page 300). One can show (Exercise 5.27) that three of the 15 linear functionals yield an orthogonal decomposition of AB. The same holds for AB^α and AB^β. Thus pseudofactors decompose each of the effects A, B, AB, AB^α and AB^β into three further components, yielding a finer decomposition than the classical one.

The analogous result holds true in any classical s^k experiment where s is a power of a prime: Pseudofactors give a finer orthogonal decomposition of $\mathbb{R}^T$ than the classical one of Sect. 5.6.

More broadly, pseudofactors are useful in $s_1 \times \cdots \times s_k$ factorials when all the s_i are powers of the same prime. A 4×8 experiment can be analyzed as a 2^5 factorial, keeping two factors belonging to the first effect and three to the second. (These would typically be denoted A_1, A_2, B_1, B_2 and B_3 if the original factors are A and B.)

Pseudofactors can also be introduced in arbitrary $s_1 \times \cdots \times s_k$ designs, factoring each s_i into a product of primes. A $3 \times 4 \times 6$ experiment with factors A, B and C will have pseudofactors B_1, B_2 and C_1 at 2 levels and C_2 (and A) at 3 levels. In this case, the method of combining subdesigns could be used on this $2^3 3^2$ pseudofactor experiment. Care must be taken to keep track of which factor a particular pseudofactor belongs to. Examples of pseudofactor designs can be found in [43, Sections 14.3, 15.4.1, 19.7], [79, Chapter 18] and [144, Section 2.1.5].

A number of authors have described the relationships between the methods we have reviewed above (and some we haven't), indicating which are more general and which produce equivalent designs; see, for example, [145] and [146] and the references therein.

5.7.2 The Problem of Confounding

We have only scratched the surface of a rather large literature, and the reader is encouraged to look into the works we have cited, and the papers that they discuss. We will limit ourselves to some general observations.

If we look to the classical symmetric case, that is, where s, the number of levels of each factor, is a prime or a power of a prime, we see the following desirable features:

(a) The block effects defined in the theory are either main effects or components of interaction. They do not overlap both a main effect and an interaction, or two interactions.
(b) Block effects are all mutually orthogonal.
(c) Each interaction is the orthogonal sum of the components contained in it. (In the 2^k case, each interaction has only one component, namely itself.)
(c) If a single blocking is used, it is easy to identify a blocking that leaves unconfounded main effects as well as interactions up to a certain order.
(d) If more than one blocking is used, it is straightforward to determine all the effects confounded with blocks. That is, there is an algebraic way to calculate the generalized interactions of the given block effects.

What makes this work, as we've seen, is the existence of a finite field $GF(s)$ that is assigned to the s levels of each factor. The properties we've listed result directly from the arithmetic of $GF(s)$ and the linear algebra of vector spaces $(GF(s))^k$.

A general theory of confounding would ideally consider all the features of the classical case, developing them where possible and proving their impossibility where necessary. Some of the former are already addressed by the methods we have described, and from the practical point of view this may suffice. But just as the classical theory goes beyond the immediate needs of the applied statistician (it is doubtful that anyone will need to design a 121^4 experiment!), a general theory will view the subject from the theoretical perspective of combinatorics. Still, we should expect this also to have useful practical ramifications.

This research must take into account, among other things, the difference between single-replicate and multiple-replicate designs. In the former, it is essential to avoid confounding a main effect (and perhaps some low-order interactions). In the latter, by contrast, one may choose a design that confounds different effects in different replications (partial confounding) in such a way that one can still make inference about all effects of interest. In either case, it is necessary to have a theory that gives good control over confounding. We note that a naïve use of modular arithmetic can unintentionally confound a main effect, as in Exercise 5.28. (It is interesting that the examples given in [149] and [91] intentionally confound main effects, as well as an interaction in the latter, although there is no discussion of replication.)

It seems likely that a general theory will consist of different approaches to an $s_1 \times \cdots \times s_k$ experiment based on different arithmetic properties of the numbers s_i. After all, the classical case does exactly that. What these cases should be, and which are especially accessible, is not clear at present.

We confront significant combinatorial obstacles when we move away from the classical case, as we can already see in $s \times s$ experiments. For example, as is well known, one cannot construct two mutually orthogonal Latin squares of order 6 [140],[22] nor is there a full set of $s - 1$ mutually orthogonal Latin squares of order s when $s = 10$ [84]. The latter, as we know, would give a complete orthogonal decomposition of interaction, at least with uniform blocksize s. At this point, the only values of s for which such a set of Latin squares is known to exist are the classical ones, $s = p^r$ for p prime. The first open case is $s = 12$.

Certain problems appear to be beyond the reach of the approaches we've discussed. For example, it is known [24] that there are pairs of mutually orthogonal Latin squares of order 10, but simply indexing the factor levels of a 10×10 experiment by $\mathbb{Z}/10$ will not work, as indicated in Exercise 5.31.

It is notable that the approaches we have reviewed often involve some arbitrary choices. For example, in indexing a set of s factor levels there may be several nonisomorphic abelian groups of order s (for example, three of order 8), and it is not clear what it is that privileges the choice of $\mathbb{Z}/s$ aside from convenience. When a theory doesn't require a canonical choice, it should at least document the effect of different choices.

The method of pseudofactors relies on the (unique) prime decomposition of the product $s_1 \cdots s_k$, and in this respect the use of pseudofactors is unambiguous. We should note, however, that it also involves some arbitrary choices. For example, there is typically more than one way to assign values of pseudofactors to levels of the original factors, but this has only a minor effect on the design and interpretation of the model. More significantly, one might also ask whether one should resort to pseudofactors to replace a factor having $s = p^r$ levels, p prime, since one could also index those levels by $GF(s)$. Here the answer can simply be that pseudofactors provide more alternatives for decomposing interaction, as we see in Example 5.76.

It is clear that the presence of an algebraic structure in a set of treatment combinations can be extremely useful in its ability to keep track of confounding patterns. Rather than imposing such a structure, though, we might consider the possibility of allowing a particular class of experiments to suggest the algebra that is needed. This is reminiscent of the problem of coordinatizing a geometry [3]. Any attempt along these lines will make explicit use of the connections between partitions and vector spaces that we have outlined in Sects. 5.2 and 5.5.1, and in

[22] Kempthorne [79, page 358] suggests that one may simply avoid a 6×6 design by choosing to use either 5 or 7 levels for the two factors.

particular the independence of partitions, which is captured in Eq. (5.6). A modest result along these lines is given in [11], where the existence of a certain complex Hadamard matrix is shown to be sufficient for a decomposition of interaction in an $a \times p$ experiment where p is a prime.

It might be instructive to investigate the classical symmetric case in light of this approach. Here the classical theory gives us a decomposition of effects in terms of components of interaction, but it's not the only one, as we've seen in Example 5.76. We are led to ask what desired properties of an s^k experiment would force us to use $GF(s)$ to index the levels of each factor. The question for other classes of experiments is, of course, even further beyond our current knowledge.

5.8 Exercises

Section 5.1

5.1 Prove: $\sum_i 1_{D_i} = 1_D$ iff $D = \cup_i D_i$ and the D_i are pairwise disjoint.

Section 5.2

5.2 Prove Lemma A.6.

5.3 (i) Prove Lemma 5.2.

Fill in the following steps in the proof of Theorem 5.5:

(ii) Prove that $\mathcal{C} \leq \mathcal{D}$ implies $U_\mathcal{C} \subseteq U_\mathcal{D}$.

(iii) Prove that $U_{\mathcal{C}\wedge\mathcal{D}} \supseteq U_\mathcal{C} \cap U_\mathcal{D}$.

(iv) Prove Eq. (5.4).

5.4 Let $\mathcal{A}$ and $\mathcal{B}$ be independent partitions of a finite set T.

(i) Prove: If $\mathcal{A}' < \mathcal{A}$ then $\mathcal{A}'$ and $\mathcal{B}$ are independent. (The probability measure need not be uniform, although that is the intended application. The finiteness of T is included only for simplicity.)

(ii) Show by example that the implication need not hold if $\mathcal{A}' > \mathcal{A}$.

5.5 Let $\mathcal{C}$, $\mathcal{D}$ and $\mathcal{E}$ be independent partitions of a finite set T. Prove:

(i) $\mathcal{C} \vee \mathcal{D}$ and $\mathcal{E}$ are independent.

(ii) $\mathcal{C}$ and $\mathcal{E}$ are conditionally independent, given $\mathcal{D}$.

5.6 Prove Proposition 5.10. (For the last statement, count dimensions, noting that each subspace $U_\mathcal{C}$ must be a subspace of U_{12}. There are other, much quicker ways to prove this inequality; see, for example, [32, page 96].)

5.7 Prove Lemma 5.15. (Find the orthogonal expansion of $P1_S$ in terms of the indicator functions 1_{D_i}, $D_i \in \mathcal{D}$. Then specialize by letting $S = CD$.)

Section 5.3

5.8 Prove Lemma 5.17(a) and (c). For the latter, separate the cases $I \cap J = \emptyset$ and $I \cap J \neq \emptyset$.

5.9 Prove parts (b) and (c) of Theorem 5.18. For part (c) use part (b) together with Eq. (5.3), Lemma 5.17(a), and induction on I. You may find it helpful to let $x_i = s_i + 1$.

5.10 Prove Corollary 5.19.

Section 5.4

5.11 Suppose we had used the contrast vectors $(2, -1, -1, 2, -1, -1)'$ and $(1, 1, -2, 1, 1, -2)'$ to represent the main effect of B in Example 5.21. Multiply each of these componentwise with the contrast vector for A and show that the resulting vectors belong to interaction. (For instance, show that they are linear combinations of the two AB vectors in the example.)

5.12 Consider the maps

$$f : \mathbb{R}^A \to \mathbb{R}^{A \times B} \quad \text{and} \quad g : \mathbb{R}^B \to \mathbb{R}^{A \times B}$$

given by

$$f : v \mapsto v \otimes 1 \quad \text{and} \quad g : w \mapsto 1 \otimes w.$$

Prove that the maps f and g are vector space isomorphisms. That is, they are one-to-one linear transformations.

5.13 Prove Proposition 5.24, parts (a), (c) and (d). (For (c) and (d), use parts (a) and (b).)

5.14 Prove Lemmas 5.28 and 5.31. For the latter, begin by showing that if $v \in \dot{U}_I$, $w \in \dot{U}_J$, and v and w are decomposable, then $v \perp w$.

5.15 Prove Proposition 5.29.

5.16 Using the methods of this section, create a basis of contrast vectors for a $3 \times 3 \times 2$ design. Calling the factors A, B and C, use as a basis of U_A and U_B the linear and quadratic contrast vectors given by $(-1, 0, 1)$ and $(1, -2, 1)$, respectively, and for U_C the vector $(-1, 1)'$. Note: The resulting contrasts for the AB interaction are called *linear-by-linear*, *linear-by-quadratic*, *quadratic-by-linear*, and *quadratic-by-quadratic* interactions.

5.17 Prove Corollary 5.33.
5.18 Prove Corollary 5.37.

Section 5.5

5.19 Consider an $a \times b$ design.

(i) If a and b are relatively prime, use Lemma 5.7 to show that every non-trivial partition of the ab treatment combinations must at least partly confound a main effect with blocks. (Show the only blocking independent of both rows and columns is the trivial partition $\{T\}$.)
(ii) More generally, show that if the partition $\mathcal{C}$ leaves main effects unconfounded with blocks, then the blocks of $\mathcal{C}$ must be a multiple of $\text{lcm}(a, b)$, the least common multiple of a and b.

(Similar results hold with more than two factors; see Corollaries 1.1.2 and 1.1.3 of [144].)

Section 5.6

5.20 Prove Lemma 5.42. (Let $\mathbf{A}$ be the matrix whose ith column is $\mathbf{a}_i$. Then the system has the form has the form $\mathbf{A}'\mathbf{t} = \mathbf{b}$. Starting with the homogeneous case ($\mathbf{b} = \mathbf{0}$), apply well-known facts from linear algebra, in particular the Rank-plus-nullity Theorem (Theorem A.103).)
5.21 Prove Lemma 5.43. For part (d), use Lemma 5.42. Alternatively, verify that the solution sets for different values of b_i are in one-to-one correspondence, and thus have equal size; the formula s^{k-j} will then drop out.
5.22 Prove Lemma 5.61. (Lemma A.6 provides one way to go. You will need Lemma 5.50.)
5.23 Consider a 4×4 experiment with factors A and B. The classical method of this section constructs three components of interaction, denoted AB, AB^α and AB^β, where $GF(4) = \{0, 1, \alpha, \beta\}$. Find these components. That is, construct three pairwise independent partitions of the 16 cells that are also independent of rows and columns, each partition having 4 blocks of size 4. (The arithmetic of $GF(4)$ is described in Sect. A.3 of the Appendix.)

Note that the three partitions also define three mutually orthogonal Latin squares (MOLS) of order 4, the maximum number of MOLS possible according to Proposition 5.10.

Section 5.6.5

5.24 Prove Corollary 5.71. To show that the columns of **N** are orthogonal, note that the complex conjugate of a column replaces ω^j by ω^{-j}, and argue that the complex inner product of two columns is therefore simply the sum the entries of another column of **N**.

5.25 (i) We claimed in the text that in the matrix **M** in Theorem 5.70, the entries of each column sum to zero. Prove this. (Proposition A.18 may help.)

(ii) The construction of the matrix **N** in Corollary 5.70 assumed that $s = p$, a prime. But there are sth roots of unity for any positive s, and certainly for any prime power. Why could we not carry out this construction when, say, $s = 4$? (Hint: Compare the group U_4 of 4th roots of unity with the additive group of $GF(4)$.)

5.26 Letting ω be a primitive 5th root of unity, create a table of complex contrasts for a 5^2 factorial experiment. Each column should be labeled with an element of the effects group.

Section 5.7

5.27 Consider the 4×4 factorial experiment with factors A and B. (You may want to refer to Problem 5.23). As in Example 5.76, let x_1 through x_4 be variables denoting the levels (0 or 1) of four pseudofactors.

(i) As we noted in the text, the AB component turns out to be given by the partition—call it $\mathcal{C}$–defined by the addition table in $GF(4)$. Let the partition $\mathcal{D}$ be defined by the linear functional $x_1 + x_3$. Show that $\mathcal{D} < \mathcal{C}$. (Recall that this holds if the blocks of $\mathcal{D}$ are unions of the blocks of $\mathcal{C}$.)

(ii) Find the other two pseudofactor components of AB. That is, find the linear functionals of x_1 through x_4 defining them.

(iii) Show that the join[23] of any two of the pseudofactor partitions is the AB partition.

5.28 Consider a 4×4 experiment with factors A and B, but suppose we use $Z/4$ instead of $GF(4)$ to index the levels of each factor. Continue to use linear equations $a_1t_1 + a_2t_2 = r$ to define partitions of the 16 cells, but with $a_i, t_i, r \in \mathbb{Z}/4$ (so that we are solving equations modulo 4). It's easy to see, for example, that the equations $t_1 = r \pmod 4$ give the rows (levels of A), and $t_2 = r \pmod 4$ the columns.

(i) Explain why the linear functional $3a_1t_1 + 3a_2t_2$ gives the same blocking as the functional $a_1t_1 + a_2t_2$.

[23] Make sure you use our definition of the join, which is based on our order, <, of partitions.

(ii) Show that the functional $t_1 + t_2$ defines a partition belonging to interaction. (Show that the partition is independent of rows and columns.)

(iii) Consider the partition $\mathcal{C}$ defined by the functional $t_1 + 2t_2$. Show that $\mathcal{C}$ belongs neither to a main effect nor to interaction. (For the latter, show that $\mathcal{C}$ is independent of one of the main effects but not the other, so can't belong to interaction.)

5.29 We noted in Example 5.74 that Kempthorne gives three partitions of a $3 \times 2 \times 2$ experiment, each of which leaves main effects unconfounded with blocks. He lists these in [79, Table 18.5]. Consider the first:

Block 1	Block 2
000	001
011	010
101	100
110	111
201	200
210	211

Show that this partly confounds the ABC interaction as well as the BC. (For example, use the method of Sect. 5.4.2 to create contrast vectors for these interactions and show that they are not orthogonal to the contrasts between the above blocks.)

5.30 Consider a 4×6 factorial experiment with factors A and B (A having 4 levels).

(i) Use Eq. (5.7) to show that if a partition is independent of rows and columns, then it must consist of two blocks of size 12.

(ii) Use the equation again to show that each block must have three cells per row and two cells per column. Find such a partition.

(iii) Find another such partition, independent of the first.

(Note: There are 15 degrees of freedom for interaction, and each partition as above defines an effect with 1 d.f., so an orthogonal decomposition of interaction by partitions, if it exists, would require 15 pairwise independent partitions.)

5.31 The entries of the addition table modulo 10 form a Latin square of order 10. The blocks are the solution sets of the equation $t_1 + t_2 = c \pmod{10}$, $c = 0, \ldots, 9$.

(i) Show that the solution sets of the equation $t_1 + 3t_2 = c \pmod{10}$ also produce a Latin square of order 10.

(ii) Show that these two Latin squares are not orthogonal. (Consider the parities of $t_1 + t_2$ and $t_1 + 3t_2$.)

Chapter 6
Fractional Factorial Designs

Abstract This chapter asks how much of the decompositions of a full factorial design can be recovered when we observe only a subset of all treatment combinations, and what we can do to control the aliasing of effects that automatically results. As in the previous chapter, we study this both in the general setting (arbitrary fractions of arbitrary factorials) and in the special setting of regular fractions in classical symmetric factorials. In the general case we see that the *strength* of the fraction controls its aliasing and its resolution, leading to a Fundamental Theorem of Aliasing. We discuss a competing approach to aliasing and resolution based on estimability and bias, and we conclude with introductions to relative aberration and to the theory of projections.

A *fractional factorial design*, or *fraction*, is an experimental design in which observations are to be made on only a subset of treatment combinations. This is used when it is difficult, due to cost or other factors, to observe all treatment combinations. Clearly, a fractional design involves loss of information, and the main issue is to choose the fraction that retains as much important information as possible. Our first example is commonly found in introductory texts on experimental design.

Example 6.1 Consider a 2^3 experiment in which the levels of each factor are indexed by $\mathbb{Z}/2$, and suppose we can only observe half the treatment combinations. If we consider the partition that confounds the ABC interaction, we see that either

J. H. Beder, *Linear Models and Design*,
https://doi.org/10.1007/978-3-031-08176-7_6

block will do. The following table rearranges Table 2.1 to show both blocks.

cell	A	B	C	AB	AC	BC	ABC
000	1	1	1	1	1	1	1
011	1	−1	−1	−1	−1	1	1
101	−1	1	−1	−1	1	−1	1
110	−1	−1	1	1	−1	−1	1
001	1	1	−1	1	−1	−1	−1
010	1	−1	1	−1	1	−1	−1
100	−1	1	1	−1	−1	1	−1
111	−1	−1	−1	1	1	1	−1

The first block of cells is the solution set of $t_1 + t_2 + t_3 = 0 \pmod 2$, the second its complement. If we only observe responses in one block, then the mean function $\mu(t)$ is restricted to that block, and contrasts are likewise restricted to just four of the eight rows of this table. In either case, we see first of all that by observing only one block we lose all information about the ABC interaction, since its contrast is lost.

The other effects are still represented by contrasts, although only of length 4. For example, if we observe only the first block, the contrast representing the main effect of C is now

$$\mu(000) - \mu(011) - \mu(101) + \mu(110).$$

But we notice something further in this fraction, namely that the restricted contrasts for C and AB are equal. Thus there is no longer any way to distinguish the main effect of C from the AB interaction. We say that C and AB are *aliases* of each other. Similarly, A is aliased with BC and B is aliased with AC. If we were to test the hypothesis that A is absent, we would be unable to know whether the result is due to A or to BC.

We do notice that the main effects are not aliased with each other. In fact, their contrasts remain mutually orthogonal when restricted to the fraction.

It is instructive to look at the second fraction. At first glance it appears that all 6 contrasts (exclusive of ABC) are different, but in fact we notice that the restricted contrast for AB is simply the negative of that for C. Thus the hypothesis that C is absent is indistinguishable from the hypothesis that AB is absent. Similarly, the hypotheses for A and BC, or for B and AC, are the same. Thus even if two restricted contrasts differ by a scalar multiple (in this case, -1), we still consider their effects to be aliased.

Factors at 2 levels are unusual in that they are represented by single contrasts. More typical are factors at 3 levels, as in the next example.

Example 6.2 Consider the 3×3 experiment of Example 5.48, and suppose we can only observe 3 of the 9 treatment combinations. To do this, we might choose one of the blocks that confounds the AB^2 component of interaction. The following table displays the contrasts for the 9 cells, rearranged in three blocks by the value of $t_1 + 2t_2 \pmod 3$.

cell	A		B		AB		AB^2	
00	1	1	1	1	1	1	1	1
11	−1	0	−1	0	0	−1	1	1
22	0	−1	0	−1	−1	0	1	1
02	1	1	0	−1	0	−1	−1	0
10	−1	0	1	1	−1	0	−1	0
21	0	−1	−1	0	1	1	−1	0
01	1	1	−1	0	−1	0	0	−1
12	−1	0	0	−1	1	1	0	−1
20	0	−1	1	1	0	−1	0	−1

In each of the three fractions the AB^2 component of interaction is lost, while the main effects and the AB component are still described by contrasts. This is analogous to what we saw in the previous example.

In the first fraction the A, B and AB effects are described by exactly the same two contrasts, and so clearly are mutually aliased. But what about the second and third fractions?

The reader can easily verify, for example, that in each fraction the restricted contrasts for B are linear combinations of those for A, and vice versa. The same holds for AB and A or for AB and B. This of course means that the hypotheses of "no A effect", "no B effect", and "no AB effect" are indistinguishable in the fraction. We thus consider all three effects to be mutually aliased, no matter which fraction is used. That is to say, the same space (in $\mathbb{R}^3$) is spanned by the contrasts for A, for B, and for AB.

Let T be the treatment combinations in a factorial experiment. Recall[1] that we view an effect as a subspace U of contrast vectors. As we have done in Chap. 5, we will find it convenient to view vectors as functions on T. In order to define aliasing in a fraction $S \subset T$, we restrict both the mean function and the contrast functions of the full factorial experiment to the subset S. Thus we let $\tilde{u}$ be the *restriction* of u

[1] See page 39.

to S, and let

$$\tilde{U} = \{\tilde{u} : u \in U\}. \tag{6.1}$$

Since addition and scalar multiplication are defined pointwise, $\tilde{U}$ is also a subspace (of $\mathbb{R}^S$, the set of real-valued functions on S). We may refer to $\tilde{c} \in \tilde{U}$ as a constant function or a contrast function in the natural way. For example, it is a contrast function on S if $\sum_{\mathbf{t} \in S} c(\mathbf{t}) = 0$.

The Euclidean inner product of functions $\tilde{u}, \tilde{v} \in \mathbb{R}^S$ is naturally given by

$$(\tilde{u}, \tilde{v}) = \sum_{t \in S} \tilde{u}(t)\tilde{v}(t). \tag{6.2}$$

(compare equation (5.1)), and functions are orthogonal in $\mathbb{R}^S$ if this equals zero.

We have informally described some effects as "lost" in a fraction. This terminology is not standard, but it is useful to adopt it:

Definition 6.3 Let S be a fraction. We will say that the effect U is

- *preserved in S* if $\tilde{U}$ consists of contrast functions,
- *completely lost in S* if $\tilde{U}$ consists entirely of constant functions, and
- *partly lost in S* otherwise.

Definition 6.4 Let S be a fraction, and let U_1 and U_2 be effects that are preserved in S. Then U_1 and U_2 are

- *unaliased in S* if $\tilde{U}_1 \perp \tilde{U}_2$,
- *completely aliased in S* if $\tilde{U}_1 = \tilde{U}_2$, and
- *partly aliased in S* otherwise.

Following the statement of Theorem 5.18 in Sect. 5.3 we suggested writing the space $\langle 1 \rangle$ of constant functions as $U_\emptyset$, and indicated that it represented the effect of the grand mean. Of course, $\tilde{U}_\emptyset$ must also consist of constant functions (on S), and so we see that an effect U is completely lost in S if it is aliased with $U_\emptyset$. There is no standard terminology for this; we may say that U is *aliased with the mean.* In regular fractions, such effects are aliased with I (the column of ones), and so we might also say that U is *aliased with the identity.*

The central question concerning fractional designs is this: *how much of the information in the full factorial design is preserved in the fraction?* The information in the full factorial design is summarized by the ANOVA decomposition of $\mathbb{R}^T$, while the corresponding result for a fraction S is that of $\mathbb{R}^S$. Table 6.1 indicates the theorem and corollaries containing these results.

For a fraction $S \subset T$, we will let π_S be the uniform probability measure on S. Note that for $B \subset S$ we have $\pi_S(B) = |B \cap S|/|S|$, so that we may also define

$$\pi_S(B) = \pi(B|S), \tag{6.3}$$

Table 6.1 Main ANOVA theorems. In this table, a fraction of a classical symmetric design is assumed to be *regular*; see Sect. 6.1 below

	Arbitrary designs	Classical symmetric designs
Full factorial	Theorem 5.18 (Eq. (5.20))	Theorem 5.46 (Eq. (5.36))
Fraction	Corollary 6.47	Corollary 6.29

the conditional probability of B given S, where $B \subset T$ and π is the uniform measure on T given earlier (Eq. (5.5)).

6.1 Aliasing in Regular Fractions

In an s^k experiment where s is a power of a prime (what we have called a classical symmetric factorial experiment), a fraction is *regular* if it is the solution set of a family of linear equations in k variables over $GF(s)$. That is, it is one block of a confounded design. Examples 6.1 and 6.2 are regular fractions for which $s = 2$. The goal of this section, summarized in Corollary 6.10, is to describe the essential properties of regular fractions in general.

As we noted in Sect. 5.6, such a solution set is a flat in the vector space

$$T = (GF(s))^k.$$

We also continue to let

$$V = (GF(s))^k$$

when we are referring to the set of coefficient vectors in linear functionals of the form (5.31), as we did throughout Sect. 5.6.

From Lemma 5.43 we see that if a regular fraction S is the solution set of r independent linear equations, then $|S| = s^{k-r}$. We often call such a fraction an s^{k-r} *design*.

Example 6.5 Consider a 2^6 factorial design with factors A through F, where we index the factor levels by 0 and 1. The solutions $(t_1, \ldots, t_6)$ to the system

$$\left.\begin{aligned} t_1 + t_2 + t_4 &= 0 \\ t_1 + t_3 + t_5 &= 0 \\ t_2 + t_3 + t_6 &= 0 \end{aligned}\right\} \pmod 2 \qquad (6.4)$$

results in the cells of a 2^{6-3} fraction, which we record along with the restricted contrasts for main effects and a couple of interactions:

cell	A	B	C	D	E	F	DE	ABD
000000	1	1	1	1	1	1	1	1
001011	1	1	−1	1	−1	−1	−1	1
010101	1	−1	1	−1	1	−1	−1	1
011110	1	−1	−1	−1	−1	1	1	1
100110	−1	1	1	−1	−1	1	1	1
101101	−1	1	−1	−1	1	−1	−1	1
110011	−1	−1	1	1	−1	−1	−1	1
111000	−1	−1	−1	1	1	1	1	1

Note that F and DE are aliased, while ABD is lost. We will say more about the alias pattern of this fraction in Sect. 6.3.

As we will see, any other choices of the right-hand side of (6.4) would result in a 2^{6-3} fraction with the same alias structure (although ABD might be a vector of -1's). By using homogeneous equations here, we have created the *principal fraction*.

As in Sect. 5.6, for each $\mathbf{a} = (a_1, \ldots, a_k) \in V$ we let $L_{\mathbf{a}}(\mathbf{t}) = a_1t_1 + \cdots + a_kt_k$. Let S be a regular fraction, say the solution set of a linear system

$$\begin{aligned} L_{\mathbf{a}_1}(\mathbf{t}) &= b_1 \\ &\vdots \\ L_{\mathbf{a}_r}(\mathbf{t}) &= b_r \end{aligned} \tag{6.5}$$

with $\mathbf{a}_1, \ldots, \mathbf{a}_r \in V$. (This is the system (5.33) with r equations.) The elements $\mathbf{t}$ of S are solutions, not only of the equations in (6.5), but of others as well:

Proposition 6.6 *Suppose the fraction S is defined by the system (6.5), and let*

$$E = \langle\, \mathbf{a}_1, \ldots, \mathbf{a}_r \,\rangle$$

(the span of the vectors $\mathbf{a}_1, \ldots, \mathbf{a}_r$).

a. *For each nonzero $\mathbf{a} \in E$ there is an element $b \in GF(s)$ such that the equation $L_{\mathbf{a}}(\mathbf{t}) = b$ is satisfied by every $\mathbf{t} \in S$.*
b. *For any basis $\mathbf{a}_1, \ldots, \mathbf{a}_r$ of E there are elements $b_1, \ldots, b_r \in GF(s)$ such that the system (6.5) defines the same fraction S.*
c. *If an equation $L_{\mathbf{a}}(\mathbf{t}) = b$ is satisfied by every $\mathbf{t} \in S$, then $\mathbf{a} \in E$.*

Because of parts (a) and (b) of this proposition, we refer to the nonzero elements of E as *defining vectors* of the regular fraction S, and E as its *defining subspace*.

Obviously E determines S uniquely; part (c) shows that S also determines E, so that we may refer to E as "the" defining subspace of S. Part (c) is the "if" part of [98, Lemma 2.6.1(b)]. It will be essential in the proof of Theorem 6.52 (Sect. 6.5).

Proof of Proposition 6.6 As before, it is convenient to write $L_{\mathbf{a}}(\mathbf{t})$ as $\mathbf{a}'\mathbf{t}$. The proofs of (a) and (b) are left as an exercise. For (c) we first consider the homogeneous case, that is, where the constants b_i and b are zero. According to statement (b) we may assume that the vectors $\mathbf{a}_1, \ldots, \mathbf{a}_r$ are linearly independent. Then S is a subspace of T of dimension $q = k - r$, by Lemma 5.42. We must show that if $\mathbf{a}'\mathbf{t} = 0$ for all $\mathbf{t} \in S$ then $\mathbf{a} \in E$. Let $E^\dagger = \{\mathbf{a} \in V\colon \mathbf{a}'\mathbf{t} = 0 \text{ for all } \mathbf{t} \in S\}$. Certainly $E^\dagger \supset E$, and we must show equality. Since $E^\dagger$ is a subspace, it suffices to show that $\dim(E^\dagger) = r$, the dimension of E. To that end, let $\mathbf{t}_1, \ldots, \mathbf{t}_q$ be a basis of S. Then $E^\dagger$ is the solution set of the system

$$\mathbf{t}_1'\mathbf{a} = 0$$

$$\vdots$$

$$\mathbf{t}_q'\mathbf{a} = 0,$$

and another application of Lemma 5.42 (with the roles of a and t reversed) shows that $E^\dagger$ has dimension $k - q$. Of course, $k - q = k - (k - r) = r$, which proves what we wanted.[2]

In the general case, suppose S is the solution set of (6.5). Let $\mathbf{t}_0 \in S$ be a particular solution, and let $S' = S - \{\mathbf{t}_0\} = \{\mathbf{u}\colon \mathbf{u} = \mathbf{t} - \mathbf{t}_0, \mathbf{t} \in S\}$. Then S' is the solution set of the homogeneous system

$$L_{\mathbf{a}_1}(\mathbf{u}) = 0$$

$$\vdots$$

$$L_{\mathbf{a}_r}(\mathbf{u}) = 0,$$

and for all $\mathbf{u} \in S'$ we also have

$$L_{\mathbf{a}}(\mathbf{u}) = 0.$$

But by the above, this implies that $\mathbf{a} \in E$. □

Fix the linear functional $L(\mathbf{t})$. In Eq. (5.34) we introduced the partition $\mathcal{B}(L)$ of T formed by the solution sets of the equations $L(\mathbf{t}) = b$ as b varies over $GF(s)$.

[2] The proof in [98, page 37] claims (in our notation) that S and E are "orthogonal complements", where $\mathbf{a} \perp \mathbf{t}$ if $\mathbf{a}'\mathbf{t} = 0$. This is true in the sense that $S = E^\perp$ (by definition of S) and $E = S^\perp$ (by the above proof). It does *not* mean that $S \cap E = \{\mathbf{0}\}$, which may be false. The idea of a dimension argument was suggested by Rahul Mukerjee (personal communication).

Now, for any fraction S let us write

$$\mathcal{B}(L, S) = \{B \cap S : B \in \mathcal{B}(L)\}. \tag{6.6}$$

Then $\mathcal{B}(L, S)$ is a partition of S. Before laying out the properties of such partitions (Theorem 6.8 below), we need to introduce some further ideas.

Recall that we defined the equivalence relation $\sim$ on V by saying that $\mathbf{b} \sim \mathbf{a}$ iff $\mathbf{b} = c\,\mathbf{a}$ for some nonzero $c \in GF(s)$. As we noted in Remark 5.63, this says that $\mathbf{a}$ and $\mathbf{b}$ lie on the same line through the origin. We now introduce two new equivalence relations on V. First, given a subspace E of V, let us write

$$\mathbf{a} \equiv \mathbf{b} \quad \text{iff} \quad \mathbf{b} - \mathbf{a} \in E, \tag{6.7}$$

and say that $\mathbf{a}$ and $\mathbf{b}$ are *equivalent modulo* E. The equivalence classes of this relation are the flats $\mathbf{a} + E$ of V, which we may call E-flats.[3] Geometrically, $\mathbf{a} \equiv \mathbf{b}$ iff $\mathbf{a}$ and $\mathbf{b}$ are in the same E-flat (Theorem A.39).

Finally, let us introduce the relation $\cong$ on V by saying that

$$\mathbf{a} \cong \mathbf{b} \quad \text{iff} \quad \begin{array}{l} \text{there is a chain of elements } \mathbf{a} = \mathbf{a}_0, \mathbf{a}_1, \ldots, \mathbf{a}_n = \mathbf{b} \\ \text{such that for each } i, \text{ either } \mathbf{a}_i \sim \mathbf{a}_{i+1} \text{ or } \mathbf{a}_i \equiv \mathbf{a}_{i+1}. \end{array} \tag{6.8}$$

We may call n the *length* of the chain. Geometrically, then, $\mathbf{a} \cong \mathbf{b}$ if one can get from $\mathbf{a}$ to $\mathbf{b}$ by a sequence of n moves, sliding either along a line or within an E-flat. We will say that $\mathbf{a}$ and $\mathbf{b}$ are *congruent* (*with respect to* E), and refer to the equivalence classes of $\cong$ as *congruence classes*.

Lemma 6.7

a. The relation $\cong$ is an equivalence relation on V.
b. Let $\mathbf{a}, \mathbf{b} \in V$. The following are equivalent:

(i) $\mathbf{b} \equiv \mathbf{c} \sim \mathbf{a}$ for some $\mathbf{c}$.
(ii) $\mathbf{b} \sim \mathbf{d} \equiv \mathbf{a}$ for some $\mathbf{d}$.
(iii) For some $c \in GF(s)^*$ and some $\mathbf{e} \in E$ we have

$$\mathbf{b} = c\,\mathbf{a} + \mathbf{e}. \tag{6.9}$$

c. If $\mathbf{a} \cong \mathbf{b}$, then $\mathbf{a}$ and $\mathbf{b}$ are connected by a chain of length at most 2.
In particular, $\mathbf{a} \cong \mathbf{b}$ if and only if (6.9) holds for some $c \in GF(s)^*$ and some $\mathbf{e} \in E$.

[3] A favorite of Mozart.

Proof Part (a) is immediate from the fact that both $\sim$ and $\equiv$ are equivalence relations. The implications in (b) are simple and are left as an exercise.

As to (c), let $\mathbf{a} \cong \mathbf{b}$; it is obvious from the transitivity of $\sim$ and $\equiv$ that any chain connecting $\mathbf{a}$ and $\mathbf{b}$ can be replaced by one in which $\sim$ and $\equiv$ alternate. Next, we claim that chains of length 3 can be replaced by chains of length 2. For suppose $\mathbf{a} \sim \mathbf{c} \equiv \mathbf{d} \sim \mathbf{b}$. Then $\mathbf{d} = b\,\mathbf{a} + \mathbf{e}$ and $\mathbf{b} = c\,\mathbf{d}$, so $\mathbf{b} = bc\,\mathbf{a} + c\,\mathbf{e}$, and so $\mathbf{b} \equiv bc\,\mathbf{a} \sim \mathbf{a}$. A similar argument holds if $\mathbf{a} \equiv \mathbf{c} \sim \mathbf{d} \equiv \mathbf{b}$.

An alternating chain of length $n > 3$ can be reduced to one of length 2 by successively replacing chains of length 3 by chains of length 2 and by collapsing any non-alternating chains that may result at each step. This proves the first statement of (c).

We have shown that if $\mathbf{a} \cong \mathbf{b}$, then $\mathbf{a}$ and $\mathbf{b}$ are connected by a chain of length 2, and so part (b) implies that (6.9) holds. Conversely, it is easy to see that of (6.9) holds then $\mathbf{a}$ and $\mathbf{b}$ are connected by a chain of length 2. This completes the proof of (c). □

Geometrically, $\mathbf{a} \cong \mathbf{b}$ iff we can get from $\mathbf{a}$ to $\mathbf{b}$ in two moves, sliding within an E-flat and along a line through the origin, in either order.

The following proposition forms the basis for what follows. Recall (6.3), the definition of π_S.

Theorem 6.8 *Let S be a regular fraction and let E be its defining subspace.*

a. If $\mathbf{a} \in E$, then $\mathcal{B}(L_{\mathbf{a}}, S) = \{S\}$, the trivial partition.
b. If $\mathbf{a} \notin E$, then $\mathcal{B}(L_{\mathbf{a}}, S)$ consists of s equal blocks (subsets of S).
c. If $\mathbf{a} \cong \mathbf{b}$, then $\mathcal{B}(L_{\mathbf{a}}, S) = \mathcal{B}(L_{\mathbf{b}}, S)$.
d. If $\mathbf{a} \ncong \mathbf{b}$, then $\mathcal{B}(L_{\mathbf{a}}, S)$ and $\mathcal{B}(L_{\mathbf{b}}, S)$ are independent partitions of S (with respect to π_S).

In particular, blockings $\mathcal{B}(L_{\mathbf{a}}, S)$ and $\mathcal{B}(L_{\mathbf{b}}, S)$ are either equal or independent.

Proof For $\mathbf{a} \in E$, Proposition 6.6(a) implies that there is a $b \in GF(s)$ such that $L_{\mathbf{a}}(\mathbf{t}) = b$ for all $\mathbf{t} \in S$, which proves (b).

For (b), let $\mathbf{a} \notin E$, and let $\mathbf{a}_1, \ldots, \mathbf{a}_r$ be a basis of E. It is easy to see that the $r+1$ vectors $\mathbf{a}, \mathbf{a}_1, \ldots, \mathbf{a}_r$ are linearly independent, so for each $b \in GF(s)$ the solution set of the system consisting of the equation $L_{\mathbf{a}}(\mathbf{t}) = b$ together with the equations (6.5) has size s^{k-r-1}, by Lemma 5.43. Since there are s choices for b, this proves (b).

Next, if $\mathbf{a} \cong \mathbf{b}$ then $\mathbf{a} \sim \mathbf{c} \equiv \mathbf{b}$ for some $\mathbf{c}$ (Lemma 6.7), so we are reduced to the case of proving $\mathcal{B}(L_{\mathbf{a}}, S) = \mathcal{B}(L_{\mathbf{b}}, S)$ if either $\mathbf{a} \sim \mathbf{b}$ or $\mathbf{a} \equiv \mathbf{b}$. If $\mathbf{a} \sim \mathbf{b}$, then $\mathcal{B}(L_{\mathbf{a}}) = \mathcal{B}(L_{\mathbf{b}})$ (Proposition 5.44), and so the result follows by taking intersections with S. So suppose $\mathbf{a} \equiv \mathbf{b}$. Then $\mathbf{a} - \mathbf{b} \in E$, so by Proposition 6.6(a), $L_{\mathbf{a}-\mathbf{b}}$ is constant on S. But $L_{\mathbf{a}-\mathbf{b}} = L_{\mathbf{a}} - L_{\mathbf{b}}$ (Lemma 5.50), so any solution set of an equation $L_{\mathbf{a}}(\mathbf{t}) = a$ is the solution set of an equation $L_{\mathbf{b}}(\mathbf{t}) = b$, and vice versa. That is, $\mathcal{B}(L_{\mathbf{a}}, S)$ and $\mathcal{B}(L_{\mathbf{b}}, S)$ consist of the same blocks. This proves (c).

To prove (d), we first note that $\mathbf{a}$ and $\mathbf{b}$ can't both be in E, since then we would have $\mathbf{a} \equiv \mathbf{b}$, so we consider two cases: Either exactly one of $\mathbf{a}$ and $\mathbf{b}$ is in E, or neither is. We need to show that (d) holds in either case.

Suppose $\mathbf{a} \in E$ and $\mathbf{b} \notin E$. Then $\mathcal{B}(L_{\mathbf{a}}, S) = \{S\}$, as we've shown. Let $B \in \mathcal{B}(L_{\mathbf{b}}, S)$. Then $\pi_S(S \cap B) = \pi_S(B) = \pi_S(S)\pi_S(B)$, so $\mathcal{B}(L_{\mathbf{a}}, S)$ and $\mathcal{B}(L_{\mathbf{b}}, S)$ are independent partitions of S.

Now suppose that neither $\mathbf{a}$ nor $\mathbf{b}$ is in E, and let $\mathbf{a}_1, \dots, \mathbf{a}_r$ be a basis of E. We claim that $\mathbf{a}_1, \dots, \mathbf{a}_r, \mathbf{a}, \mathbf{b}$ are linearly independent. For suppose there are constants $c_1, \dots, c_r, c, d \in GF(s)$ such that

$$\sum_{i=1}^{r} c_i \mathbf{a}_i + c\mathbf{a} + d\mathbf{b} = 0.$$

If both c and d are nonzero then letting $\mathbf{e} = -\sum_i c_i \mathbf{a}_i$ we have

$$c\mathbf{a} + d\mathbf{b} = \mathbf{e} \in E,$$

so that

$$\mathbf{b} = -(c/d)\mathbf{a} + (1/d)\mathbf{e}.$$

But then $\mathbf{b} \cong \mathbf{a}$ (Lemma 6.7), a contradiction. Similarly, if exactly one of c and d is nonzero, then either $\mathbf{a}$ or $\mathbf{b}$ belongs to E, also contradicting assumptions. Thus $c = d = 0$, so that

$$\sum_i c_i \mathbf{a}_i = 0,$$

and so $c_1 = \cdots = c_r = 0$. This establishes the linear independence of $\mathbf{a}_1, \dots, \mathbf{a}_r, \mathbf{a}, \mathbf{b}$.

Now let $B_1 \in \mathcal{B}(L_{\mathbf{a}})$ and $B_2 \in \mathcal{B}(L_{\mathbf{b}})$. Then it follows from Lemma 5.43 that $|B_1 \cap S| = s^{k-r-1} = |B_2 \cap S|$ and $|B_1 \cap B_2 \cap S| = s^{k-r-2}$, so that $\pi_S(B_1) = \pi_S(B_2) = 1/s$ and $\pi_S(B_1 \cap B_2) = 1/s^2 = \pi_S(B_1)\pi_S(B_2)$. This proves (d). □

In terms of restricted contrasts, we observe the following (notation as in Sect. 5.5, $\tilde{U}$ defined as in Eq. (6.1)):

Lemma 6.9 *Let S be a fraction (not necessarily regular) of an s^k factorial experiment.*[4]

a. $\tilde{U}_{\mathcal{B}(L_{\mathbf{a}})}$ consists of constant functions (on S) iff $\mathcal{B}(L_{\mathbf{a}}, S) = \{S\}$.
b. $\tilde{U}_{\mathcal{B}(L_{\mathbf{a}})}$ consists of contrast functions (on S) iff $\mathcal{B}(L_{\mathbf{a}}, S)$ consists of s blocks of equal size.

[4] We assume, of course, that s is a prime or prime power.

Proof The partition $\mathcal{B}(L_{\mathbf{a}})$ consists of s blocks of equal size (Proposition 5.44), say $B_1, \ldots, B_s$. Any function $c \in U_{\mathcal{B}(L_{\mathbf{a}})}$ is constant on each block B_i. Thus each $\tilde{c} \in \tilde{U}_{\mathcal{B}(L_{\mathbf{a}})}$ is constant on each set $B_i \cap S$—that is, on the blocks of $\mathcal{B}(L_{\mathbf{a}}, S)$. Let us denote these constants generically by $c_1, \ldots, c_s$, so that $c(t) = c_i$ for all $t \in B_i$. Since the blocksizes are equal we have $\sum_i c_i = 0$.

Now $\mathcal{B}(L_{\mathbf{a}}, S) = \{S\}$ if and only if $S \subset B_i$ for some i (easy proof). If this holds, then for each $c \in U_{\mathcal{B}(L_{\mathbf{a}})}$ we have $c(t) \equiv c_i$ for all $t \in S$. Conversely, if it doesn't hold then there are distinct i, j such that $S \cap B_i \neq \emptyset$ and $S \cap B_j \neq \emptyset$, so that $c(t)$ takes at least two values (c_i and c_j) on S. This proves (a).

To prove (b), we note that c is a contrast function on S iff $\sum_{t \in S} c(t) = 0$. Now, for $c \in U_{\mathcal{B}(L_{\mathbf{a}})}$ we have

$$\sum_{t \in S} c(t) = \sum_i c_i |B_i \cap S|.$$

For the moment, let us write $\mathbf{c} = (c_1, \ldots, c_s)'$ and $\mathbf{d} = (d_1, \ldots, d_s)'$ where $d_i = |B_i \cap S|$, and let U be the set of all $\mathbf{c} \in \mathbb{R}^s$ such that $\sum_i c_i = 0$. Then $\sum_{t \in S} c(t) = 0$ for all $c \in U_{\mathcal{B}(L_{\mathbf{a}})}$ means that

$$\mathbf{d} \perp \mathbf{c} \text{ for all } \mathbf{c} \in U, \tag{6.10}$$

that is, if $\mathbf{d} \perp U$. But $U = \mathbf{1}^{\perp}$, the orthocomplement of $\mathbf{1}$ in $\mathbb{R}^s$, so (6.10) holds if and only if $\mathbf{d}$ is a scalar multiple of $\mathbf{1}$—in other words if and only if $d_1 = \cdots = d_s$. This proves (b). □

Lemma 6.9 will be useful to us in Sect. 6.8. With this lemma, the following is an immediate consequence of Theorem 6.8:

Corollary 6.10 *Let $U_{\mathcal{B}(L_{\mathbf{a}})}$ be the block effect for the partition $\mathcal{B}(L_{\mathbf{a}})$ of T. Let S be a regular fraction and let E be its defining subspace.*

a. If $\mathbf{a} \in E$, then $\tilde{U}_{\mathcal{B}(L_{\mathbf{a}})}$ consists of constant functions.
b. If $\mathbf{a} \notin E$, then $\tilde{U}_{\mathcal{B}(L_{\mathbf{a}})}$ consists of contrast functions.
c. If $\mathbf{a} \cong \mathbf{b}$, then $\tilde{U}_{\mathcal{B}(L_{\mathbf{a}})} = \tilde{U}_{\mathcal{B}(L_{\mathbf{b}})}$.
d. If $\mathbf{a} \not\cong \mathbf{b}$, then $\tilde{U}_{\mathcal{B}(L_{\mathbf{a}})} \perp \tilde{U}_{\mathcal{B}(L_{\mathbf{b}})}$.

In particular, $\tilde{U}_{\mathcal{B}(L_{\mathbf{a}})}$ and $\tilde{U}_{\mathcal{B}(L_{\mathbf{b}})}$ are either equal or orthogonal.

Note that part (d) follows immediately from the elementary Lemma 5.7, applied to functions on S. In the terminology that we have introduced, Corollary 6.10 says:

a. If $\mathbf{a} \in E$, then $U_{\mathcal{B}(L_{\mathbf{a}})}$ is completely lost in S.
b. If $\mathbf{a} \notin E$, then $U_{\mathcal{B}(L_{\mathbf{a}})}$ is preserved in S.
c. If $\mathbf{a} \cong \mathbf{b}$, then $U_{\mathcal{B}(L_{\mathbf{a}})}$ and $U_{\mathcal{B}(L_{\mathbf{b}})}$ are completely aliased in S.
d. If $\mathbf{a} \not\cong \mathbf{b}$, then $U_{\mathcal{B}(L_{\mathbf{a}})}$ and $U_{\mathcal{B}(L_{\mathbf{b}})}$ are unaliased in S.

Thus *in a regular fraction, two effects (main effects or components of interaction) become either completely aliased or unaliased.*

In a regular fraction of an s^k factorial experiment, some of the $(s^k - 1)/(s - 1)$ distinct effects are lost, and the rest are divided up into *alias sets*, that is, maximal sets containing mutually aliased effects. It is of interest to know how many there are of each, and how they may be computed. This is the content of the following result.

Corollary 6.11 *Let the fraction S be defined by (6.5), where $\mathbf{a}_1, \ldots, \mathbf{a}_r$ are linearly independent in V, and let $E = \langle \mathbf{a}_1, \ldots, \mathbf{a}_r \rangle$. Then:*

a. $(s^r - 1)/(s - 1)$ *effects are lost in S.*
b. For any $\mathbf{a} \in V\backslash E$, the alias set of $U_{\mathcal{B}(L_\mathbf{a})}$ contains s^r distinct effects, indexed uniquely by the vectors in $\mathbf{a} + E$.
c. There are $(s^{k-r} - 1)/(s - 1)$ alias sets in S.

The effect $U_{\mathcal{B}(L_\mathbf{a})}$ is indexed by the vector $\mathbf{a}$. As we know, the same effect could be indexed by more than one vector (i.e., by any nonzero scalar multiple of $\mathbf{a}$). By saying that a set of effects is uniquely indexed by a set of vectors, we mean that the vectors are in one-to-one correspondence with the effects.

Before launching into the proof of this corollary, we consider two quick illustrations.

Example 6.12 Let us use the linear functional $L_\mathbf{a}(t_1, t_2, t_3) = t_1 + t_2 + t_3$ to define a 1/2-fraction of a 2^3 experiment, so that $\mathbf{a} = (1, 1, 1)$. (There are two possible fractions, but either one will give the same result.) Here $T = V = (\mathbb{Z}/2)^3$ and $E = \langle (1, 1, 1) \rangle = \{(0, 0, 0), (1, 1, 1)\}$. Recalling our multiplicative notation we see that the ABC interaction is lost. Each alias set will consist of 2 effects, and we expect the number of alias sets to be $(2^{3-1} - 1)/(2 - 1) = 3$.

Of the 6 elements of $V\backslash E$ we need to choose two such that together with $(1, 1, 1)$ they form a basis of V. If we choose $(1, 0, 0)$ and $(0, 1, 0)$, then the three alias sets will be represented by them and their sum, $(1, 1, 0)$. Over $\mathbb{Z}/2$ the relation $\sim$ is trivial (the only scalars are 0 and 1), and so we need only consider the relation $\equiv$. We find (modulo 2) that

$$\begin{aligned}
(1, 0, 0) + (1, 1, 1) &= (0, 1, 1), \quad \text{so } (1, 0, 0) \equiv (0, 1, 1), \\
(0, 1, 0) + (1, 1, 1) &= (1, 0, 1), \quad \text{so } (0, 1, 0) \equiv (1, 0, 1), \\
(1, 1, 0) + (1, 1, 1) &= (0, 0, 1), \quad \text{so } (1, 1, 0) \equiv (0, 0, 1).
\end{aligned}$$

Thus the alias sets are $\{A, BC\}$, $\{B, AC\}$, and $\{C, AB\}$. This is exactly what we found in Example 6.1.

Example 6.13 We consider the 1/3-fraction of a 3^2 experiment determined by the linear functional $L(t_1, t_2) = t_1 + 2t_2$ in $\mathbb{Z}/3$. (There are three possible fractions, all giving the same alias patterns.) Now $T = V = (\mathbb{Z}/3)^2$ and $E = \langle (1, 2) \rangle = \{(0, 0), (1, 2), (2, 1)\}$. The AB^2 component of interaction is lost in the fraction, and we expect $(3^{2-1})/(3 - 1) = 1$ alias set, which may be represented by any element of $V\backslash E$, say $(1, 0)$. We verify this by finding the following (over $\mathbb{Z}/3$):

$$\begin{aligned}(1, 0) + E &= \{(1, 0), (2, 2), (0, 1)\} \\ &\sim \{(1, 0), (1, 1), (0, 1)\}\end{aligned}$$

That is, $(1, 0) \cong (0, 1) \cong (1, 1)$, so that, in our earlier notation, A, B and the interaction component AB are all aliased in the fraction. This is of course what we observed in Example 6.2.

Proof of Corollary 6.11 We proceed by determining the congruence classes of V, that is, the equivalence classes of V under the relation $\cong$. We then apply the relation $\sim$ to find the effects determined by each class.

We first observe that E itself is a congruence class. We verify this by noting that the elements of E are equivalent under $\equiv$ and thus under $\cong$, and that if $\mathbf{e} \in E$ and either $\mathbf{a} \sim \mathbf{e}$ or $\mathbf{a} \equiv \mathbf{e}$, then $\mathbf{a} \in E$. According to Corollary 6.10, the effects determined by vectors in E^*, and only those vectors, are lost in S. Lemma 5.57 now gives us (a).

For $\mathbf{a} \notin E$, the congruence class of $\mathbf{a}$ is a (disjoint) union C of E-flats, namely

$$C = \bigcup_{c \in GF(s)^*} (c\mathbf{a} + E), \tag{6.11}$$

as we see from Lemma 6.7. The effects determined by the vectors of C are the aliases of the effect $U_{\mathcal{B}(L_\mathbf{a})}$, but since C is closed under (nonzero) scalar multiplication, different vectors in C may determine the same effect. Now

$$|C| = \sum_{c \in GF(s)^*} |c\mathbf{a} + E| = \sum_{c \in GF(s)^*} |E| = (s - 1)s^r,$$

but the relation $\sim$ partitions C into $|C|/(s - 1) = s^r$ sets, each of which determines a unique effect. This establishes that the alias set of $U_{\mathcal{B}(L_\mathbf{a})}$ contains s^r effects. To conclude the proof of (b) we must show that the vectors in $\mathbf{a} + E$ index these effects uniquely. But these vectors cannot be equivalent with respect to $\sim$, for if $\mathbf{b}_1, \mathbf{b}_2 \in \mathbf{a} + E$ and $\mathbf{b}_2 = c\mathbf{b}_1$, then $(c - 1)\mathbf{b}_1 \in E$, and since $\mathbf{b}_1 \notin E$ we must have $c = 1$ and thus $\mathbf{b}_1 = \mathbf{b}_2$. Thus the elements of $\mathbf{a} + E$ represent distinct effects, and since $|\mathbf{a} + E| = |E| = s^r$, they represent all the effects in the alias set determined by $\mathbf{a}$. This establishes (b).

Finally, the number of alias sets in S is the number of sets C of form (6.11). Say this number is m. We have partitioned the s^k elements of V into E and sets of the latter form. But $|E| = s^r$ and $|C| = (s - 1)s^r$, so

$$s^k = s^r + m(s - 1)s^r = s^r(1 + m(s - 1),$$

so

$$m = (s^{k-r} - 1)/(s - 1),$$

as asserted. □

Remark 6.14 A regular fraction is defined by a system of equations of the form (6.5). It is crucially important to note that all our results, from Theorem 6.8 on, have been *independent of the particular constants* $b_1, \ldots, b_r$ of (6.5). Each of the s^r choices for these constants will determine a fraction, but *the alias structure of these fractions is the same.*

Remark 6.15 In Remark 5.63 we noted that the nonzero equivalence classes of the relation $\sim$ in the set $V = (GF(s))^k$—the lines through the origin—are the points of the *projective geometry* $PG(k-1, s)$, and thus each of the corresponding block effects, namely main effects and components of interaction, may be identified with a point in this geometry. Corollary 6.11 hints at something similar. Each nonzero element $\mathbf{a} \in E$ determines an effect that is lost in the fraction S, and if $\mathbf{b} \sim \mathbf{a}$ ($\mathbf{b} = c\mathbf{a}$) then $\mathbf{b}$ determines the same effect. Thus each line through the origin of E may be identified with one of the effects that is lost in the fraction. These lines (often called *defining pencils*) are the points of $PG(r-1, s)$. In fact, one finds regular fractions described in the literature as projective spaces; see, for example, [98, Section 2.7]. However, it would appear that use of the relation $\sim$ allows us to prove any result of interest by affine methods, so that projective geometry is not used in an essential way.

Remark 6.16 The first exposition of fractional designs and aliasing appears to be that of Finney [54], who applied Fisher's group-theoretic analysis of confounding [58, 59] and introduced the defining subgroup, discussed below. A very different approach, introduced a few years later by Box and Wilson [29], identifies aliasing with bias due to lack of fit. The relationship between these concepts of aliasing is discussed in Sect. 6.7.

6.1.1 Multiplicative Notation Again: The Defining Subgroup

In Sect. 5.6.4 we introduced the effects group G to calculate generalized interactions and to control confounding in classical symmetric factorial designs. We can use it in similar fashion to calculate aliases in regular fractions.

The group arose by writing the linear algebra of V multiplicatively, summarized in Proposition 5.66 (especially the map ϕ_2). Addition became multiplication, and scalar multiplication became exponentiation. We have already converted linear independence into the condition (5.42) in G, and the equivalence relation $\sim$ into the relation (5.43) on G. Continuing in this vein, we extend the translation:

- A subspace $E \subset V$ corresponds to a subgroup $H \subset G$ with the property that $F^c \in H$ for every $F \in H$ and $c \in GF(s)$. Such a subgroup is called a *stable subgroup*. As is common in the statistical literature, we will generally refer to H simply as a *subgroup*.[5]
- Suppose the subgroup $H \subset G$ corresponds to the subspace $E \subset V$. Then the relation (6.7) on V defines a corresponding one on G: If F_1 and F_2 are in G, then

$$F_1 \equiv F_2 \quad \text{iff} \quad F_2 F_1^{-1} \in H,$$

  and we say that F_1 and F_2 are *equivalent modulo* H. The equivalence classes of this relation are, of course, the *cosets* of H in G.

Applying these ideas specifically to the effects group G and a given regular fraction S, we then have the following:

- Corresponding to Lemma 6.7, the relation $\cong$ is defined in the obvious way: $F_1 \cong F_2$ if there is an element $F \in G$ such that $F_1 \sim F \equiv F_2$ (or, equivalently, such that $F_1 \equiv F \sim F_2$). Alternatively, this means that $F_2 = F_1^c F$ for some $F \in H$ and $c \in GF(s)^*$. When this holds, F_1 and F_2 are aliased in S.
- If $F_i \in G$ corresponds to $\mathbf{a}_i \in V, i = 1, \ldots, r$, and if $\mathbf{a}_1, \ldots, \mathbf{a}_r$ are a basis of the subspace E, then the corresponding subgroup of G is

$$H = \{F_1^{c_1} \cdots F_r^{c_r} : c_i \in GF(s)\}.$$

  If $\mathbf{a}_1, \ldots, \mathbf{a}_r$ defines a regular fraction by (6.5), then H is known as the *defining subgroup of the fraction*, and its nonzero elements are *defining words*. The words $F_1, \ldots, F_r$ are said to *generate* H. There are many choices of generators of H, but any set of independent generators of H will always have r elements ($r = \dim(E)$).

  Corollary 6.10 says that the effects represented by the elements of H are completely lost in the fraction S, while those not in H are preserved.

Corollary 6.11 gives us some useful counts, along with a recipe for finding the effects that are lost in a given fraction and for computing alias sets. We may translate this recipe into our multiplicative framework as follows. Let $F_1, \ldots, F_r$ be independent words defining the fraction, and let H be the subgroup that they generate.

a. The $(s^r - 1)/(s - 1)$ lost effects are given by the words of the form $F_1^{c_1} \cdots F_r^{c_r}$ where $(c_1, \ldots, c_r)$ is monic.

[5] If s is prime, then $GF(s) = \mathbb{Z}/s$ and all subgroups of G are stable subgroups. The adjective "stable" is necessary in other cases; see Remark 5.67. Other adjectives, such as "admissible", are also used.

b. If $F \notin H$, then the s^r effects aliased with F are given by the s^r words in the coset FH. These words are usually not all monic, but they can be reduced to monic form in the usual way (raising to an exponent in $GF(s)$).

   In order to compute the aliases of the effect F, it is typical to list the elements of H in the form of an equation

$$I = F_1 = \cdots = F_r = F_1^2 = \cdots = F_1F_2 = \cdots \tag{6.12}$$

   where we use = to mean ≡, and then to multiply through by F. Equation (6.12) is often called the *defining equation* of the fraction.[6]

c. Choose words $F_1', \ldots, F_\ell' \notin H$, $\ell = k - r$, so that $F_1, \ldots, F_r, F_1', \ldots, F_\ell'$ are independent. Then a set of unique representatives of the $(s^\ell - 1)/(s - 1)$ alias sets is the set of words of the form $(F_1')^{c_1} \cdots (F_\ell')^{c_\ell}$ where $(c_1, \ldots, c_\ell)$ is monic.

To illustrate, we begin by redoing Examples 6.12 and 6.13:

Example 6.17 In Example 6.12 we have chosen a 2^{3-1} fraction defined by ABC, so that ABC is lost. Then the defining equation is

$$I = ABC.$$

Multiplying this by A, B and C in turn and using the fact that $A^2 = B^2 = C^2 = I$ gives us

$$A = BC$$
$$B = AC$$
$$C = AB$$

This gives us the alias structure of the fraction, as we have already seen.

Example 6.18 Example 6.13 presents a 3^{2-1} design defined by AB^2, so that AB^2 is lost. Since $A^3 = B^3 = I$, so that $(AB^2)^2 = A^2B$, the defining equation is

$$I = AB^2 = A^2B$$

and so the alias set of A is

$$A = A^2B^2 = B.$$

[6] But see Remark 6.20 below.

Noting that

$$A^2B^2 \sim AB,$$

we see that A, B and the AB component of interaction are aliased in this fraction, as we saw earlier. There is no need to go further, since we have accounted for both main effects and both components of interaction. Multiplying the defining equation by B (or by AB) will lead to the same conclusion.

Example 6.13 is artificial, and the fraction is obviously undesirable as the two main effects are aliased with each other. A more realistic and reasonable example is the following, discussed briefly in [151, Section 6.4].

Example 6.19 Consider a regular 3^{5-2} design (1/9 of a 3^5 factorial experiment) generated by $F_1 = ABD^2$ and $F_2 = AB^2CE^2$.

In this fraction, $(3^2-1)/(3-1) = 4$ effects are lost. Aside from F_1 and F_2, they are

$$F_1F_2 = A^2CD^2E^2 \sim AC^2DE \quad \text{and} \quad F_1F_2^2 = B^2C^2C^2E \sim BCDE^2.$$

The defining group H has $3^2 = 9$ elements, as does each alias set. If we write H in the order $\{F_1, F_2, F_1^2, F_2^2, F_1F_2, F_1F_2^2, F_1^2F_2, F_1^2F_2^2\}$, then the defining equation is

$$\begin{aligned} I &= ABD^2 = AB^2CE^2 = A^2B^2D = A^2BC^2E \\ &= A^2CD^2E^2 = B^2C^2D^2E = BCDE^2 = AC^2DE. \end{aligned} \tag{6.13}$$

Multiplying through by A gives

$$\begin{aligned} A &= A^2BD^2 = A^2B^2CE^2 = B^2D = BC^2E \\ &= CD^2E^2 = AB^2C^2D^2E = ABCDE^2 = A^2C^2DE, \end{aligned}$$

and squaring as necessary we have

$$\begin{aligned} A &= AB^2D = ABC^2E = BD^2 = BC^2E \\ &= CD^2E^2 = AB^2C^2D^2E = ABCDE^2 = ACD^2E^2. \end{aligned}$$

Similarly, the aliases of B are

$$\begin{aligned} B &= AB^2D^2 = ACE^2 = AD^2 = ABCE^2 \\ &= AB^2C^2DE = CDE^2 = BC^2D^2E = ASBC^2DE. \end{aligned}$$

Remark 6.20 We have adopted terminology that is consistent with the underlying mathematics. In particular, we have included all defining words (not just the monic ones) in the defining equation. As we have seen, this is the equation that we need in order to compute aliases. But terminology varies in the literature. In [96] and [151] the defining equation in a 3^{k-r} design includes only reduced (i.e., monic) words, and in fact the set of monic defining words (along with I) is sometimes called the defining subgroup in [151] even though it is technically not the whole group.

Of course, this difference is irrelevant for two-level designs ($s = 2$).

6.2 The Resolution of a Regular Fraction

Example 6.21 Consider a 2^{5-1} fraction (1/2 of a 2^5 factorial experiment) with defining relation

$$I = ABCDE.$$

Here

$$\begin{aligned} A &= BCDE, \\ AB &= CDE, \end{aligned}$$

and, in general, each main effect is aliased with a 4–factor interaction, and each 2–factor interaction is aliased with a 3–factor interaction. In particular, every main effect is *un*aliased with every 2– and 3–factor interaction, and 2–factor interactions are unaliased with each other.

The defining word $ABCDE$ acts as a kind of fulcrum in these calculatons. Its length, 5, plays a direct roll:

- No p–factor effect in aliased with an effect having fewer than $5 - p$ factors.
- For each p there are effects of lengths p and $5 - p$ that *are* aliased.

We say that this fraction has resolution 5. The general definition of resolution is given below.

In the above example, every effect is represented by a word $A^{c_1} B^{c_2} \cdots F^{c_6}$ in the effects group, where $c_i = 0$ or 1, and the number of letters in the word is the number of nonzero exponents c_i. Recall that the *support* of $\mathbf{a} = (a_1, \ldots, a_k)'$ is the set

$$\text{supp}(\mathbf{a}) = \{i : a_i \neq 0\}.$$

Definition 6.22 Let $\mathbf{a} \in (GF(s))^k$. The *Hamming weight* (or *Hamming length*) of $\mathbf{a}$ is $\ell(\mathbf{a}) = |\,\text{supp}(\mathbf{a})|$.

That is, $\ell(\mathbf{a})$ (often denoted $\text{wt}(\mathbf{a})$) is the number of nonzero components of $\mathbf{a}$.

Lemma 6.23 *Let* $\mathbf{a} = (a_1, \ldots, a_k)$ *and* $\mathbf{b} = (b_1, \ldots, b_k)$ *be vectors in* $(GF(s))^k$, *and assume* $\ell(\mathbf{a}) < \ell(\mathbf{b})$. *Let* I *and* J *be the support of* $\mathbf{a}$ *and* $\mathbf{b}$, *respectively. Then*

$$\ell(\mathbf{a} + \mathbf{b}) \geq \ell(\mathbf{b}) - \ell(\mathbf{a}), \tag{6.14}$$

with equality iff $I \subset J$ *and* $a_i + b_i = 0$ *for every* $i \in I$.

Proof Certainly $\mathrm{supp}(\mathbf{a} + \mathbf{b}) \subset I \cup J$. Let

$$K = \{i : a_i \neq 0, b_i \neq 0, a_i + b_i = 0\}.$$

Then $\mathrm{supp}(\mathbf{a} + \mathbf{b}) = (I \cup J) \backslash K$, so

$$\begin{aligned} \ell(\mathbf{a} + \mathbf{b}) &= |I \cup J| - |K| \\ &= |I| + |J| - |I \cap J| - |K|. \end{aligned}$$

Given $\ell(\mathbf{a})$ and $\ell(\mathbf{b})$, this is minimized when both $|I \cap J|$ and $|K|$ are maximized. But since we have assumed $|I| < |J|$, $|I \cap J|$ is maximized iff $I \subset J$, in which case $I \cap J = I$. On the other hand, $K \subset I \cap J$, so $|K|$ is maximized iff $K = I \cap J = I$. In this case, $\min \ell(\mathbf{a} + \mathbf{b}) = |I| + |J| - |I| - |I| = |J| - |I| = \ell(\mathbf{b}) - \ell(\mathbf{a})$. □

The Hamming weight of a vector has a counterpart in the effects group. Let $F = A_1^{c_1} \cdots A_k^{c_k}$. Then the number of letters in the word F is the Hamming weight $\ell(\mathbf{c})$ where $\mathbf{c} = (c_1, \ldots, c_k)'$. We refer to this as the *wordlength* of F, and we will denote it $\ell(F)$ as well. Context will make it clear whether we are referring to a word or a vector.

Note that if $\mathbf{a} \sim \mathbf{b}$ then $\ell(\mathbf{a}) = \ell(\mathbf{b})$, and similarly

$$F_1 \sim F_2 \text{ implies } \ell(F_1) = \ell(F_2). \tag{6.15}$$

Theorem 6.24 *Let* R *be the minimum length of all the non-identity words in the defining subgroup of a regular fraction, and let* $p < R$.

a. *If* $\ell(F_1) = p$ *and* $\ell(F_2) < R - p$, *then the effects* F_1 *and* F_2 *are unaliased.*
b. *There are words* F_1 *and* F_2 *with* $\ell(F_1) = p$ *and* $\ell(F_2) = R - p$ *such that the effects* F_1 *and* F_2 *are aliased.*
c. *If* R *is even, then there are words* F_1 *and* F_2 *with* $\ell(F_1) = \ell(F_2) = R/2$ *whose effects are unaliased.*

Proof Let $F = A_1^{e_1} \cdots A_k^{e_k}$ be a defining word, and let $F_1 = A_1^{a_1} \cdots A_k^{a_k}$ have length p. Let $\mathbf{e} = (e_1 \ldots, e_k)$ and $\mathbf{a} = (a_1, \ldots, a_k)$. Then by (6.14),

$$\ell(F_1 F) = \ell(\mathbf{a} + \mathbf{e}) \geq \ell(\mathbf{e}) - \ell(\mathbf{a}) = \ell(\mathbf{e}) - p \geq R - p.$$

Therefore, if $\ell(F_2) < R - p$ then $F_2 \neq F_1 F$ for any defining word F, and so F_1 and F_2 must be unaliased. This proves (a).

To construct F_1 and F_2 as in (b), let $F = A_1^{e_1} \cdots A_k^{e_k}$ be a defining word of length R, let $\mathbf{e} = (e_1, \ldots, e_k)$, let $J = \text{supp}(\mathbf{e})$, and choose any $I \subset J$ such that $|I| = p$. Define

$$\begin{aligned} a_i &= -e_i,\ i \in I, \\ &= \quad 0 \text{ otherwise,} \end{aligned}$$

and put $\mathbf{a} = (a_1, \ldots, a_k)$. Then $\ell(\mathbf{a}) = p$, and by Lemma 6.23

$$\ell(\mathbf{a} + \mathbf{e}) = \ell(\mathbf{e}) - \ell(\mathbf{a}) = R - p.$$

Put $F_1 = A_1^{a_1} \cdots A_k^{a_k}$ and $F_2 = F_1 F$. Then F_1 and F_2 are aliased and have lengths p and $R - p$, respectively, as desired.

The proof of (c) is left as an exercise. □

Resolution was first defined by Box and Hunter [27, page 319]:

Definition 6.25 A fractional factorial design is said to have *resolution* R if no p–factor effect is aliased with another effect having fewer than $R - p$ factors.

Thus an integer R is the resolution of a given fraction if it satisfies condition (a) of Theorem 6.24. Note that according to this definition, a fraction of resolution R also has resolution R' for $R' < R$. The theorem is thus making a statement about the *maximum resolution* of a regular fraction, namely:

Corollary 6.26 *Among the non-identity words in the defining subgroup of a regular fraction, minimum wordlength = maximum resolution.*

Note that one needs to consider all the defining words of the fraction, not just its generators. By (6.15) it suffices to consider only the monic words.

Maximum resolution is typically denoted by Roman numerals, and indicated as a subscript. For example, the fraction in Example 6.21 is of type 2_V^{5-1}. The term "resolution" is often used to mean maximum resolution. Indeed, immediately before giving their definition in [27] Box and Hunter explain resolutions 3, 4 and 5 in just this way; for example, a design has resolution 5 if

> no main effect or two-factor interaction is confounded [aliased] with any other main effect or two-factor interaction, *but two-factor interactions are confounded with three-factor interactions* (emphasis added).

Example 6.27 We began Sect. 6.1 by constructing a regular 2^{6-3} fraction with factors A through F, defined by a system (6.4) of three linear equations (Example 6.5). The equations used the linear functions $t_1 + t_2 + t_4$, $t_1 + t_3 + t_5$ and $t_2 + t_3 + t_6$, so that the words ABD, ACE and BCF define the fraction. The full defining relation for the fraction is thus

$$I = ABD = ACE = BCF = BCDE = ACDF = ABEF = DEF,$$

from which we see that the design has resolution III. The defining effects are lost in the fraction, while the aliases of F, for example, are

$$F = ABDF = ACEF = BC = BCDEF = ACD = ABEF = DE.$$

as the reader can verify. (We had already observed that F and DE are aliased.) We leave it as an exercise to describe all the alias relations for this fraction.

The next example indicates how aliases and resolution are applied in practice.

Example 6.28 Consider a 2_{IV}^{4-1} fractional factorial with factors A, B, C and D and defining relation $I = ABCD$. According to Theorem 6.24, the main effects together with a subset of the two-factor interactions are mutually unaliased. In fact, the alias relations for these interactions are

$$AB = CD$$
$$AC = BD$$
$$AD = BC,$$

so $\{AB, AC, AD\}$ such a subset.

The following table presents a simulated data set in such a fraction with two observations (Y) per cell (a total of 16 observations). Note that the cell $xyzw$ satisfies $x + y + z + w = 0 \mod 2$.

cell	Y	cell	Y	cell	Y	cell	Y
0000	1.97, 1.81	0011	2.59, 1.71	0101	2.70, 1.90	0110	−0.74, 2.64
1001	−4.13, −3.78	1010	−4.16, −4.85	1100	0.02, −0.55	1111	−1.21, −0.69

The ANOVA table looks like this:

Source	SS (adj)	df	MS	F	p-value
A	71.953	1	71.9528	81.89	0.000
B	10.417	1	10.4168	11.86	0.009
C	1.351	1	1.3514	1.54	0.250
D	0.544	1	0.5439	0.62	0.454
AB	16.140	1	16.1403	18.37	0.003
AC	0.005	1	0.0053	0.01	0.940
AD	0.761	1	0.7613	0.87	0.379
Error	7.029	8	0.8786		
Total	108.201	15			

In order to omit all the aliases, *we have made the assumption that all interactions not listed are actually absent*. This is a typical practice. Note, incidentally, that the adjusted sums of squares are additive due to two things: the fact that the seven effects listed are mutually unaliased, and the balance of the design.

The example above illustrates an important way in which resolution is used: namely, to quantify how much of the ANOVA of the full factorial experiment is recovered in the fractional design. In general, how much of the ANOVA decomposition (5.36) of Theorem 5.46 can we recover? We may summarize the answer in the following result. We continue to let $T = V = (GF(s))^k$, where T is the set of treatment combinations and V is the set of coefficient vectors of linear functionals (5.31).

Corollary 6.29 *Let R be the minimum length of all the words in the defining subgroup of a regular fraction $S \subset T$. Then we have*

$$\mathbb{R}^S \supset \langle \mathbf{1} \rangle \oplus_{\mathbf{a}\in\mathcal{E}} \tilde{U}_{\mathcal{B}_{\mathbf{a}}} \quad \textit{(orthogonal sum)}, \tag{6.16}$$

where $\mathcal{B}_{\mathbf{a}} = \mathcal{B}(L_{\mathbf{a}})$ and where $\mathcal{E}$ is a set of representatives $\mathbf{a}$ of the $\sim$-equivalence classes in $V^* = V \backslash \{\mathbf{0}\}$ such that $\ell(\mathbf{a}) < R/2$.

If R is even, then there is a nonempty set $\mathcal{F}$ of representatives $\mathbf{a}$ with $\ell(\mathbf{a}) = R/2$ such that

$$\mathbb{R}^S \supset \langle \mathbf{1} \rangle \oplus_{\mathbf{a}\in\mathcal{E}} \tilde{U}_{\mathcal{B}_{\mathbf{a}}} \oplus_{\mathbf{a}\in\mathcal{F}} \tilde{U}_{\mathcal{B}_{\mathbf{a}}}. \tag{6.17}$$

The corollary asserts two things:

- In the fraction S, the effects (main effects and components of interaction) involving fewer than $R/2$ factors are unaliased, and so may be included together in an analysis of variance.
- When R is even, there is also a nonempty set of effects involving $R/2$ factors that may be included as well. (By Theorem 6.24(b) this set cannot include all such effects.)

Thus the fraction of resolution R can "*resolve*" main effects and interactions in a fraction up to order roughly $R/2$. The proof of the corollary is straightforward and is left as an exercise.

It is important to understand that we are not *really* recovering any effects from the full factorial experiment. It is only by convention that we identify a contrast $\mathbf{c}'\boldsymbol{\mu}$ with its restriction $\tilde{\mathbf{c}}'\tilde{\boldsymbol{\mu}}$. In the ANOVA table above we should probably write $\tilde{A}$ rather than A, and so on, but no one does this. It is certainly reasonable to take the restricted contrast

$$\mu(000) + \mu(011) - \mu(101) - \mu(110)$$

as a proxy for the main effect of A in the 2^{3-1} experiment of Example 6.1, since it contrasts high and low levels of A.

Remark 6.30 We make a few further comments about terminology.

1. Because of Theorem 6.24 and Corollary 6.26, it is not uncommon to *define* the resolution of a regular fraction as the minimum wordlength in the defining subgroup—see [151], for example. This raises the question of how we would extend the concept of resolution to nonregular fractional designs. We will address this question in Sect. 6.5
2. Resolution is often defined in terms of estimability of various contrasts; see, for example, [98] or [110]. *This is clearly a different meaning of resolution.* We will discuss this in Sect. 6.7.
3. Combinatorial group theorists define wordlength differently, since they count repeated letters. Thus the length of the word AB^2 would be 3 rather than 2 since $AB^2 = ABB$. This simply reflects the difference between the questions being asked by the group theorist (for whom nonabelian groups are a central interest) and those asked by the statistician.

6.3 Construction of Regular Fractions

In Example 6.5 (Sect. 6.1) we constructed a regular 2^{6-3} fraction with factors A through F, with defining words ABD, ACE and BCF. We gave its full defining relation and one of its alias sets in Example 6.27.

The fraction was constructed in a spreadsheet by creating the 64 cells of the full 2^6 factorial along with their contrasts and then extracting the 8 cells satisfying equations (6.4).[7] But after a brief look at the table in that example we note two things:

- The contrasts for A through C in this fraction are those of a complete 2^3 factorial.
- The contrasts for D through F can be constructed from A through C; for example, $D = AB$, $E = AC$ and $F = BC$.

This suggests that we could have constructed the fraction easily in two steps:

1. Create the main effect contrasts of a full 2^3 factorial. Label them A through C.
2. Create D, E and F from these using the defining relations.

This method is described in elementary texts on experimental design. One sometimes labels the last r columns to indicate the defining relations used—e.g., $D{=}AB$, $E{=}AC$ and $F{=}BC$ in this example.

Two questions arise: Does the method work in general for 2^{k-r} fractions, and if so, why? And does the method work for regular s^{k-r} fractions where $s > 2$? We will answer these questions simultaneously.

[7] The whole process was carried out in Minitab.

We start by noting that the fraction above is principal. Let's test our idea with a *non*-principal fraction using the same defining words, say that given by

$$\left.\begin{aligned} t_1 + t_2 + t_4 &= 0 \\ t_1 + t_3 + t_5 &= 1 \\ t_2 + t_3 + t_6 &= 1 \end{aligned}\right\} \pmod 2. \tag{6.18}$$

The resulting fraction is this:

cell	A	B	C	D	E	F
000011	1	1	1	1	−1	−1
001000	1	1	−1	1	1	1
010110	1	−1	1	−1	−1	1
011101	1	−1	−1	−1	1	−1
100101	−1	1	1	−1	1	−1
101110	−1	1	−1	−1	−1	1
110000	−1	−1	1	1	1	1
111011	−1	−1	−1	1	−1	−1

We still have $D = AB$ in this table, as before, but we do not quite have $E = AC$ or $F = BC$, as we did in the principal fraction. Instead, $E = -AC$ and $F = -BC$. To see why, we should solve (6.18) for t_4, t_5 and t_6:

$$D = AB \quad \text{because} \quad t_4 = t_1 + t_2 \pmod 2,$$

using the fact that $-x = x \pmod 2$. Similarly,

$$\begin{aligned} E = -AC \quad &\text{because} \quad t_5 = 1 + t_1 + t_3 \pmod 2 \\ \text{and } F = -BC \quad &\text{because} \quad t_6 = 1 + t_2 + t_3 \pmod 2. \end{aligned}$$

Thus rather than working with the effects group, we should work directly with linear equations over $\mathbb{Z}/2$, or over $GF(s)$ in the general case. This is the key.

To construct a regular s^{k-r} fraction with r defining equations, then, we go through the following steps. All constants and variables are in $GF(s)$.

1. Write down the r independent defining equations in the form (6.5), namely

$$\begin{aligned} a_{11}t_1 + \cdots + a_{1k}t_k &= b_1 \\ \vdots \qquad\qquad & \quad \vdots \\ a_{r1}t_1 + \cdots + a_{rk}t_k &= b_r, \end{aligned} \tag{6.19}$$

2. Rewrite the system (6.19) in the following form:

$$
\begin{array}{llllll}
b_{11}t_1 + \cdots + b_{1,k-r}t_{k-r} + t_{k-r+1} & & & = c_1 \\
b_{21}t_1 + \cdots + b_{2,k-r}t_{k-r} & + t_{k-r+2} & & = c_2 \\
\vdots \qquad\qquad \vdots & & \ddots & \vdots \\
b_{r1}t_1 + \cdots + b_{r,k-1}t_{k-r} & & + t_k & = c_r,
\end{array}
\tag{6.20}
$$

3. Create a complete s^p factorial design with $p = k - r$, using as symbols the elements of $GF(s)$. Display it as an array in which each row is a cell of the complete s^p design. Label the columns $t_1, \ldots, t_{k-r}$.
4. For each $j > k - r$, solve the equation for t_j in (6.20). Using this expression for t_j, compute column j from columns $t_1, \ldots, t_{k-r}$. With the additional columns, each row is a cell of the fractional design. Relabel the columns $A_1, \ldots, A_k$ if desired.

This can be done as long as Step 2 can, and it always can:

Proposition 6.31 *If the system (6.19) consists of independent equations, it can be brought into the form (6.20) by elementary row operations.*

The proof uses the familiar method of *Gaussian elimination*. In matrix form it is a sequence of elementary row operations[8] that effect the transformation

$$
\left[\begin{array}{ccc|c}
a_{11} & \cdots & a_{1k} & b_1 \\
\vdots & & \vdots & \vdots \\
a_{r1} & \cdots & a_{rk} & b_k
\end{array}\right]
\rightarrow
\left[\begin{array}{ccccc|c}
b_{11} & \cdots & b_{1,k-r} & 1 & & c_1 \\
\vdots & & \vdots & & \ddots & \vdots \\
b_{1r} & \cdots & b_{r,k-r} & & 1 & c_r
\end{array}\right]
$$

In this case the arithmetic operations are over the finite field $GF(s)$ rather than $\mathbb{R}$ or $\mathbb{C}$. Proposition 6.31 is needed merely to show that the defining equations can always be put into the form (6.20). In applications it is not usually necessary to apply Gaussian elimination in order to do this.

Example 6.32 Let us use this method to construct the 3^{4-2} fraction on factors A, B, C and D defined by the equations

$$
\left.\begin{array}{l}
t_1 + t_2 + 2t_3 = 0 \\
t_1 + 2t_2 + 2t_4 = 2
\end{array}\right\} \pmod 3.
\tag{6.21}
$$

The defining words for this fraction are ABC^2 and AB^2D^2, which we may read off from the left-hand side of (6.21). Adding t_3 to the first equation and $t_4 + 1$ to the

[8] The row operations are the interchange of two rows (equations), multiplication of a row by a nonzero constant, and replacing a row by the sum of itself and a multiple of another row.

second gives

$$\left.\begin{aligned} t_1 + \ t_2 \qquad &= t_3 \\ t_1 + 2t_2 + 1 &= t_4 \end{aligned}\right\} \text{ (mod 3).} \tag{6.22}$$

(Note how these equations reflect the aliases $C = AB$ and $D = AB^2$.) We now create the cells of a complete 3^2 factorial design in two columns, labeled t_1 and t_2, and then use (6.22) to create the columns for t_3 and t_4. The result is the following:

t_1	t_2	t_3	t_4
0	0	0	1
0	1	1	0
0	2	2	2
1	0	1	2
1	1	2	1
1	2	0	0
2	0	2	0
2	1	0	2
2	2	1	1
A	B	C	D

The 9 cells of this fraction are given by the rows of this array. The columns are relabeled A through D for clarity.

Remark 6.33 In this example, the aliases $C = AB$ and $D = AB^2$ suggest that we might be able to construct the *principal* fraction having these defining relations by multiplying columns, as we can do with regular 2^{k-r} fractions. To do this, we must introduce the cube roots of unity, namely $1, \omega$ and ω^2, as discussed in Sect. 5.6.5 ($\omega = \exp(2\pi i/3) = (-1+i\sqrt{3})/2$). We create the first two columns, labelled A and B, containing the cells of a complete 3^2 design but using these new symbols rather than 0, 1 and 2. We then create columns $C = AB$ and $D = AB^2$ by multiplication, using the fact that $\omega^3 = 1$. The reader is invited to carry this out in Exercise 6.9.

This method works for constructing s^{k-r} fractions when s is prime (in which case one indexes the levels of each factor by powers of a primitive sth root of unity).

6.4 An Unexpected Pattern

While the material in this section is of independent interest, its main result, Theorem 6.35, will be used only in Sect. 6.7, which is devoted to an alternative approach to fractional designs.

In a regular 2^{3-1} design defined by the relation $I = ABC$, the alias relations are $A = BC$, $B = AC$, and $C = AB$. Consider the full 2^3 factorial design, with its contrast columns ($+1$ assigned to level 0 and -1 to level 1 of each factor), as in Table 2.1. Adding the columns in each alias set, we find the following:

cell	I	A	B	C	AB	AC	BC	ABC	$A+BC$	$B+AC$	$C+AB$
000	1	1	1	1	1	1	1	1	2	2	2
001	1	1	1	−1	1	−1	−1	−1	0	0	0
010	1	1	−1	1	−1	1	−1	−1	0	0	0
011	1	1	−1	−1	−1	−1	1	1	2	−2	−2
100	1	−1	1	1	−1	−1	1	−1	0	0	0
101	1	−1	1	−1	−1	1	−1	1	−2	2	−2
110	1	−1	−1	1	1	−1	−1	1	−2	−2	2
111	1	−1	−1	−1	1	1	1	−1	0	0	0

Note that the three sum columns are nonzero exactly on the cells 000, 011, 101 and 110. Moreover, the nonzero cells in $A + BC$ are a contrast vector belonging the restriction of A (and of BC) to those cells, and similarly for the other two sums. In other words, adding the contrasts in a given alias set results in a contrast having two properties:

a. Its support is the principal fraction defined by $I = ABC$.
b. Restricted to that fraction, it belongs to the effects in that alias set. In fact, it is double the restriction of those contrasts to the fraction.

We leave it as an exercise to show that these sums would be supported on the non-principal fraction if we associated -1 with level 0 and $+1$ with level 1.

This pattern for regular two-level fractions has been known for a long time. It is the basis for a practice of some writers to express alias sets with expressions like $A + BC$ and $AB + CD$ (see, for example, [62]).

The idea of "summing contrasts over an alias set" has been extended to regular s^{k-r} fractions with $s \geq 3$. The extension, which we now describe, is a bit delicate. Recall that we have written $L_{\mathbf{a}}(\mathbf{t}) = a_1 t_1 + \cdots + a_k t_k$, where $a_i, t_i \in GF(s)$ (equation (5.31)). It will be convenient to express this in the form

$$L_{\mathbf{a}}(\mathbf{t}) = \mathbf{a}'\mathbf{t},$$

where $\mathbf{a} = (a_1, \ldots, a_k)'$ and $\mathbf{t} = (t_1, \ldots, t_k)'$. For each $\mathbf{a}$ the function $L_{\mathbf{a}}$ defines a blocking $\mathcal{B}(L_{\mathbf{a}})$ and a corresponding effect $U_{\mathcal{B}(L_{\mathbf{a}})}$. We continue to distinguish V, the set of coefficient vectors $\mathbf{a}$, from T, the set of treatment combinations $\mathbf{t}$, although both sets equal $(GF(s))^k$.

Let us fix the fraction S to be the set of solutions $\mathbf{t}$ to the system

$$\begin{aligned} L_{\mathbf{a}_1}(\mathbf{t}) &= 0 \\ &\vdots \\ L_{\mathbf{a}_r}(\mathbf{t}) &= 0 \end{aligned} \tag{6.23}$$

with $\mathbf{a}_1, \ldots, \mathbf{a}_r \in V$, and let $E = \langle \mathbf{a}_1, \ldots, \mathbf{a}_r \rangle$ (the span of these vectors). Thus S is a principal fraction. According to Corollary 6.11(b), if $\mathbf{a} \in V \backslash E$ then the aliases of the effect $U_{\mathcal{B}(L_{\mathbf{a}})}$ are the effects $U_{\mathcal{B}(L_{\mathbf{a}+\mathbf{b}})}$ with $\mathbf{b} \in E$. The set of elements $\mathbf{a} + \mathbf{b}$ is denoted $\mathbf{a} + E$.

Lemma 6.34 *Let S be a regular fraction given by (6.23), and let $E = \langle \mathbf{a}_1, \ldots, \mathbf{a}_r \rangle$ with $\mathbf{a}_i$ linearly independent. Fix $\mathbf{a}_0 \in V \backslash E$ and $\mathbf{t} \in T$.*

a. If $\mathbf{t} \in S$, then the value of $L_{\mathbf{a}}(\mathbf{t})$ is constant as $\mathbf{a}$ varies over $\mathbf{a}_0 + E$.
b. If $\mathbf{t} \in T \backslash S$, then the expression $L_{\mathbf{a}}(\mathbf{t})$ takes on each value in $GF(s)$ the same number (s^{r-1}) of times, as $\mathbf{a}$ varies over $\mathbf{a}_0 + E$.

Proof In both cases we use the fact that if $\mathbf{a} = \mathbf{a}_0 + \mathbf{b} \in \mathbf{a}_0 + E$ then

$$L_{\mathbf{a}}(\mathbf{t}) = L_{\mathbf{a}_0}(\mathbf{t}) + L_{\mathbf{b}}(\mathbf{t}). \tag{6.24}$$

First assume $\mathbf{t} \in S$. Then $L_{\mathbf{b}}(\mathbf{t}) = 0$ for all $\mathbf{b} \in E$, since this is true for $\mathbf{b} \in \{\mathbf{a}_1, \ldots, \mathbf{a}_r\}$ (easy proof). Thus if $\mathbf{a} \in \mathbf{a}_0 + E$ then $L_{\mathbf{a}}(\mathbf{t}) = L_{\mathbf{a}_0}(\mathbf{t})$, which establishes (a).

In proving (b) we make use of the fact that

$$L_{\mathbf{b}}(\mathbf{t}) = \mathbf{b}'\mathbf{t} = L_{\mathbf{t}}(\mathbf{b}), \tag{6.25}$$

Now $\mathbf{t} \in T \backslash S$, so in particular, $\mathbf{t} \neq \mathbf{0}$, and so Lemma 5.43(c) implies that for each $c \in GF(s)$ we have

$$|\{\mathbf{b} \in E \colon L_{\mathbf{t}}(\mathbf{b}) = c\}| = |B(L_{\mathbf{t}}, c)| = s^{r-1},$$

as $\dim E = r$. Now by (6.25) it follows that

$$|\{\mathbf{b} \in E \colon L_{\mathbf{b}}(\mathbf{t}) = c\}| = s^{r-1},$$

that is, the expression $L_{\mathbf{b}}(\mathbf{t})$ takes on each value $c \in GF(s)$ exactly s^{r-1} times as $\mathbf{b}$ ranges over E. But for any fixed c_0 the sum $c_0 + c$ takes on every value in $GF(s)$ when c does, and so by (6.24) the expression $L_{\mathbf{a}}(\mathbf{t})$ takes every value in $GF(s)$ exactly s^{r-1} times, as claimed. □

To state our main result, consider the following way of constructing a contrast function on T. Fix an enumeration $c_0, c_1, \ldots, c_{s-1}$ of the elements of $GF(s)$. Let

$\ell_0, \ell_1, \ldots, \ell_{s-1}$ be real numbers that sum to 0. Given $\mathbf{a} \in V$, define the function $c_{\mathbf{a}}(\mathbf{t})$ by

$$c_{\mathbf{a}}(\mathbf{t}) = \ell_i \quad \text{if} \quad L_{\mathbf{a}}(\mathbf{t}) = c_i. \tag{6.26}$$

That is, $c_{\mathbf{a}}$ is constant on each block of $\mathcal{B}(L_{\mathbf{a}})$, the constant being ℓ_i for some i, and is a contrast function because

$$\sum_{\mathbf{t} \in T} c_{\mathbf{a}}(\mathbf{t}) = s^{k-1} \sum_i \ell_i = 0.$$

In other words, $c_{\mathbf{a}} \in U_{\mathcal{B}(L_{\mathbf{a}})}$.

Theorem 6.35 *Let S be a regular fraction given by (6.23), let $E = \langle \mathbf{a}_1, \ldots, \mathbf{a}_r \rangle$ with $\mathbf{a}_i$ linearly independent, and let $\mathbf{a}_0 \in V \backslash E$. Fix $c_0, \ldots, c_{s-1}$ and $\ell_0, \ldots, \ell_{s-1}$ as above, and for each $\mathbf{a} \in \mathbf{a}_0 + E$ define the contrast function $c_{\mathbf{a}}$ by (6.26). Then*

$$\begin{aligned} \textstyle\sum_{\mathbf{a}} c_{\mathbf{a}}(\mathbf{t}) &= s^r c_{\mathbf{a}_0}(\mathbf{t}), \quad \mathbf{t} \in S \\ &= 0, \qquad\qquad\quad \mathbf{t} \in T \backslash S, \end{aligned}$$

summing over $\mathbf{a} \in \mathbf{a}_0 + E$.

The proof of this theorem is an application of Lemma 6.34 and is left as an exercise. It is not clear who first formulated and proved it. An early exposition is given in [33, page 104]. For a more recent statement and proof, see [45, Lemma 8.2.4] or [98, Lemma 2.4.3].

We have noted that a contrast function $c_{\mathbf{a}}$ defined by (6.26) belongs to $U_{\mathcal{B}(L_{\mathbf{a}})}$, and that each vector $\mathbf{a} \in \mathbf{a}_0 + E$ indexes an effect $U_{\mathcal{B}(L_{\mathbf{a}})}$ that is aliased with $U_{\mathcal{B}(L_{\mathbf{a}_0})}$. It is thus natural to adopt the following terminology:

- The contrast functions $c_{\mathbf{a}}$ are *aliases of the contrast function* $c_{\mathbf{a}_0}$;
- The corresponding contrast *vectors* $\mathbf{c}_{\mathbf{a}}$ are aliases of $\mathbf{c}_{\mathbf{a}_0}$;
- The contrasts $\mathbf{c}'_{\mathbf{a}}\boldsymbol{\mu}$ are aliases of $\mathbf{c}'_{\mathbf{a}_0}\boldsymbol{\mu}$;

One sometimes also refers to the indexing vector $\mathbf{a}$ as an *alias of the vector* $\mathbf{a}_0$ [98, page 26].

It is important to note just how specialized the assumptions of Theorem 6.35 are. In order to be aliased, the contrast functions $c_{\mathbf{a}}$ must take on exactly the same values $\ell_0, \ldots, \ell_{s-1}$, and must correspond to the elements $c_0, \ldots, c_{s-1} \in GF(s)$ according to equation (6.26). It is in this sense that the theorem is "summing contrasts over an alias set." The theorem does not view arbitrary functions $c \in U_{\mathcal{B}(L_{\mathbf{a}})}$ and $d \in U_{\mathcal{B}(L_{\mathbf{a}_0})}$ as aliased contrast functions.

Example 6.36 Table 6.2 illustrates Theorem 6.35 in the principal 3^{3-1} fraction defined by $t_1 + t_2 + t_3 = 0 \pmod 3$. Here we work over $GF(3) = \mathbb{Z}/3$. Now

Table 6.2 Illustration of Theorem 6.35 in the principal regular 3^{3-1} fraction with defining relation $I = ABC$, vectors $\mathbf{a}$ belonging to the alias set of A, and corresponding contrast vectors $\mathbf{c_a}$. See Example 6.36 for details.

	$\mathbf{a} =$			$\mathbf{c_a} =$			
cell	100	211	022	$\mathbf{c}_{100}$	$\mathbf{c}_{211}$	$\mathbf{c}_{022}$	sum
000	0	0	0	-3	-3	-3	-9
001	0	1	2	-3	1	2	0
002	0	2	1	-3	2	1	0
010	0	1	2	-3	1	2	0
011	0	2	1	-3	2	1	0
012	0	0	0	-3	-3	-3	-9
020	0	2	1	-3	2	1	0
021	0	0	0	-3	-3	-3	-9
022	0	1	2	-3	1	2	0
100	1	2	0	1	2	-3	0
101	1	0	2	1	-3	2	0
102	1	1	1	1	1	1	3
110	1	0	2	1	-3	2	0
111	1	1	1	1	1	1	3
112	1	2	0	1	2	-3	0
120	1	1	1	1	1	1	3
121	1	2	0	1	2	-3	0
122	1	0	2	1	-3	2	0
200	2	1	0	2	1	-3	0
201	2	2	2	2	2	2	6
202	2	0	1	2	-3	1	0
210	2	2	2	2	2	2	6
211	2	0	1	2	-3	1	0
212	2	1	0	2	1	-3	0
220	2	0	1	2	-3	1	0
221	2	1	0	2	1	-3	0
222	2	2	2	2	2	2	6

$t_1 + t_2 + t_3 = (1, 1, 1)\mathbf{t}$, so

$$E = \langle\, (1, 1, 1)' \,\rangle = \{(0, 0, 0)', (1, 1, 1)', (2, 2, 2)'\},$$

and so the aliases of the vector $\mathbf{a}_0 = (1, 0, 0)'$ (which defines the main effect of A) are $(2, 1, 1)'$ and $(0, 2, 2)'$. The table gives three contrast vectors, $\mathbf{c}_{100}$, $\mathbf{c}_{211}$ and $\mathbf{c}_{022}$, that take the values $\ell = -3, 1, 2$, corresponding respectively to the elements $c = 0, 1, 2$ of $GF(3)$. We see that $\mathbf{c}_{100} + \mathbf{c}_{211} + \mathbf{c}_{022}$ is a vector that is 3ℓ for cells $\mathbf{t}$ belonging to the fraction and zero for the other cells.

Note that the aliases of $\mathbf{a}_0$ are not in monic form: $(2, 1, 1)'$ corresponds to A^2BC, and $(0, 2, 2)'$ to B^2C^2.

6.5 Aliasing and Resolution in Arbitrary Fractions

In Sects. 6.1 and 6.2 we saw how to derive the alias structure of a regular fraction and to find its resolution. How would we extend these results to fractions of more general factorial experiments?

This question faces many of the same issues that arose in dealing with confounding, which we reviewed in Sect. 5.7. A key obstruction is the lack of systems of "components of interaction" such as that provided by finite field theory in classical symmetric experiments (Sect. 5.6).

However, we can extend the notion of resolution to arbitrary fractions without assuming any algebraic structure on T. What allows us to do this is that *we have taken care to define aliasing only in terms of contrast vectors* (Definitions 6.3 and 6.4). This allows us to apply the original definition of resolution (Definition 6.25) to such fractions. The reader should review those definitions (pages 222 and 238).[9]

6.5.1 *Restriction Maps*

The operations of restriction and projection are central to what follows. Here we deal briefly with the former.

For the moment, let T be an arbitrary set and let $S \subset T$. Recall (Sect. 5.1) that $\mathbb{R}^T$, the set of functions from T to $\mathbb{R}$, is an algebra; of course $\mathbb{R}^S$ is as well. Both $\mathbb{R}^T$ and $\mathbb{R}^S$ contain a function which is constantly 1, and we will use 1 to denote both functions.

Given $S \subset T$, let $r(v) = \tilde{v}$, where $\tilde{v}$ is the restriction of the function v to S. We call r the *restriction map* (with respect to S).

Proposition 6.37 *Let $S \subset T$. The restriction map $r : \mathbb{R}^T \to \mathbb{R}^S$ is a surjective linear transformation such that $r(uv) = r(u)r(v)$ and $r(1) = 1$.*

The proposition says that r is an *algebra homomorphism*, and that it maps $\mathbb{R}^T$ *onto* $\mathbb{R}^S$. Its proof is left as an exercise.

Of course, there is a different restriction map for each $S \subset T$, and so we should probably write r_S for the map restricting functions to S. In general we will always fix a particular subset S, and "the" restriction map r will refer to this subset.

[9] Much of the material in this section is taken from [12],[13] and [16].

6.5.2 Strength and Aliasing

Consider the following matrix (the vertical lines are inserted merely for ease of reading):

$$\begin{pmatrix} 0&1&2&3&4&5&6&7&0&1&2&3&4&5&6&7&0&1&2&3&4&5&6&7&0&1&2&3&4&5&6&7\\ 0&0&0&0&0&0&0&0&1&1&1&1&1&1&1&1&2&2&2&2&2&2&2&2&3&3&3&3&3&3&3&3\\ 0&0&1&1&2&2&3&3&1&1&2&2&3&3&0&0&2&2&3&3&0&0&1&1&3&3&0&0&1&1&2&2 \end{pmatrix}$$

The 32 columns represent the cells of a 1/4-fraction of an $8 \times 4 \times 4$ factorial experiment. The levels of the first factor are indexed by the symbols $0, 1, \ldots, 7$, and by $0, 1, 2, 3$ for the other two factors. The reader may check that the matrix satisfies the following conditions:

- The submatrix consisting of rows 1 and 2 contains one copy of a complete 8×4 factorial design. The same holds for rows 1 and 3.
- The submatrix consisting of rows 2 and 3 contains two copies of a complete 4×4 design.

This matrix, and the fractional design it represents, is said to have strength 2. Each submatrix is said to be the projection of the design on two of the three factors. The matrix is referred to as an *orthogonal array*.

Consider a factorial experiment with treatment combinations $T = A_1 \times \cdots \times A_k$, and a fractional design $S \subset T$. If we write the elements of a design S as columns, then we may represent S as a $k \times N$ orthogonal array O. The *projection* of O on j factors is the $j \times N$ submatrix consisting of the rows corresponding to those factors. As in our example, this submatrix may have repeated columns. Thus it is natural to define an *orthogonal array* to be a *subset of* $A_1 \times \cdots \times A_k$ *with repeated columns*, so that the projection of an orthogonal array is an orthogonal array.

Definition 6.38 Let O be an orthogonal array on $A_1 \times \cdots \times A_k$. We say that O has *strength* $t \geq 1$ if for any subsequence $I = \{i_1, \ldots, i_t\} \subset \{1, \ldots, k\}$ of size t there is a positive integer λ_I such that the projection of O on the factors indexed by I consists of λ_I copies of the Cartesian product $A_{i_1} \times \cdots \times A_{i_t}$. We say that the fraction S has *strength* t if the corresponding array O does.

In particular, a Cartesian product (that is, a full factorial design) with m factors has strength t for all $t \leq m$. It follows easily that if S has strength t then it has strength t' for every $t' < t$. We will usually be interested in the *maximum* strength of a fraction. A fraction not having strength 1 will be said to have strength 0.

It follows from Definition 6.38 that if S is a fraction of size N and strength $t \geq 1$ then for each I of size t we have

$$N = \lambda_I \prod_{i \in I} s_i .$$

Table 6.3 A 16-run orthogonal array of strength 2. Elements are the columns. Of the 12 distinct ordered quadruples, four appear twice. See Remark 6.39 for details

0	0	1	1	1	1	0	0	0	0	0	0	1	1	1	1
0	0	0	0	1	1	1	1	0	0	1	1	0	0	1	1
0	0	1	1	0	0	1	1	0	1	0	1	0	1	0	1
0	1	0	1	0	1	0	1	0	0	1	1	1	1	0	0

In the symmetric case ($s_i = s$ for all i), $N = \lambda_I s^t$ for every I of size t, so that λ_I is the same for all such I. The common value $\lambda = N/s^t$ is called the *index* of the orthogonal array.

Remark 6.39 The combinatorial parameter *strength* was introduced by Rao [111] for symmetric factorial designs and extended by him to arbitrary factorials in [114]. He initially referred to fractions as *arrays*. The term *orthogonal array* was introduced soon after, and is used in a more general way to allow the k-tuples to repeat.[10] We have chosen to represent such arrays as $k \times N$ matrices for ease of presentation, but many authors write them as $N \times k$ matrices. In either case, the k-tuples are often called the *runs* of the design, and N counts the number of runs including multiplicities. For a given orthogonal array, the nonnegative function

$$O(\mathbf{t}) = \text{the number of times } \mathbf{t} \text{ appears in the array}$$

is called the *counting function* (or, sometimes, the *indicator function*) of the array, so that $N = \sum_{\mathbf{t} \in T} O(\mathbf{t})$.

We have reserved the term *fraction* for orthogonal arrays that are ordinary subsets; for these, $O(\mathbf{t}) = 0$ or 1. These are also called *simple* orthogonal arrays. The arrays in Rao's original paper [111] are simple.

An orthogonal array is called *symmetric* if $s_i = s$ for all i, and otherwise *asymmetric* or *mixed-level*. In the symmetric case, one typically assumes that the sets of levels A_k are all the same, so that the array has just s symbols.

Table 6.3 displays an orthogonal array with 16 runs based on 4 factors, each having 2 levels. The array has strength 2, and is the juxtaposition of two 2^{4-1} fractions of strength 2, having defining relations $I = ABC$ and $I = ABD$, respectively. It is not hard to see that the juxtaposition of two orthogonal arrays on k factors at s levels and strength t_1 and t_2 is an orthogonal array of strength $t \geq \min(t_1, t_2)$ (Exercise 6.15). For the array in Table 6.3, $O(0000) = 2$, $O(0001) = 1$, and $O(1111) = 0$.

A standard reference on orthogonal arrays is [72].

[10] A set in which each element is repeated with some multiplicity is called a *multiset*. A subset of a set T in which each element is repeated is called a *multisubset* of T. Thus an orthogonal array is a multisubset of a set $A_1 \times \cdots \times A_k$. As with arrays, a multiset has a counting function.

There is a matrix-free way to describe strength that will be useful for us. For each $I = \{i_1, \ldots, i_m\} \subset \{1, \ldots, k\}$, $i_1 < \cdots < i_m$, there is a *projection map*

$$P_I\colon A_1 \times \cdots \times A_k \to A_{i_1} \times \cdots \times A_{i_m}$$

such that

$$(t_1, \ldots, t_k) \mapsto (t_{i_1}, \ldots, t_{i_m}). \tag{6.27}$$

Then another way to say that the fraction $S \subset A_1 \times \cdots \times A_k$ has strength t is to say that *if* $I = \{i_1, \ldots, i_t\}$ *then the projection map* P_I*, restricted to* S*, is a* λ_I*-to-1 map onto* $A_{i_1} \times \cdots \times A_{i_t}$.

Recall the definition of the join $\vee_{i\in I}\mathcal{A}_i$ of a set of partitions $\mathcal{A}_i$, where $\mathcal{A}_i$ consists of the blocks determined by the levels of the ith factor (Sect. 5.3). It will be convenient to introduce the symbol $\perp\!\!\!\perp$ to denote independence with respect to the uniform probability measure π on T (the measure was introduced in Sect. 5.2). If $\mathcal{C}$ is a partition of T, then $S \perp\!\!\!\perp \mathcal{C}$ means that $S \perp\!\!\!\perp C$ for every $C \in \mathcal{C}$.

Proposition 6.40 *Let* $T = A_1 \times \cdots \times A_k$ *and* $S \subset T$*, and let* π *be the uniform probability measure on* T*. Then* S *has strength* t *iff* $S \perp\!\!\!\perp \vee_{i\in I}\mathcal{A}_i$ *for every* $I \subset \{1, \ldots, k\}$ *of size* t*.*

Proof Assume that S has strength t. We must show that $\pi(S \cap C) = \pi(S)\pi(C)$, or equivalently

$$|S \cap C||T| = |S||C|, \tag{6.28}$$

for every I of size t and every block $C \in \vee_{i\in I}\mathcal{A}_i$.

Fix $I = \{i_1, \ldots, i_t\}$. It is easy to see that the *level sets* of the projection map P_I are precisely the blocks of $\vee_{i\in I}\mathcal{A}_i$. For consider $\mathbf{r} = (r_1, \ldots, r_t) \in A_{i_1} \times \cdots \times A_{i_t}$; the inverse image of $\mathbf{r}$ is a set C of the form $B_1 \times \cdots \times B_k$ where the sets B_i are exactly of the form (5.16), and every block $C \in \vee_{i\in I}\mathcal{A}_i$ arises in this way. From (5.16) we have $|C| = \prod_{i\in I^c} s_i$.

On the other hand, if S has strength t then the number of pre-images of $\mathbf{r}$ that lie in S is precisely λ_I, since P_I is λ_I-to-1 on S. The set of such pre-images is $S \cap C$, so that $|S \cap C| = \lambda_I$.

We have already established that $|S| = \lambda_I \prod_{i\in I} s_i$, and of course $|T| = \prod_{i=1}^k s_i$. But then $|S \cap C||T| = \lambda_I \prod_{i=1}^k s_i = \lambda_I \prod_{i\in I} s_i \prod_{i\in I^c} s_i = |S||C|$, which establishes (6.28).

Conversely, fix $S \subset T$, and suppose that (6.28) holds for every $I \subset \{1, \ldots, k\}$ of size t and every block $C \in \vee_{i\in I}\mathcal{A}_i$. To show that t = the strength of S, it suffices to show that P_I maps S onto $A_{i_1} \times \cdots \times A_{i_t}$ in λ-to-1 manner for some λ. Now fix I, so that the terms $|T|$, $|S|$ and $|C|$ in (6.28) are fixed (the blocks C all have the same size). Then $\lambda = |S \cap C|$ is the same for every block C, and is nonzero. Since it is nonzero, $S \cap C \neq \emptyset$. But every $\mathbf{r} \in A_{i_1} \times \cdots \times A_{i_t}$ determines a block C, and since $S \cap C \neq \emptyset$ we see that every such $\mathbf{r}$ has a pre-image in S. On the other hand, P_I maps the elements of C, and in particular the elements of $S \cap C$, onto a single element of $A_{i_1} \times \cdots \times A_{i_t}$, and $S = \cup_C (S \cap C)$ (disjoint union), so P_I indeed maps S onto $A_{i_1} \times \cdots \times A_{i_t}$ in a λ-to-1 manner, as claimed. □

We note that if $\mathcal{C}$ is a partition of T, then

$$S \perp\!\!\!\perp \mathcal{C} \quad \text{iff} \quad S \perp\!\!\!\perp B \text{ whenever } B \text{ is a union of blocks of } \mathcal{C}. \tag{6.29}$$

Since $J \subset I$ implies $\vee_{i \in J} \mathcal{A}_i < \vee_{i \in I} \mathcal{A}_i$ (in the sense of *refinement*), it follows from (6.29) that $S \perp\!\!\!\perp \vee_{i \in I} \mathcal{A}_i$ implies $S \perp\!\!\!\perp \vee_{i \in J} \mathcal{A}_i$. This gives another proof that if S has strength t then it has strength t' for every $t' < t$.

Rao's primary goal in [111] and [114] was to recover as much as possible of Theorem 5.18 in the fraction S, and that is our next goal as well. For the moment let T be an arbitrary finite set. As in Sect. 5.2 we put

$$M_{\mathcal{C}} = \{w \in \mathbb{R}^T \colon w \text{ is constant on each block of } \mathcal{C}\}$$

for any partition $\mathcal{C}$ of T. (We referred to $M_{\mathcal{C}}$ as the *incidence space* of $\mathcal{C}$.) Then $w \in M_{\mathcal{C}}$ iff $w^{-1}(y)$ is a union of blocks of $\mathcal{C}$ for any $y \in \mathbb{R}$.

Lemma 6.41 *Let T be finite, $S \subset T$, and $\mathcal{C}$ a partition of T such that $S \perp\!\!\!\perp \mathcal{C}$. If $w \in M_{\mathcal{C}}$, then $\sum_{s \in S} w(s) = \pi(S) \sum_{s \in T} w(s)$.*

Proof Let the range of w be $\{y_1, \ldots y_m\}$, and let $A_j = w^{-1}(y_j)$. Then A_j is a union of blocks of $\mathcal{C}$, and so

$$\begin{aligned}\sum_{s \in S} w(s) &= \sum_{j=1}^{m} \sum_{s \in S \cap A_j} w(s) = \sum_{j=1}^{m} y_j |S \cap A_j| = \sum_{j=1}^{m} y_j\, \pi(S \cap A_j)\, |T| \\ &= \sum_{j=1}^{m} y_j\, \pi(S) \pi(A_j)\, |T| = \pi(S) \sum_{j=1}^{m} y_j |A_j| = \pi(S) \sum_{s \in T} w(s).\end{aligned}$$

□

Recall the (Euclidean) inner product of functions, (u, v), given by equation (5.1), and the definition of the restriction map in Sect. 6.5.1.

Proposition 6.42 *Let T be finite, $S \subset T$, and $\mathcal{C}$ a partition of T such that $S \perp\!\!\!\perp \mathcal{C}$. Then the restriction map r*

a. preserves orthogonality on $M_{\mathcal{C}}$. More precisely, if $u, v \in M_{\mathcal{C}}$ then $r(u) \perp r(v)$ (in $\mathbb{R}^S$) iff $u \perp v$ (in $\mathbb{R}^T$).
b. maps $M_{\mathcal{C}}$ one-to-one into $\mathbb{R}^S$.

Proof Applying the lemma to the pointwise product $w = uv$, we see that

$$(r(u), r(v)) = \pi(S)(u, v) \tag{6.30}$$

for all $u, v \in M_{\mathcal{C}}$ (inner products in $\mathbb{R}^S$ and $\mathbb{R}^T$, respectively). Thus $r(u) \perp r(v)$ iff $u \perp v$, as claimed. Moreover, from (6.30) we have in particular that $\|u\|^2 = \|r(u)\|^2/\pi(S)$ (norms respectively in $\mathbb{R}^T$ and $\mathbb{R}^S$). But then $u = 0$ if (and only if) $r(u) = 0$, and so r, viewed as a linear transformation on the vector space $M_{\mathcal{C}}$, has trivial nullspace. In other words, r is one-to-one on $M_{\mathcal{C}}$. □

The next result is the analog of part (a) of Theorem 5.18, and is fundamental to all that follows.

Theorem 6.43 (Fundamental Theorem of Aliasing) *Let $T = A_1 \times \cdots \times A_k$, and let $S \subset T$ be a fraction of strength $t \geq 1$. Let $I, J \subset \{1, \ldots, k\}$ with $|I \cup J| \leq t$. If $I \neq J$, then $\tilde{U}_I \perp \tilde{U}_J$.*

If $1 \leq |I| \leq t$ then $\tilde{U}_I$ consists of contrast functions.

Proof The general statement follows from Theorem 5.18(a) and Proposition 6.42(a) by taking $\mathcal{C} = \vee_{i \in I \cup J} \mathcal{A}_i$. The second statement follows by applying Proposition 6.42(a) to $M_{\mathcal{C}}$ where $\mathcal{C} = \vee_{i \in I} \mathcal{A}_i$ and noting that $U_I \subset M_{\mathcal{C}}$, $1 \in M_{\mathcal{C}}$, and $U_I \perp 1$. □

Example 6.44 Consider a fraction S of strength 5 in a factorial experiment with factors A, B, C, D, E, F. Here all 4-factor interactions are unaliased in S with every main effect. The $A \times B \times C \times D \times E$ interaction is unaliased with the main effects of A, B, C, D and E, though it may be aliased with the main effect of F.

Theorem 6.43 says that the effects U_I and U_J are unaliased in the fraction S as long as $|I \cup J|$ does not exceed the strength of S. If $|I|$ and $|J|$ are nearly equal then, roughly speaking, the strength of S has to be twice $|I|$ to guarantee that the orthogonality of U_I and U_J is preserved in the fraction. The next corollary spells this out (the proof is left as an exercise). We denote by $[x]$ the greatest integer not exceeding x.

Corollary 6.45 *Assuming the conditions of Theorem 6.43, let $e = [t/2]$, and let I and J be distinct subsets of $\{1, \ldots, k\}$. Then any of the following conditions implies that $\tilde{U}_I \perp \tilde{U}_J$:*

a. $|I| \leq e$ and $|J| \leq e$.
b. t is odd ($= 2e + 1$), $|I| = e + 1$ and $|J| \leq e$.
c. t is odd, $|I| = |J| = e + 1$ and $I \cap J \neq \phi$.

Example 6.46 To illustrate the corollary, consider again the fraction in Example 6.44. Here $e = 2$, and we can conclude things like this:

a. Main effects are unaliased in S. So are two-factor interactions, and main effects with two-factor interactions.

b. Three-factor interactions are unaliased with main effects and with two-factor interactions.
c. The $A \times B \times C$ and $C \times D \times E$ interactions are unaliased in S. However, the corollary makes no claim about the $A \times B \times C$ and $D \times E \times F$ interactions. (This will be discussed in the next section.)

The next result contains the analogs of parts (b) and (c) of Theorem 5.18. We let $\oplus$ denote orthogonal sum, as before.

Corollary 6.47 *Assume the conditions of Theorem 6.43.*

a. If $e = [t/2]$ and $\mathcal{E}$ is the family of all nonempty $I \subset \{1, \ldots, k\}$ of size at most e, then

$$\mathbb{R}^S \supset \langle 1 \rangle \oplus_{I \in \mathcal{E}} \tilde{U}_I.$$

If in addition t is odd then

$$\mathbb{R}^S \supset \langle 1 \rangle \oplus_{I \in \mathcal{E} \cup \mathcal{F}} \tilde{U}_I,$$

where $\mathcal{F}$ is an intersecting family of subsets of size $e + 1$ of $\{1, \ldots, k\}$.
b. $\dim \tilde{U}_I = \prod_{i \in I}(s_i - 1)$ *whenever* $0 < |I| \leq t$.

($\mathcal{F}$ is an *intersecting family* if $I \cap J \neq \emptyset$ for all $I, J \in \mathcal{F}$.)
Proof (a) The subspaces $\tilde{U}_I$ are all contained in $\mathbb{R}^S$. Their orthogonality follows from Corollary 6.45.

(b) Note that for any I, the linear transformation r maps U_I onto $\tilde{U}_I$ and that $U_I \subset M_{\mathcal{C}}$ where $\mathcal{C} = \vee_{i \in I} \mathcal{A}_i$. But if $|I| \leq t$, then Proposition 6.42(b) shows that r is an isomorphism on U_I, so that $\dim \tilde{U}_I = \dim U_I$, and the conclusion follows from Theorem 5.18(c). □

Example 6.48 Consider once more the fraction in Example 6.44. According to Corollary 6.47, its ANOVA table can contain all main effects and two-factor interactions, plus the ten three-factor interactions $A \times B \times C$, $A \times B \times D, \ldots,$ $A \times E \times F$ that all involve A. The corresponding sequential and adjusted sums of squares will be equal if the fraction is observed in an equireplicate experiment.

The set $\mathcal{F} = \{\{A, B, C\}, \{A, B, D\}, \ldots, \{A, E, F\}\}$ is an example of an intersecting family.

We might certainly ask whether there is a larger intersecting family we could have used in Example 6.48. The answer is no: The Erdős-Ko-Rado Theorem [52] asserts that any intersecting family $\mathcal{F}$ would have to satisfy $|\mathcal{F}| \leq \binom{k-1}{e}$ (the so-called *EKR inequality*). Moreover, the example of $\mathcal{F}$ above is the only way to construct such a maximal family, according to a theorem of Hilton and Milnor [4, Theorem 5.6.2].

Counting dimensions in the displays in Corollary 6.47 is what gives us *Rao's inequalities for orthogonal arrays*. As an example, in a fraction S of strength 2 we have

$$N \geq 1 + \sum_{i=1}^{k} (s_i - 1),$$

where $N = |S|$. In general these inequalities give a lower bound for N, the size of the fraction. For symmetric designs with s levels, they give a relationship between the four parameters N, k, s and t of the design. We leave it as an exercise to write out the inequalities in general.

Remark 6.49 The Rao inequalities hold for orthogonal arrays, that is, designs in which some or all k-tuples are allowed to repeat. Proofs for the symmetric case may be found in [20] and [72, Sec. 2.2], and for the mixed-level case in [47] and [72, Sec 9.2]. Our proof of Corollary 6.47 applies only to *simple* orthogonal arrays, that is, subsets (fractions) of Cartesian products. We have made use of Rao's approach [111, 112], adding clarification and detail as necessary. Theorem 6.43 is original [12, 13].

6.5.3 Resolution

We have said (Definition 6.25) that S has *resolution R* if, for each p, every p-factor effect is unaliased with every effect having fewer than $R - p$ factors. The reader may have already sensed the idea of resolution in the examples of Sect. 6.5.2. We now make that explicit by relating resolution to strength.

One piece of this connection is an easy corollary of the Fundamental Theorem:

Proposition 6.50 *Let $T = A_1 \times \cdots \times A_k$ and let $S \subset T$. If S has strength $t \geq 1$ then it has resolution $t + 1$.*

Proof Suppose S has strength t, and let I and J be distinct subsets of $\{1, \ldots, k\}$ such that

$$|I| = p \text{ and } |J| \leq t - p.$$

By Theorem 6.43, $\tilde{U}_I \perp \tilde{U}_J$. Thus no interaction of p factors is aliased with any interaction of at most $t - p$ factors. But this means that S has resolution $t + 1$. □

Proposition 6.50 implies that if S has *maximum* strength t then S has resolution $R \geq t + 1$. We now show that R cannot exceed $t + 1$.

Theorem 6.51 *If a simple fraction has maximum strength $t \geq 1$, then it has maximum resolution $t + 1$.*

Proof In view of the remarks preceding the theorem, we just need to show that a fraction S of maximum strength t does not have resolution $t+2$. To do this, we must produce $I, J \subset \{1, \ldots, k\}$ such that $|J| < t+2-|I|$ but $\tilde{U}_I \not\perp \tilde{U}_J$.

We will use $(\cdot, \cdot)$ to denote inner products in either $\mathbb{R}^T$ or $\mathbb{R}^S$—see equations (5.1) and (6.2).

Since S does not have strength $t+1$, there exists a set $K \subset \{1, \ldots, k\}$ such that $|K| = t+1$ and $S \not\perp\!\!\!\perp \mathcal{C}_K$, where $\mathcal{C}_K = \bigvee_{i \in K} \mathcal{A}_i$. That means there exists a block $B \in \mathcal{C}_K$ such that $S \not\perp\!\!\!\perp B$.

Now $|K| \geq 2$, so we may write $K = I \cup J$, where both I and J are nonempty and $I \cap J = \emptyset$. Since $K = I \cup J$, we have $\mathcal{C}_K = \mathcal{C}_I \vee \mathcal{C}_J$ by Lemma 5.17, so there exist $B' \in \mathcal{C}_I$ and $B'' \in \mathcal{C}_J$ such that $B = B' \cap B''$.

Let $u = 1_{B'} - \pi(B')1$ and $v = 1_{B''} - \pi(B'')1$. Then $u \in U_{\mathcal{C}_I}$ and $v \in U_{\mathcal{C}_J}$. Using equation (5.19) we have the orthogonal sums

$$u = \sum_{I' \subseteq I} u_{I'}, \quad v = \sum_{J' \subseteq J} v_{J'},$$

where $u_{I'} \in U_{I'}$ and $v_{J'} \in U_{J'}$. Now if $I' \subset I$ and $J' \subset J$, then $I' \neq J'$ (in fact they are disjoint), and in particular $(u_{I'}, u_{J'}) = 0$. Moreover, if $I' \neq I$ or $J' \neq J$, then $|I' \cup J'| \leq t$, and thus $(\tilde{u}_{I'}, \tilde{v}_{J'}) = 0$ by the Fundamental Theorem (Theorem 6.43). Hence $(\tilde{u}, \tilde{v}) = (\tilde{u}_I, \tilde{v}_J)$. We will show that $(\tilde{u}, \tilde{v}) \neq 0$. Then $(\tilde{u}_I, \tilde{v}_J) \neq 0$, and thus $\tilde{U}_I \not\perp \tilde{U}_J$. Now

$$\begin{aligned}
(\tilde{u}, \tilde{v}) &= \textstyle\sum_{s \in S} u(s)v(s) \\
&= \textstyle\sum_{s \in S} (1_{B'}(s) - \pi(B')1)(1_{B''}(s) - \pi(B'')1) \\
&= |B' \cap B'' \cap S| - \pi(B')|B'' \cap S| - \pi(B'')|B' \cap S| + |S|\pi(B')\pi(B'') \\
&= |T|\,[\pi(B' \cap B'' \cap S) - \pi(B')\pi(B'' \cap S) - \pi(B'')\pi(B' \cap S) + \pi(S)\pi(B')\pi(B'')].
\end{aligned}$$

Since S has strength t, it is independent of both $\mathcal{C}_I$ and $\mathcal{C}_J$ (Proposition 6.40), and so we have $\pi(B' \cap S) = \pi(B')\pi(S)$ and $\pi(B'' \cap S) = \pi(B'')\pi(S)$. Moreover, since $I \cap J = \emptyset$, we have $\mathcal{C}_I \perp\!\!\!\perp \mathcal{C}_J$ by Lemma 5.17 , and thus $\pi(B' \cap B'') = \pi(B')\pi(B'')$. Therefore,

$$\begin{aligned}
(\tilde{u}, \tilde{v}) &= |T|\,[\pi(B' \cap B'' \cap S) - \pi(B')\pi(B'')\pi(S)] \\
&= |T|\,[\pi(B \cap S) - \pi(B')\pi(B'')\pi(S)] \\
&= |T|\,[\pi(B \cap S) - \pi(B' \cap B'')\pi(S)] \\
&= |T|\,[\pi(B \cap S) - \pi(B)\pi(S)] \\
&\neq 0,
\end{aligned}$$

since $S \not\perp\!\!\!\perp B$. □

For regular fractions the converse of Theorem 6.51 also holds.

Theorem 6.52 *If a regular fraction has maximum resolution R, then it has maximum strength $R-1$.*

Table 6.4 The 12-run Plackett-Burman design described in Example 6.53. Columns A through K give the contrasts for main effects in this fraction, while the rows of those columns encode its 12 cells or treatment combinations. If we code the levels by 0 and 1 instead of 1 and -1, then the first run is the cell (01011100010) (reproduced from [13])

run	1	A	B	C	D	E	F	G	H	I	J	K	AB	AC	…	JK
1	1	1	−1	1	−1	−1	−1	1	1	1	−1	1	−1	1	…	−1
2	1	−1	1	−1	−1	−1	1	1	1	−1	1	1	−1	1	…	1
3	1	1	−1	−1	−1	1	1	1	−1	1	1	−1	−1	−1	…	−1
4	1	−1	−1	−1	1	1	1	−1	1	1	−1	1	1	1	…	−1
5	1	−1	−1	1	1	1	−1	1	1	−1	1	−1	1	−1	…	−1
6	1	−1	1	1	1	−1	1	1	−1	1	−1	−1	−1	−1	…	1
7	1	1	1	1	−1	1	1	−1	1	−1	−1	−1	1	1	…	1
8	1	1	1	−1	1	1	−1	1	−1	−1	−1	1	1	−1	…	−1
9	1	1	−1	1	1	−1	1	−1	−1	−1	1	1	−1	1	…	1
10	1	−1	1	1	−1	1	−1	−1	−1	1	1	1	−1	−1	…	1
11	1	1	1	−1	1	−1	−1	−1	1	1	1	−1	1	−1	…	−1
12	1	−1	−1	−1	−1	−1	−1	−1	−1	−1	−1	−1	1	1	…	1

Clearly such a fraction cannot have strength R, since then it would have resolution $R + 1$, by Theorem 6.51. So to prove this we just need to show that it has strength $R - 1$. We defer the proof to Sect. 6.9, where it will follow quickly from Corollary 6.81.

Whether Theorem 6.52 holds for arbitrary fractions appears to be unknown.

Example 6.53 Table 6.4 describes a 12-run fraction of a 2^{11} factorial experiment on factors A through K. The rows of columns A through K specify the 12 treatment combinations in the fraction. This is a nonregular fraction (12 is not a power of 2), and cannot have strength 3 (12 is not a multiple of 8). One may check that columns A through K are mutually orthogonal contrast vectors, so that the fraction does have strength 2 and therefore resolution 3.

This fraction is a *Plackett-Burman design*. It is obtained by cyclically permuting the 11×1 column vector $[1, -1, 1, -1, -1, -1, 1, 1, 1, -1, 1]'$ and then adding a row of -1's, resulting in the design given in columns A through K of the table. The generating vector is taken from [93, equation (2.1)].[11]

The interaction columns AB through JK may be computed by componentwise multiplication of the corresponding main effects contrasts, since this is true in the full (2^{11}) factorial and since restriction respects pointwise multiplication (Proposition 6.37).

We have added a column of 1's, denoted by 1 (rather than by I, which is one of the factors). The 12×12 matrix $\mathbf{H}$ consisting of columns 1 through K has the property that $\mathbf{H}'\mathbf{H} = 12\mathbf{I}$, which summarizes the fact that each of the columns A

[11] The Plackett-Burman design described here and displayed in Table 6.4 is the one analyzed in [93], but is not the one displayed in [93, Table 1].

through K has six 1's and six -1's and that the columns are mutually orthogonal. It also defines $\mathbf{H}$ as a *Hadamard matrix* of order 12 (see Remark 2.16).

We will revisit this example in Sect. 6.7 (Example 6.60).

6.6 Aliasing and Confounding

The terms "aliased" and "confounded" are often used interchangeably in the design literature. It is Kempthorne [78, pages 264ff.] who first explained the relationship. A brief summary of this may be found in [79, Section 21.2].

In one direction the connection is easy to see. Consider a confounded design in which the set of treatment combinations $A_1 \times \cdots \times A_k$ is partitioned into blocks $B_1, \ldots, B_r$. We introduce a "pseudofactor" R that is at level j for all treatments in block j. We now have a fractional factorial experiment with $k+1$ factors $A_1, \ldots, A_k, R$. It is fractional because not all combinations of these factors occurs—for example, the treatment combinations in block 1 do not occur when R is at level 2. Effects which were originally confounded with blocks are now aliased with R.

This relationship can be seen more clearly in a classical s^k factorial experiment (s a prime or prime power). Kempthorne [79] considers a 3^3 design in which the blocks are the solution sets of $t_1 + t_2 + t_3 = b \pmod 3$, where $b = 0, 1, 2$. This confounds the ABC interaction. Kempthorne introduces a pseudofactor D, and a variable t_4, so that the blocks are given (modulo 3) by the system

$$t_1 + t_2 + t_3 = 0,\ t_4 = 0,$$
$$t_1 + t_2 + t_3 = 1,\ t_4 = 1,$$
$$t_1 + t_2 + t_3 = 2,\ t_4 = 2.$$

Since this implies that $t_1 + t_2 + t_3 = t_4 \pmod 3$, we can rewrite this system in the form

$$t_1 + t_2 + t_3 + 2t_4 = 0,$$

so that our design is a principal 3^{4-1} fraction, with defining relation $D = ABC$, or $I = ABCD^2$. We could even write down the alias structure of the design, although this is not generally of interest with respect to confounding.

In any case, this indicates that "confounding with blocks" can be viewed as aliasing (in the preceding example, D is aliased with ABC). However, one does not usually say that an effect is "aliased with blocks".

It is in the other direction that the terms "aliased" and "confounded" are most often used synonymously. That is, if effects F and G are aliased in a fraction, one often reads that they are confounded with each other. To justify this, one would have to show that it is always possible to write a fractional factorial as a confounded design. It is not clear whether this is true.

6.7 Aliasing, Estimability and Bias

As the reader will note, we have developed our main results without reference to estimability. Our emphasis has instead been on testing and the analysis of variance (see especially Example 6.28 and Corollaries 6.29 and 6.47). Yet the basic concepts in fractional designs are often framed in terms of estimability. Let us take a moment to explore this approach.

Consider the 2^3 experiment of Table 2.1 (page 38). The contrasts for the three main effects (for factors A, B and C) are

$$\psi_A = \mu_{000} + \mu_{001} + \mu_{010} + \mu_{011} - \mu_{100} - \mu_{101} - \mu_{110} - \mu_{111}, \tag{6.31}$$

$$\psi_B = \mu_{000} + \mu_{001} - \mu_{010} - \mu_{011} + \mu_{100} + \mu_{101} - \mu_{110} - \mu_{111}, \text{ and} \tag{6.32}$$

$$\psi_C = \mu_{000} - \mu_{001} + \mu_{010} - \mu_{011} + \mu_{100} - \mu_{101} + \mu_{110} - \mu_{111}. \tag{6.33}$$

If we observe one response Y_{ijk} to each treatment combination, we would we estimate ψ_A by

$$\hat{\psi}_A = Y_{000} + Y_{001} + Y_{010} + Y_{011} - Y_{100} - Y_{101} - Y_{110} - Y_{111},$$

and similarly for ψ_B and ψ_C. If there are more than one observation per cell, the random variables Y are replaced by cell averages.

Now suppose we only observe the principal fraction $S = \{000, 011, 101, 110\}$ in a regular 2^{3-1} fraction with defining relation $I = ABC$. On the face of it, the contrasts (6.31)–(6.33) cannot be estimated in S. The problem, of course, is that we lack estimates for half of the terms in these expressions. In fact, without further assumptions the only contrasts in cell means that are estimable in S are those that involve only the four cells in S. In general, we say that a contrast is *estimable in a fraction* if it is a linear function of cell means involving only cells belonging to S.

The literature treats this essentially as a missing data problem, which is handled in effect by *imputation* of the missing cells. We impose linear constraints on the model in such a way that the means $\mu(\mathbf{t})$ for $\mathbf{t} \notin S$ may be expressed in terms of those for $\mathbf{t} \in S$, so that a given contrast can be written entirely in terms of cells belonging to S. But what constraints? The following example illustrates one solution.

Example 6.54 In the case of our 2^{3-1} fraction, suppose we assume that the BC effect is absent, that is, that

$$\mu_{000} - \mu_{001} - \mu_{010} + \mu_{011} + \mu_{100} - \mu_{101} - \mu_{110} + \mu_{111} = 0.$$

This implies that

$$\mu_{001} + \mu_{010} - \mu_{100} - \mu_{111} = \mu_{000} + \mu_{011} - \mu_{101} - \mu_{110}. \quad (6.34)$$

Substituting the left-hand side of (6.34) into ψ_A gives

$$\psi_A = 2(\mu_{000} + \mu_{011} - \mu_{101} - \mu_{110}), \quad (6.35)$$

which is estimable from the cells in the fraction S.

The reader will note that BC is the alias of A, and we have shown that the contrast ψ_A is estimable in S if we assume that the BC interaction is absent. The idea of setting the BC contrast to zero actually comes from Theorem 6.35, which says that if we add together a set of aliased contrast vectors, the result is a contrast vector $\mathbf{c}$ whose components vanish outside of the fraction S, so that the contrast $\mathbf{c}'\boldsymbol{\mu}$ is estimable in S. (The theorem also explains the multiple 2 that appears in (6.35).) Thus, if we wish to estimate a contrast belonging to a particular effect in a principal s^{k-r} fraction, we would set all its aliases to zero.

Example 6.55 Now let S be the principal 3^{3-1} fraction in Example 6.36, defined by $I = ABC$, and let $\mathbf{c} = \mathbf{c}_{100} + \mathbf{c}_{211} + \mathbf{c}_{022}$. Then according to Table 6.2,

$$\mathbf{c}'\boldsymbol{\mu} = -9(\mu_{000} + \mu_{012} + \mu_{021}) + 3(\mu_{102} + \mu_{111} + \mu_{120}) + 6(\mu_{201} + \mu_{210} + \mu_{222}).$$

This contrast contains only the means of cells in S, and so it is estimable in S. But

$$\mathbf{c}'\boldsymbol{\mu} = \mathbf{c}'_{100}\boldsymbol{\mu} + \mathbf{c}'_{211}\boldsymbol{\mu} + \mathbf{c}'_{022}\boldsymbol{\mu},$$

and so if we assume that

$$\mathbf{c}'_{211}\boldsymbol{\mu} = 0 \text{ and } \mathbf{c}'_{022}\boldsymbol{\mu} = 0, \quad (6.36)$$

then $\mathbf{c}'_{100}\boldsymbol{\mu}$ is estimable in S.

Of course, the particular $\mathbf{c}'_{100}\boldsymbol{\mu}$ that we've used is only one contrast belonging to the main effect of A, and assuming (6.36) would not guarantee the estimability of any other contrast for that effect.[12] To do that, we'd need to pick another (independent) $\mathbf{c}_{100}$ belonging to A, construct *its* two aliases, and set those two contrasts to zero. This would guarantee the estimability of all the contrast belonging to A, since the set of such contrasts has dimension 2. In fact, with a little work (see Exercise 6.12) we can show that this is equivalent to simply saying that the aliases of A, namely AB^2C^2 and BC, are absent.

[12] Recall that the subscript 100 indicates only the blocking function L_{100} that defines the main effect of A. The contrast vector $\mathbf{c}_{100}$ is also determined by a choice of constants λ_i, one for each level of A, and there are many such choices.

The preceding examples are special cases of a general result that is an immediate consequence of Theorem 6.35. Let us say that an effect is *estimable* if every contrast belonging to that effect is estimable.

Theorem 6.56 *Given a principal regular fraction S, let F be an effect that is preserved in S. Then F is estimable in S if all its aliases are absent.*

This result is stated along with its converse in Lemma 8.2.5 of [45] and Theorem 2.4.2 of [98]. However, the converse is not true without further assumptions, as the following example shows.

Example 6.57 Returning to the 2^{3-1} fraction S considered in Example 6.54, suppose that instead of assuming (6.34), i.e., that the BC interaction is absent, we assume

$$\mu_{001}+\mu_{010}-\mu_{100}-\mu_{111}=\mu_{000}-\mu_{101}. \tag{6.37}$$

With this constraint, we would have

$$\psi_A = 2\mu_{000}+\mu_{011}-2\mu_{101}-\mu_{110},$$

which is estimable in the S, with estimator

$$\hat{\psi}_A = 2Y_{000}+Y_{011}-2Y_{101}-Y_{110}.$$

In fact, there are any number of non-standard constraints we could have applied instead of (6.37) that would do much the same thing. The converse of Theorem 6.56 presumably restricts the admissible constraints, for example requiring them to have natural or standard interpretations.

Similar reasoning would seem to let us estimate defining effects, which are lost in a fraction. For example, in the 2^{3-1} fraction above with defining effect ABC, we could technically estimate

$$\psi_{ABC}=\mu_{000}-\mu_{001}-\mu_{010}+\mu_{011}-\mu_{100}+\mu_{101}+\mu_{110}-\mu_{111}, \tag{6.38}$$

by imposing another constraint on the cell means, but such constraints would not have natural interpretations or would be otherwise unacceptable. See, for example, Exercise 6.19.

Resolution

A typical definition of resolution is the following, adapted from a classic text [110, Definition 7.1]:

Definition R A factorial design is said to be of *resolution* R if all factorial effects up to order k are estimable, where k is the greatest integer less than $R/2$, under the assumption that all factorial effects of order $R-k$ and higher are zero.

This clearly differs from Definition 6.25 in that the assumption that high-order effects are zero is now part of the definition. This makes the concept of resolution model-dependent. It also allows fractions to have resolution R even if they have strength less than $R-1$, as an example shows.[13]

Example 6.58 Once again we consider the principal 2^{3-1} fraction $S = \{000, 011, 101, 110\}$ in Example 6.54. The assumption that all interactions are absent may be written succinctly as

$$\begin{bmatrix} 1 & 1 & -1 & -1 & -1 & -1 & 1 & 1 \\ 1 & -1 & 1 & -1 & -1 & 1 & -1 & 1 \\ 1 & -1 & -1 & 1 & 1 & -1 & -1 & 1 \\ 1 & -1 & -1 & 1 & -1 & 1 & 1 & -1 \end{bmatrix} \boldsymbol{\mu} = \mathbf{0}, \tag{6.39}$$

where $\boldsymbol{\mu} = [\mu_{000}, \mu_{001}, \mu_{010}, \mu_{011}, \mu_{100}, \mu_{101}, \mu_{110}, \mu_{111}]'$. We may solve this system for the means of the four cells not in the fraction (straighforward using Gaussian elimination). The reader may check that this gives

$$\mu_{001} = (1/2)(\mu_{000} + \mu_{011} + \mu_{101} - \mu_{110})$$

$$\mu_{010} = (1/2)(\mu_{000} + \mu_{011} - \mu_{101} + \mu_{110})$$

$$\mu_{100} = (1/2)(\mu_{000} - \mu_{011} + \mu_{101} + \mu_{110})$$

$$\mu_{111} = (1/2)(-\mu_{000} + \mu_{011} + \mu_{101} + \mu_{110})$$

Substituting these back into (6.31)–(6.33), we see that ψ_A is given by (6.35), and similarly

$$\psi_B = 2(\mu_{000} - \mu_{011} + \mu_{101} - \mu_{110}) \text{ and}$$

$$\psi_C = 2(\mu_{000} - \mu_{011} - \mu_{101} + \mu_{110}),$$

all of which are estimable in S. Thus, according to Definition R this fraction has Resolution III, as it does according to Definition 6.25.

Where these two definitions diverge can be seen if instead we choose a nonregular fraction of size 4. Indeed, we can solve the system (6.39) for *any* four cell means. Thus, if our chosen fraction is $\{000, 001, 010, 100\}$, then assuming that interactions are absent, we may solve (6.39) for $\mu_{011}, \mu_{101}, \mu_{110}$ and μ_{111}. The

[13] This point is noted in [72, page 281], where an additional assumption is given.

result may be written succinctly as

$$\begin{bmatrix} \mu_{011} \\ \mu_{101} \\ \mu_{110} \\ \mu_{111} \end{bmatrix} = \begin{bmatrix} -1 & 1 & 1 & 0 \\ -1 & 1 & 0 & 1 \\ -1 & 0 & 1 & 1 \\ -2 & 1 & 1 & 1 \end{bmatrix} \begin{bmatrix} \mu_{000} \\ \mu_{001} \\ \mu_{010} \\ \mu_{100} \end{bmatrix}. \tag{6.40}$$

Using (6.40) to replace $\mu_{011}, \mu_{101}, \mu_{110}$ and μ_{111} in the expressions (6.31)–(6.33) gives us the A-, B- and C-contrasts

$$\left.\begin{aligned} \psi_A &= 4(\mu_{000} - \mu_{100}), \\ \psi_B &= 4(\mu_{000} - \mu_{010}), \\ \psi_C &= 4(\mu_{000} - \mu_{001}), \end{aligned}\right\} \tag{6.41}$$

which are estimable in this fraction—for example, ψ_A has the estimator $4(Y_{000} - Y_{100})$. Thus, according to Definition R the fraction $\{000, 001, 010, 100\}$ has Resolution III, though Theorem 6.51 implies that it doesn't even have Resolution II. (We leave the preceding computations as an exercise.)

Aliasing and Bias

Consider a linear model

$$\mathrm{E}(\mathbf{Y}) = \mathbf{X}\boldsymbol{\beta}, \tag{6.42}$$

and partition $\boldsymbol{\beta}$ so that

$$\boldsymbol{\beta} = \begin{bmatrix} \boldsymbol{\beta}_1 \\ \boldsymbol{\beta}_2 \end{bmatrix},$$

where $\boldsymbol{\beta}_2$ consists of parameters that are not of interest. Partitioning the columns of $\mathbf{X}$ correspondingly, we may write our model as

$$\mathrm{E}(\mathbf{Y}) = \mathbf{X}_1\boldsymbol{\beta}_1 + \mathbf{X}_2\boldsymbol{\beta}_2. \tag{6.43}$$

If $\boldsymbol{\beta}_2$ were absent, the least squares estimate of $\boldsymbol{\beta}_1$ would be

$$\hat{\boldsymbol{\beta}}_1 = (\mathbf{X}_1'\mathbf{X}_1)^{-1}\mathbf{X}_1'\mathbf{Y}.$$

This is unbiased for $\boldsymbol{\beta}_1$ if $\boldsymbol{\beta}_2 = \mathbf{0}$, but otherwise we have

$$\begin{aligned} \mathrm{E}(\hat{\boldsymbol{\beta}}_1) &= \boldsymbol{\beta}_1 + (\mathbf{X}_1'\mathbf{X}_1)^{-1}\mathbf{X}_1'\mathbf{X}_2\boldsymbol{\beta}_2 \\ &= \boldsymbol{\beta}_1 + \mathbf{A}\boldsymbol{\beta}_2, \end{aligned} \tag{6.44}$$

say. Box and Wilson [29] called $\mathbf{A}$ an *alias matrix*. It is also known, naturally, as a *bias matrix*.

It is common to apply this to a fractional design in terms of the factor-effects model. Thus in the above, $\boldsymbol{\beta}$ is the vector of of factor-effects parameters of the full factorial experiment, and $\boldsymbol{\beta}_1$ consists of the parameters of interest (typically those representing main effects and possibly low-order interactions). The the assumption that certain (high-order) interactions are absent can then be written as $\boldsymbol{\beta}_2 = \mathbf{0}$. Now let $\mathbf{Y}$ be the vector of observations in the given fraction. The Box-Wilson approach posits a model of the form (6.42), which we may write in the form (6.43) above. A couple of examples will illustrate this.

Example 6.59 Let us reproduce the top half of the table in Example 6.1, corresponding to the principal 2^{3-1} fraction that we have been discussing:

cell	I	A	B	C	AB	AC	BC	ABC
000	1	1	1	1	1	1	1	1
011	1	1	−1	−1	−1	−1	1	1
101	1	−1	1	−1	−1	1	−1	1
110	1	−1	−1	1	1	−1	−1	1

Here we have added a column of ones, denoted I. Let $\mathbf{X}$ be the matrix of columns I through ABC, let $\boldsymbol{\beta}$ be the vector of factor-effects parameters defined in equation (2.36), and let $\mathbf{Y} = (Y_{000}, Y_{011}, Y_{101}, Y_{110})'$ be the vector of observations, one per cell, then

$$\mathrm{E}(\mathbf{Y}) = \mathbf{X}\boldsymbol{\beta} \tag{6.45}$$

(this is the "top half" of equation (2.38)). We write this in the form (6.43), where $\mathbf{X}_1$ consists of columns I, A, B and C, and $\mathbf{X}_2$ the columns AB, AC, BC and ABC. Since the columns of $\mathbf{X}_1$ are orthogonal, we see that

$$\mathbf{X}_1'\mathbf{X}_1 = 4\mathbf{I}.$$

(That is, $\mathbf{X}_1$ is a Hadamard matrix of order 4.) Thus the alias matrix for this design is

$$\mathbf{A} = (1/4)\mathbf{X}_1'\mathbf{X}_2 = \begin{pmatrix} 0 & 0 & 0 & 1 \\ 0 & 0 & 1 & 0 \\ 0 & 1 & 0 & 0 \\ 1 & 0 & 0 & 0 \end{pmatrix}.$$

The (i, j)th element of this matrix is the dot product of column i of $\mathbf{X}_1$ with column j of $\mathbf{X}_2$. The zeros indicate lack of aliasing (orthogonal columns), while the ones indicate complete aliasing (two equal columns—note that I and ABC are considered aliases here). These agree with what we already know about this fraction. It is in this way that $\mathbf{A}$ gives us information about the alias structure of the fraction.

Example 6.60 Consider the Plackett-Burman design in Example 6.53.

As in Example 6.59 we let $\mathbf{Y}$ be the 12×1 vector of observations of this fraction, one per treatment combination. We take $\mathbf{X}_1$ to be composed of the 12 columns 1 through K of Table 6.4, and $\mathbf{X}_2$ the 55 columns AB through JK. Assuming that all interactions of three or more factors are absent, we write our model in the form (6.43). Since $\mathbf{X}_1$ (earlier denoted $\mathbf{H}$) is a Hadamard matrix of order 12, we have

$$\mathbf{X}_1'\mathbf{X}_1 = 12\,\mathbf{I}, \tag{6.46}$$

so that the alias matrix is

$$\mathbf{A} = (1/12)\,\mathbf{X}_1'\mathbf{X}_2. \tag{6.47}$$

The matrix $\mathbf{A}$ is 55×12 and will not be displayed here (see [93, Table 3]), but we can say a lot about its entries. The columns of $\mathbf{X}_2$—the interaction vectors—belong to $\mathbb{R}^{12}$. But the columns $\mathbf{x}_1, \ldots, \mathbf{x}_{12}$ of $\mathbf{X}_1$ are already a basis for $\mathbb{R}^{12}$—in fact, an orthogonal basis. Let $\mathbf{v}$ be the AB column of $\mathbf{X}_2$, and write

$$\mathbf{v} = \sum_{i=1}^{12} a_i \mathbf{x}_i. \tag{6.48}$$

Then $\mathbf{x}_j'\mathbf{v} = 12\,a_j$, so the jth coefficient of (6.48) is

$$a_j = (1/12)\mathbf{x}_j'\mathbf{v}.$$

Thus the coefficients a_j are given by $(1/12)\mathbf{X}'\mathbf{v}$. By direct calculation,

$$\begin{aligned}(1/12)\mathbf{X}'\mathbf{v} &= (1/12)[0, 0, 0, -4, 4, 4, -4, -4, 4, -4, -4, -4]' \\ &= (1/3)[0, 0, 0, -1, 1, 1, -1, -1, 1, -1, -1, -1]'.\end{aligned} \tag{6.49}$$

Then we may write (6.48) as

$$AB = (1/3)[-C + D + E - F - G + H - I - J - K].$$

Thus the alias of AB is a linear combination of the effects C through K. In the language of Definition 6.4, AB is *partly aliased* with each of these main effects.

A similar calculation will give the aliases of each two-factor interaction. If $\mathbf{v}_j$ is the jth interaction, then the coefficients of the alias relation will be given by the vector $(1/12)\mathbf{X}'\mathbf{v}_j$. But this is the jth column of the alias matrix $\mathbf{A}$. As in Example 6.59, $\mathbf{A}$ describes the aliasing in the fraction.

The zero components of $\mathbf{X}'\mathbf{v}$ in (6.49) carry special information. In particular, two of the zeros indicate that the AB interaction is unaliased with the main effects of A and B. We leave it as an exercise to explain the other zeros that occur in the alias matrix in this example.

The reader may have noticed a problem arising in these two examples. In Example 6.59, the vector $\mathbf{Y}$ has four components, so $\mathrm{E}(\mathbf{Y})$ contains four parameters, but the vector $\boldsymbol{\beta}$ in equation (6.45) is 8×1. Thus unless $\boldsymbol{\beta}_2 = \mathbf{0}$, the model is overparametrized. Similarly, in Example 6.53 $\mathrm{E}(\mathbf{Y})$ is 11×1, but in the equation $\mathrm{E}(\mathbf{Y}) = \mathbf{X}\boldsymbol{\beta}$ the vector $\boldsymbol{\beta}$ is 67×1. Thus in these examples the model specifies a parameter vector $\boldsymbol{\beta}$ that is not identifiable. In particular, it is not clear that we can view the parameters in $\boldsymbol{\beta}$ as representing the effects that we intend. Yet the matrix $\mathbf{X}_1'\mathbf{X}_2$ clearly summarizes information about the aliasing structure of the fraction!

It may be objected that we can always make $\boldsymbol{\beta}$ identifiable by imposing appropriate constraints. But it is not clear what constraints we should impose. Of course, assuming $\boldsymbol{\beta}_2 = \mathbf{0}$ will work, but that would eliminate the very bias that we claim exists.

The difficulty disappears if we simply choose not to identify aliasing with bias. There is nothing in our definition of aliasing that indicates such a connection. Nor would abandoning this view prevent us from computing matrix products such as $\mathbf{X}_1'\mathbf{X}_2$.

6.8 Relative Aberration

In resolution IV designs there is no aliasing among main effects or between main effects and two-factor interactions, but we do expect some mutual aliasing between two-factor interactions. Since these interactions are next in importance to main effects, we would prefer to minimize this aliasing. In [62] Fries and Hunter compared three 2_{IV}^{7-2} fractional factorial designs with respect to this. The results are described in Table 6.5.

Clearly, design (c) is preferable. Fries and Hunter describe it as having the least *aberration* among the three designs. Could there exist a design that is even better than (c)? For this, we have to go further. Fries and Hunter observe that mutual aliasing between two-factor interactions is a direct result of the presence of a defining word of length 4, and we see that design (a) has three such words, while design (b) has two and (c) has only one. Among all resolution IV designs having one defining word of length 4, we should minimize the number of words of length 5, and so on.

The relevant information about a design is summarized in its *wordlength pattern*: For design (c), it is $(0, 0, 0, 1, 2, 0, 0)$, meaning that there is one defining word of length 4, two of length 5, and none of any other length (the maximum length is 7). Similarly, the wordlength pattern of design (a) is $(0, 0, 0, 3, 0, 0, 0)$, and that of (b) is $(0, 0, 0, 2, 0, 1, 0)$. The first place where they differ is in the fourth

Table 6.5 Mutual aliasing of two-factor interactions in three different 2^{7-2}_{IV} fractional factorial designs. Adapted from [62, Table 1].

Design	(a)	(b)	(c)
Defining relation	$I = ABCF$ $= BCDG = ADFG$	$I = ABCF$ $= ADEG = BCDEFG$	$I = ABCDF$ $= ABCEG = DEFG$
Alias sets among two-factor interactions	$AB = CF$	$AB = CF$	$DE = FG$
	$AC = BF$	$AC = BF$	$DF = EG$
	$AD = FG$	$AD = EG$	$DG = EF$
	$AG = DF$	$AE = DG$	
	$BD = CG$	$AF = BC$	
	$BG = CD$	$AG = DE$	
	$AF = BC = DG$		

coordinate, where design (c) is smallest. Of course, all 2^{7-2}_{IV} designs have at least one defining word of length 4 (minimum wordlength = maximum resolution). Thus a design with even less aberration would need to have a wordlength pattern of form $(0, 0, 0, 1, x, y, z)$ where $x = 0$ or 1. With a bit more work we can show that such a design cannot exist, so that design (c) is a *minimum aberration* design (Exercise 6.21). Note that interchanging E and F in the defining words of design (c) will yield another minimum aberration design, so such designs are not unique.

One can similarly compare regular s^{k-r} designs of a given resolution. Given two s^{k-r} fractions of resolution R, we look at the number of defining words of length R for each, and choose the fraction for which this number is smaller. We note that this number might be the same for both, in which case we can look at the number of defining words of length $R + 1$, and so on. For s prime, this was first described by Franklin [61].

Recall that the *defining words* of a fraction are the non-identity elements of the defining subgroup.

Definition 6.61 The *wordlength pattern* of a regular fraction S on k factors is the k-tuple $W(S) = (W_1(S), \ldots, W_k(S))$, where $W_i(S)$ is the number of defining words of length i.

Example 6.62 Consider the 3^{5-2} design of Example 6.19, generated by the defining words ABD^2 and AB^2CE^2. From the defining equation (6.13), page 235, we see that the wordlength pattern of the fraction is $(0, 0, 2, 6, 0)$.

Let us say that the word $A_1^{a_1} \cdots A_k^{a_k}$ *contains* A_j if $a_j > 0$. We may also say that A_j *occurs* or *appears in* the word.

Lemma 6.63 *Given a regular s^{k-r} design on the factors $A_1, \ldots, A_k$, with wordlength pattern $(W_1, \ldots, W_k)$:*

a. If the design has maximum resolution R, then $W_1 = \cdots = W_{R-1} = 0 < W_R$.
b. We have $\sum_{i=1}^{k} W_i = s^r - 1$.

c. *We have* $\sum_{i=1}^{k} iW_i = \sum_{j=1}^{k} f_j$, *where* f_j *is the number of defining words containing* A_j.

Part (a) restates Corollary 6.26, while (b) comes from the fact that the defining subgroup has s^r elements. Part (c) is left as an exercise.

We note that the length of a word $A_1^{a_1} \cdots A_k^{a_k}$ is the Hamming weight of the vector $\mathbf{a} = (a_1, \ldots, a_k)$, that is, the number of nonzero components of $\mathbf{a}$. Thus we may equivalently consider the Hamming weights of defining *vectors*[14] instead of the lengths of defining words. In this case the wordlength pattern is known as the *weight distribution* of the design.

Definition 6.64 Let S_1 and S_2 be regular s^{k-r} fractions, with wordlength patterns $W(S_1)$ and $W(S_2)$. We say that S_1 has *less aberration* than S_2 if $W(S_1) < W(S_2)$ with respect to lexicographic order.

If a s^{k-r} fraction S has the property that no other s^{k-r} fraction has less aberration, we say that S has *minimum aberration.*

Lexicographic ordering on wordlength patterns means that $W(S_1) < W(S_2)$ if there is an ℓ such that $W_i(S_1) = W_i(S_2)$ for $i \leq \ell - 1$ and $W_\ell(S_1) < W_\ell(S_2)$.

Unlike resolution, there is no number called "the aberration" of a design. Rather, aberration is used to compare designs, typically of the same resolution. The reader will note that Definition 6.64 makes no mention of resolution. That's because Lemma 6.63(a) makes this unnecessary: Greater resolution implies less aberration, and conversely, if S_1 has less aberration than S_2 then resolution(S_1) $\geq$ resolution(S_2).

The following two results are among several that help us to narrow down the search for minimum aberration designs. The proofs are adapted from [98].

Lemma 6.65 *Let* S *be a regular* s^{k-r} *design on the factors* $A_1, \ldots, A_k$. *If* S *has minimum aberration, then every letter appears in at least one defining word.*

Proof Assume *per contra* that some letter, say A_j, does not appear in any defining word. We will show that there exists another s^{k-r} fraction S^* with less aberration than S.

Now S is the solution set of a system of equations (6.5) given by linearly independent defining vectors $\mathbf{a}_1, \ldots, \mathbf{a}_r \in E$, where E is the defining subspace of S. By assumption, all the vectors in E have zero in the jth component. To construct S^*, let $\mathbf{a}_1^* \in (GF(s))^k$ be the same as $\mathbf{a}_1$ except for having 1 as its jth component. Then $\mathbf{a}_1^*, \mathbf{a}_2, \ldots, \mathbf{a}_r$ are also linearly independent, and so they define another regular s^{k-r} fraction S^*. We claim that $W(S^*) < W(S)$.

Let $E^* = \langle \mathbf{a}_1^*, \mathbf{a}_2, \ldots, \mathbf{a}_r \rangle$ be the defining subspace of S^*. The vectors $\mathbf{a} \in E$ and $\mathbf{a}^* \in E^*$ correspond one-to-one via

$$\mathbf{a} = c_1\mathbf{a}_1 + c_2\mathbf{a}_2 + \cdots + c_r\mathbf{a}_r \quad \longleftrightarrow \quad \mathbf{a}^* = c_1\mathbf{a}_1^* + c_2\mathbf{a}_2 + \cdots + c_r\mathbf{a}_r.$$

[14] See page 224.

Of the vectors in E with $c_1 \neq 0$, let $\mathbf{a}$ have lowest Hamming weight, say ℓ. This vector corresponds to a vector $\mathbf{a}^* \in E^*$ of Hamming weight $\ell + 1$, which means that E^* has at least one fewer vector of weight ℓ. Vectors $\mathbf{a}$ of lower weight have $c_1 = 0$, so E and E^* have the same weight distribution of vectors of weight $< \ell$. This means that $W(S^*) < W(S)$, as claimed. □

Proposition 6.66 *Let S be a regular s^{k-r} design on factors $A_1, \ldots, A_k$, and let f_j be the number of defining words containing A_j. If $f_j > 0$ for all j, then:*

a. $f_j = s^{r-1}(s-1)$ *for all* j.
b. If S has wordlength pattern $(W_1, \ldots, W_k)$, then

$$\sum_{i=1}^{k} i W_i = k s^{r-1}(s-1). \tag{6.50}$$

In particular, if S has minimum aberration then (a) and (b) hold.

Proof The assumption about f_j means that each letter appears in at least one defining word, so the last statement follows immediately from Lemma 6.65. Also, part (b) follows from (a) and Lemma 6.63(c). Thus it remains to prove (a). To prove this, we claim that the number of defining words *not* containing A_j is $s^{r-1} - 1$, so that $f_j = s^r - 1 - (s^{r-1} - 1) = s^{r-1}(s-1)$.

Suppose that S is the solution set of a system of equations of the form (6.5) given by the linearly independent vectors $\mathbf{a}_1, \ldots, \mathbf{a}_r$. The general defining vector is then $c_1\mathbf{a}_1 + c_2\mathbf{a}_2 + \cdots + c_r\mathbf{a}_r$, and an equivalent form of our claim is that $s^{r-1} - 1$ of these vectors have a zero in the jth coordinate. Proof of this claim is left as an exercise. □

Example 6.67 Consider the three 2^{7-2}_{IV} designs discussed at the beginning of this section. Design (a) already fails the test of Lemma 6.65, so it can't have minimum aberration. The reader can check that design (b) satisfies (6.50), which shows that this condition, while necessary, is not sufficient to conclude minimum aberration.

Design (c) also satisfies the condition (6.50), but as we see, that is not enough by itself to conclude that it is a minimum aberration design.

There has been a great deal of research on the necessary and sufficient conditions for a design to have minimum aberration, and on methods of constructing such designs. Mukerjee and Wu [98] give in-depth survey of this field with respect to regular designs. They also note that some results have roots going back to the 1940's.

Remark 6.68 We conclude with a couple of observations.

- We have chosen to compute the wordlength pattern from the entire set of defining words, but it is often computed from counting only the reduced (monic) words; see, e.g., [98, Example 2.5.1]. If we did this, the wordlength pattern of Example 6.62 would be (0, 0, 1, 3, 0), counting only the words ABD^2, AB^2CE^2, $BCDE^2$, and AC^2DE.

Now, the length of a word is unchanged by exponentiation: In an s-level (s^{k-r}) design, if a word F has length d, so does F^a for any nonzero $a \in GF(s)$, so that our word count is $s-1$ times as big as if we limited ourselves to monic words. Therefore, this would not alter the hierarchy of designs imposed by relative aberration. Of course, this distinction does not arise in a 2-level design.

In making our choice we are following Xu and Wu [152]; see in particular their comment, page 1068. They craft their definition so that is consistent with their generalization of wordlength pattern, which we are about to study.

- Because of the non-uniqueness of minimum aberration designs, some authors use the term "minimal" instead of "minimum" [72]. On the other hand, wordlength patterns are linearly ordered according to Definition 6.64, and so two minimum aberration regular s^{k-r} designs must have the same wordlength pattern, which provides an argument for the term "minimum".

6.8.1 *In Nonregular Designs*

In 2^k Factorials

Let us return to the 2^{3-1} fraction we examined in Example 6.59, with an additional line:

cell	A	B	C	AB	AC	BC	ABC
000	1	1	1	1	1	1	1
011	1	−1	−1	−1	−1	1	1
101	−1	1	−1	−1	1	−1	1
110	−1	−1	1	1	−1	−1	1
sum	0	0	0	0	0	0	4

The sums are 0 for those contrasts that are preserved in the fraction. The sum of 4 indicates that ABC is a defining word. Let us apply this idea to two more complicated examples, one regular, the other not.

Example 6.69 The following gives the contrast vectors for the principal 2^{4-2} fraction with defining equation $I = ABC = BCD = AD$:

cell	A	B	C	D	AB	AC	AD	BC	BD	CD	ABC	ABD	ACD	BCD	$ABCD$
0000	1	1	1	1	1	1	1	1	1	1	1	1	1	1	1
0110	1	−1	−1	1	−1	−1	1	1	−1	−1	1	−1	−1	1	1
1011	−1	1	−1	−1	−1	1	1	−1	−1	1	1	1	−1	1	−1
1101	−1	−1	1	−1	1	−1	1	−1	1	−1	1	−1	1	1	−1
sum	0	0	0	0	0	0	4	0	0	0	4	0	0	4	0

The nonzero sums belong precisely to the three defining words. In addition, we may read off some information about aliasing from the zero sums. For example, the fact that sum$(ABD) = 0$ (in the obvious notation) indicates that columns AB and D are orthogonal, meaning that those effects are unaliased. This is because $ABD = (AB)(D)$ componentwise, and so sum$(ABD) = AB \cdot D$. Similarly, the fact that sum$(ABC) = 4$ reflects the fact that $AB = C$—in other words, that AB and C are completely aliased.

In [138] Tang introduced the term *J-characteristics* for the sums we have computed.[15] In the preceding example, for instance, we may write $J_{AB} = 0$ and $J_{ABC} = 4$.

Example 6.70 Consider the Plackett-Burman design of Table 6.4. Here is a small selection of the $2^{11} - 1 = 2047$ contrasts for main effects and interactions. Their J-characteristics are given in the bottom line.

A	B	$\cdots$	K	AB	ABC	ABD	$ABCD$	$ABCDE$	$ABCDF$	$FGHIJK$	$AB\cdots JK$
1	−1	⋯	1	−1	−1	1	1	−1	−1	1	−1
−1	1	⋯	1	−1	1	1	−1	1	−1	−1	−1
1	−1	⋯	−1	−1	1	1	−1	−1	−1	1	−1
−1	−1	⋯	1	1	−1	1	−1	−1	−1	1	−1
−1	−1	⋯	−1	1	1	1	1	1	−1	−1	−1
−1	1	⋯	−1	−1	−1	−1	−1	1	−1	−1	−1
1	1	⋯	−1	1	1	−1	−1	−1	−1	1	−1
1	1	⋯	1	1	−1	1	−1	−1	1	1	−1
1	−1	⋯	1	−1	−1	−1	−1	1	−1	−1	−1
−1	1	⋯	1	−1	−1	1	1	1	−1	−1	−1
1	1	⋯	−1	1	−1	1	−1	1	1	−1	−1
−1	−1	⋯	−1	1	−1	−1	1	−1	−1	1	−1
0	0	⋯	0	0	−4	4	−4	0	−8	0	−12

The zero sums belong to effects that are preserved in the fraction. They also tell us, for example, that AB is not aliased with CDE (since $AB \cdot CDE = J_{ABCDE} = 0$). On the other hand, the fact that $J_{ABCDEFGHIJK} = -12$ reflects the fact that this effect (the unique 11-factor interaction) is lost in the fraction, as we see from the constancy of the column entries. In fact, no column sum can exceed 12 in absolute value, and a sum of ± 12 will always indicate an effect that is completely lost in the fraction.

[15] As Tang indicates, this is a modification of an earlier definition of J-characteristic given in joint papers [44, 139] with L. Y. Deng.

What is new here is the presence of intermediate sums between 0 and ± 12. We might say that these effects are "partly lost" in the fraction, and indicate other effects that are partly aliased.

We have defined the J-characteristics of a fraction S by summing columns over the cells $\mathbf{t} \in S$. When there are k factors, say $A_1, \ldots, A_k$, each effect is defined by a subset of factors, or equivalently by a subset $a \subset \{1, \ldots, k\}$; for example, $a = \{1, 2\}$ represents the interaction of A_1 and A_2. Let $\mathbf{c}_a$ be the contrast vector (in the full factorial) representing the effect indicated by a. We define

$$J_a = \sum_{\mathbf{t} \in S} c_a(\mathbf{t}) \tag{6.51}$$

to be the J-characteristic of that effect, where $c_a(\mathbf{t})$ is $\mathbf{t}$-th component of $\mathbf{c}$.

To indicate dependence on the fraction S, we write $J_a(S)$. It is also a convention to write, e.g., J_1 for $J_{\{1\}}$ and J_{12} for $J_{\{1,2\}}$. Note that J_a is defined only up to scalar multiple; in particular, if the entries of $\mathbf{c}_a$ are all ± 1, as we will assume, then its J-characteristic is only determined up to sign.

Formula (6.51) is not exactly how Deng and Tang expressed J_a. Rather, we note that once we fix the main-effect contrasts $\mathbf{c}_1, \ldots \mathbf{c}_k$, the other contrasts may be determined as coordinatewise products: $\mathbf{c}_a = \prod_{i \in a} \mathbf{c}_i$. (This is true in the full 2^k factorial; that it is true for fractions follows from Proposition 6.37, as we have pointed out.) We may therefore write

$$J_a = \sum_{\mathbf{t} \in S} \prod_{i \in a} \mathbf{c}_i(\mathbf{t}). \tag{6.52}$$

This is the way the J-characteristics are defined in [138], and will be the basis for its generalization below.

A primary purpose of introducing J-characteristics was to express wordlength patterns in terms of them. As in Example 6.70 we have $0 \leq |J_a| \leq n$, where $n = |S|$, so the numbers J_a^2/n^2 are between 0 and 1. Moreover, in regular fractions the only possible values are 0 and 1, and the value 1 occurs if and only if $J_a = n$, that is, iff the effect indexed by s is a defining word. Therefore, the number of defining words of length j in a regular 2^{k-r} fraction may be given by

$$W_j = \sum_{|a|=j} J_a^2/n^2, \tag{6.53}$$

the sum taken over subsets $a \subset \{1, \ldots, k\}$ of size j. We may take this as a definition of W_j in the nonregular case, and simply define the *generalized* wordlength pattern of the fraction S to be $W(S) = (W_1, \ldots, W_k)$. We understand from their definition that the numbers W_j may be fractions. With this, we can extend Definition 6.64 to nonregular designs:

Definition 6.71 Let S_1 and S_2 be fractions of the same size, with *generalized* wordlength patterns $W(S_1)$ and $W(S_2)$. We say that S_1 has *less aberration* than S_2 if $W(S_1) < W(S_2)$ with respect to lexicographic order.

If a fraction S has the property that no other fraction of its size has less aberration, we say that S has *minimum aberration.*

At this point, we have only defined generalized wordlength patterns to fractions of 2^k factorial experiments. We now explore extending these patterns to other designs.

In p^k Factorials

Equations (6.51), (6.52) and (6.53) can be extended to fractions of p^k factorial designs, p prime, if we represent every effect by a *complex* contrast vector as described in Sect. 5.6.5. We give a quick review of this topic; the reader is referred to that section for details.

We now use $GF(p) = \mathbb{Z}/p = \{0, 1, \ldots, p-1\}$ as the index set for the levels of each factor. The elements of $(\mathbb{Z}/p)^k$ serve two purposes:

a. They are the treatment combinations $\mathbf{t}$ of the experiment.
b. They determine the elements of the effects group: If $\mathbf{a} = (a_1, \ldots, a_k)$, then the corresponding effect is $A_1^{a_1} \cdots A_k^{a_k}$. **In this section we will denote this effect by** $\mathbf{a}$. The effects are thus $\mathbf{a}_0, \ldots, \mathbf{a}_{q-1}$, where $q = p^k$.

Each $\mathbf{a}$ determines a column of values $\mathbf{a}'\mathbf{t}$ where $\mathbf{t}$ runs over all treatment combinations. These values of course lie in $\mathbb{Z}/p$. We transform this column to a complex contrast vector by replacing $j \in \mathbb{Z}/p$ by the number ω^j, where $\omega = e^{2\pi i/p}$, a primitive pth root of unity. (In the binary case we have $j = 0$ or 1, and $\omega = -1$.) The columns of Table 5.5 are the complex contrast vectors for the full p^k factorial design.

The $\mathbf{t}$-th component of the contrast vector $c_{\mathbf{a}}$ for effect $\mathbf{a}$ is given by

$$c_{\mathbf{a}}(\mathbf{t}) = \omega^{\mathbf{a}'\mathbf{t}}.$$

Substituting this into (6.51) gives us

$$J_{\mathbf{a}} = \sum_{\mathbf{t} \in S} \omega^{\mathbf{a}'\mathbf{t}}. \tag{6.54}$$

This is the J-characteristic of the effect $\mathbf{a}$ for an arbitrary fraction $S \subset (\mathbb{Z}/p)^k$. Again, we may write $J_{\mathbf{a}}(S)$ if we need to indicate the fraction. As we observed earlier (equation (5.47)), if $\mathbf{t} = (t_1, \ldots, t_k)$ and $\mathbf{a} = (a_1, \ldots, a_k)$, then

$$c_{\mathbf{a}}(\mathbf{t}) = \prod_i \omega^{a_i t_i}, \tag{6.55}$$

so that

$$J_{\mathbf{a}} = \sum_{\mathbf{t} \in S} \prod_{i} \omega^{a_i t_i}. \tag{6.56}$$

This is the generalization of (6.52). Note that $J_{\mathbf{a}}$ is complex-valued.

The key property of J-characteristics carries over from the two-level case:

Proposition 6.72 *Let $S \subset (\mathbb{Z}/p)^k$ be a fraction of size n from a p^k factorial experiment, p a prime. The J-characteristics of S satisfy*

$$0 \leq |J_{\mathbf{a}}| \leq n \quad \textit{for all} \quad \mathbf{a} \in (\mathbb{Z}/p)^k. \tag{6.57}$$

Moreover,

a. $|J_{\mathbf{a}}| = n$ iff the effect $\mathbf{a}$ is completely lost in S.
b. $J_{\mathbf{a}} = 0$ iff the effect $\mathbf{a}$ is preserved in S.

If S is regular, these are the only possibilities.

Proof Since $|\omega| = 1$, we see from (6.54) that

$$|J_{\mathbf{a}}| = |\sum_{\mathbf{t} \in S} \omega^{\mathbf{a}'\mathbf{t}}| \leq \sum_{\mathbf{t} \in S} 1 = n.$$

This proves (6.57).

For the remainder of this proof, let us fix the complex contrast vector $\mathbf{c_a}$, with components $c_{\mathbf{a}}(\mathbf{t}), \mathbf{t} \in (\mathbb{Z}/p)^k$. As we know from Sect. 5.6.5, the components of $\mathbf{c_a}$ determine the blocking $\mathcal{B}(L_{\mathbf{a}})$. Therefore, the components restricted to $\mathbf{t} \in S$ determine the blocks of $\mathcal{B}(L_{\mathbf{a}}, S)$ (defined by (6.6)). From Lemma 6.9 we see that we need to show:

a. $\mathcal{B}(L_{\mathbf{a}}, S) = \{S\}$ iff $|J_{\mathbf{a}}| = n$.
b. $\mathcal{B}(L_{\mathbf{a}}, S)$ consists of p equal-sized blocks iff $J_{\mathbf{a}} = 0$.

As we know from Theorem 6.8, these are the only possibilities if S is regular.

Proof of (a): The blocking $\mathcal{B}(L_{\mathbf{a}}, S)$ consists of just a single block, namely S itself, if and only if the components $c_{\mathbf{a}}(\mathbf{t}), \mathbf{t} \in S$, are all equal. Thus it suffices to show that $|J_{\mathbf{a}}| = n$ iff the quantities

$$\omega^{\mathbf{a}'\mathbf{t}}, \mathbf{t} \in S \tag{6.58}$$

are equal.

Without loss of generality, we may assume that the cells of the full factorial are numbered so that the cells of S are $\mathbf{t}_1, \ldots, \mathbf{t}_n$. Clearly, if the numbers (6.58) are equal then $J_{\mathbf{a}} = n\omega^{\mathbf{a}'\mathbf{t}_1}$, so $|J_{\mathbf{a}}| = n$. Conversely, suppose that they are not equal; without loss of generality, suppose for convenience that $\mathbf{a}'\mathbf{t}_1 \neq \mathbf{a}'\mathbf{t}_2 \pmod{p}$. Then the complex numbers $\omega^{\mathbf{a}'\mathbf{t}_1}$ and $\omega^{\mathbf{a}'\mathbf{t}_2}$ are nonzero, and neither is a positive multiple of the other. Thus from the "equality" part of the triangle inequality[16] we have

$$|\omega^{\mathbf{a}'\mathbf{t}_1} + \omega^{\mathbf{a}'\mathbf{t}_2}| < |\omega^{\mathbf{a}'\mathbf{t}_1}| + |\omega^{\mathbf{a}'\mathbf{t}_2}|.$$

But then

$$|J_{\mathbf{a}}| < |\omega^{\mathbf{a}'\mathbf{t}_1}| + |\omega^{\mathbf{a}'\mathbf{t}_2}| + \sum_{i=3}^{n} |\omega^{\mathbf{a}'\mathbf{t}_i}| = n.$$

Proof of (b): The blocking $\mathcal{B}(L_{\mathbf{a}}, S)$ consists of p equal-sized blocks if and only if the components $c_{\mathbf{a}}(\mathbf{t})$, $\mathbf{t} \in S$, take on the values $1, \omega, \ldots, \omega^{p-1}$ equally often. Let n_j be the number of times that the value ω^j occurs among these components. Then $\mathcal{B}(L_{\mathbf{a}}, S)$ consists of p equal-sized blocks iff $n_0 = \cdots = n_{p-1}$. On the other hand,

$$J_{\mathbf{a}} = \sum_{j=0}^{p-1} n_j \omega^j = f(\omega),$$

say, so the numbers n_j are equal iff $f(\omega)$ is a constant multiple of $1 + \omega + \cdots + \omega^{p-1} = \Phi_p(\omega)$, where $\Phi_p(x) = 1 + x + \ldots + x^{p-1}$. Thus we must show that $f(\omega)$ is a constant multiple of $\Phi_p(\omega)$ iff $f(\omega) = 0$.

Now $\Phi(\omega) = (1 - \omega^p)/(1 - \omega) = 0$, so certainly if $f(\omega)$ is a multiple of $\Phi_p(\omega)$ then $f(\omega) = 0$. To see the converse, we note that $\Phi_p(x)$ is the minimal polynomial of ω over the rationals (Proposition A.15), so that if $f(\omega) = 0$ then $f(x) = \Phi_p(x)q(x)$ for some polynomial q (Theorem A.12). But f has degree (at most) $p - 1$, and Φ has degree $p - 1$, so q must be a constant. Thus $f(x) = q\Phi(x)$ for all x, and in particular for $x = \omega$, as we needed to show. □

From (6.57) we see that $0 \leq |J_{\mathbf{a}}|^2/n^2 \leq 1$ for all $\mathbf{a} \in (\mathbb{Z}/p)^k$, the values 1 and 0 occuring according to parts (a) and (b) of the proposition. The value is 1 in a *regular* fraction iff **a** represents a defining word, since these words are precisely those that are completely lost in the fraction. The value is 0 iff **a** represents an effect that is preserved in the fraction.

To define the generalized wordlengths W_j in this context, we modify (6.53) slightly:

$$W_j = \sum_{\ell(\mathbf{a})=j} |J_{\mathbf{a}}|^2/n^2, \tag{6.59}$$

the sum being taken over all $\mathbf{a} \in (\mathbb{Z}/p)^k$ of Hamming weight j. Note that in a *regular* fraction W_j is the number of defining words of length j. Also, if $p = 2$

[16] See Example A.54.

then $\ell(\mathbf{a})$ is the number of 1's in $\mathbf{a} = (a_1, \ldots, a_k)'$; the set $a = \{i : a_i = 1\}$ is the original subscript of J_a in (6.51)–(6.53) for fractions of 2^k experiments.

We note that $W_j = 0$ iff all effects of wordlength j in the effects group are preserved in the fraction. This raises the question of whether the generalized wordlength pattern can be used to identify the resolution, which for regular fractions is the first index j for which $W_j > 0$. That is indeed the case, but a proof would take us beyond the scope of this text. We will return to this in a moment.

In Arbitrary Factorials

In [152] Xu and Wu extended the notion of generalized wordlength pattern to arbitrary fractions of arbitrary factorial experiments, and thereby extended the notion of relative (and minimum) aberration to all fractions. Here's their approach.

Consider a $s_1 \times \cdots \times s_k$ experiment. Index the levels of the ith factor by the cyclic group $\mathbb{Z}/s_i$, so that the set of treatment combinations is

$$T = (\mathbb{Z}/s_1) \times \cdots \times (\mathbb{Z}/s_k).$$

This makes T an abelian group. By analogy with the p^k case, we also put

$$G = (\mathbb{Z}/s_1) \times \cdots \times (\mathbb{Z}/s_k)$$

and allow G to formally play the role of the effects group. It turns out that for our purposes the interpretation of G is immaterial.

For any s let $\omega_s = e^{2\pi i/s}$, a primitive sth root of unity. Paralleling equation (6.55), we create a vector $\mathbf{c_a}$ for each $\mathbf{a} \in G$. Its $\mathbf{t}$-th component is

$$c_{\mathbf{a}}(\mathbf{t}) = \prod_i \omega_{s_i}^{a_i t_i}, \tag{6.60}$$

where again $\mathbf{t} = (t_1, \ldots, t_k)$ and $\mathbf{a} = (a_1, \ldots, a_k)$. One can show (Exercise 6.24) that $\mathbf{c_a}$ is indeed a contrast vector in the full factorial design. The J-statistics of a given fraction S are now defined by summing over $\mathbf{t} \in S$, as before, giving a modified version of (6.56):

$$J_{\mathbf{a}} = \sum_{\mathbf{t} \in S} \prod_i \omega_{s_i}^{a_i t_i}. \tag{6.61}$$

This definition also applies when S is an *orthogonal array* if we understand the sum in (6.61) to allow repeated terms. A more precise way to say this is to write

$$J_{\mathbf{a}} = \sum_{\mathbf{t} \in S} O(\mathbf{t}) \prod_i \omega_{s_i}^{a_i t_i},$$

where $O(\mathbf{t})$ is the *counting function* of the array. In any case, we may then define the generalized wordlengths W_i by (6.59), exactly as before. Now the definitions of relative and minimum aberration (Definition 6.71) may be applied directly to the generalized wordlength patterns $(W_1, \ldots, W_k)$.

The following two results, which we present without proof, are of central importance. The first establishes something we noticed in the case of p^k factorials earlier:

Theorem 6.73 ([152, Theorem 3]) *The generalized wordlength pattern of a regular fraction is equal to its usual wordlength pattern.*

Recall that an orthogonal array is a fraction in which some runs are repeated.

Theorem 6.74 ([152, Theorem 4(ii)]) *The generalized wordlength pattern of an orthogonal array S satisfies*

$$W_1 = \ldots = W_t = 0 < W_{t+1} \tag{6.62}$$

if and only if S has maximum strength t.

For simple fractions (i.e., having no repeated runs), this theorem combined with Theorem 6.51 allows us to conclude the following, in answer to a question we raised earlier:

Corollary 6.75 *If the generalized wordlength pattern of a fraction S satisfies (6.62) then S has maximum resolution $t + 1$.*

The assignment of cyclic groups $\mathbb{Z}/s$ to index the levels of a factor may seem odd in one respect: When dealing with classical s^k factorial designs we used the finite field $GF(s)$, which has a different structure from $\mathbb{Z}/s$ when s is a prime power but not a prime. This leads to the question of how sensitive Theorems 6.73 and 6.74 are to the choice of groups. To allow for groups (of appropriate orders) other than cyclic ones, we need to replace the functions $\chi_a(t) = \omega_s^{at}$ by *group characters*, which takes us beyond the scope of this text.[17] We simply mention two points:

Theorem 6.76 ([17, Theorem 2.2 and Example 3.1]) *The generalized wordlength pattern of an orthogonal array is invariant with respect to the choice of abelian groups used to index the levels of the factors, but the J-characteristics do depend on this choice.*

Theorem 6.77 ([15, Theorem 4.3]) *Theorem 6.74 still holds if we index the levels of the factors by arbitrary abelian groups, and even by nonabelian groups if the counting function of the array is constant on conjugacy classes of G.*

Some Reflections

In developing our theory for fractional p^k designs, we interpreted J-characteristics and generalized wordlength patterns directly based on the theory for complex

[17] The functions $\chi_a(t) = \omega_s^{at}$ are themselves characters of $\mathbb{Z}/s$, as is noted in the literature.

contrasts developed in Sect. 5.6.5. Each contrast clearly represents an element of the effects group in an explicit fashion. The J-characteristics of a (possibly nonregular) fraction tell us exactly which effects are preserved and which are completely lost in the fraction, and can tell us which effects are mutually unaliased. Similarly, $W_j = 0$ tells us something globally about all the effects involving j factors.

In moving to fractions of arbitrary designs, we simply extended the formulas for $J_{\mathbf{a}}$ and W_j by analogy. In doing this, though, we lose interpretability. In particular:

- One would like to have a result like Proposition 6.72, but the vector $\mathbf{a} \in G$ no longer represents an effect in an obvious way, and it is not clear what effect the values $c_{\mathbf{a}}(\mathbf{t})$ encode. In fact, in this general case *we do not have an effects group to speak of*. In the case of classical symmetric fractions, these connections are very precise, as we know, and it would be desirable to develop a similar theory for arbitrary fractions.

  This question is complicated by the fact that the contrasts $\mathbf{c}_{\mathbf{a}}$ and the value of $J_{\mathbf{a}}$ depend on the use of cyclic groups to index levels of each factor, and as we have noted, this choice is arbitrary.
- Recall that in the original example of Fries and Hunter, and in regular fractions in general, the wordlengths W_j actually count words, and the comparison of wordlength patterns is based on underlying aliasing patterns. But in the case of nonregular fractions *there are no words*. It is imperative to determine just what the numbers W_j represent in nonregular fractions, and why it makes sense to compare wordlength patterns for nonregular fractions.

The literature makes some attempt to deal with these questions, but compared with what we know in the case of regular fractions these efforts are less than satisfactory. They often fall back on approaches we analyzed in Sect. 6.7, with their attendant difficulties. A close reading of the literature sometimes reveals vagueness at critical points, or statements begging for explanation (for example, models of response variables involving complex coefficients). A statement such as our Corollary 6.75 assumes a specific approach to resolution, and the reader needs to know at least what that approach is.

The theory of regular fractions is a benchmark toward which a general theory should aim. The purpose of these remarks is to indicate the work that remains in order to achieve this.

6.9 Projections

When we say that a fraction S has (maximum) strength t, we are describing the structure of the arrays we get when projecting S on t or fewer factors (Definition 6.38). But it is of both theoretical and practical interest to know the structure when we project on *more* than t factors.

The practical interest arises in so-called *screening experiments*. These are fractional factorial experiments with a large number of factors, with the assumption that only a few of the factors are "active". Various special methods have been developed to detect the active factors (since one generally has just one observation per treatment combination). Once these factors are identified, the fraction is then projected onto them, and the data re-analyzed.[18] The reader is referred to [42] for a recent survey of this topic.

We begin with a simple example that exhibits the main features of the general situation.

Example 6.78 Consider the principal 2^{4-1}_{III} fraction with defining equation $I = ABC$ (the fourth factor is D). The fraction is the solution set to the equation $t_1 + t_2 + t_3 = 0$ in $(\mathbb{Z}/2)^4$:

t_1	t_2	t_3	t_4
0	0	0	0
0	0	0	1
0	1	1	0
0	1	1	1
1	0	1	0
1	0	1	1
1	1	0	0
1	1	0	1

If we project this fraction on the first three factors (columns), we get two copies of the principal 2^{3-1}_{III} fraction with defining relation $I = ABC$. If we project instead on the last three factors, we get the full 2^3 factorial design on factors B, C and D.

In the first case, the defining word of the projected design is the same as that in the parent design. This can only happen when the defining relation involves only the factors on which we project. The second case occurs when we project on B, C and D, and there are no defining words in the parent design involving only these factors.

The main result of this section is that the projections of regular fractions consist either of copies of a complete factorial design or copies of a regular fraction. Roughly speaking, *projections of regular fractions are regular.* The proof is based on joint work with W. Diestelkamp.

We begin with some notation. If $\mathbf{v} = (v_1, \ldots, v_k)'$ and $\emptyset \neq I \subset \{1, \ldots, k\}$, then $\mathbf{v}_I$ is the subvector consisting of the components $v_i, i \in I$. The deleted components form the vector $\mathbf{v}_{I^c}$. For example, if $\mathbf{v} = (a, b, c, d)'$ and $I = \{1, 3\}$, then $\mathbf{v}_I = (a, c)'$ and $\mathbf{v}_{I^c} = (b, d)'$. Note that $\mathbf{v}_I = P_I(\mathbf{v})$ where P_I is the projection map of $A_1 \times \cdots \times A_k$ onto a subproduct $A_{i_1} \times \cdots \times A_{i_m}$ described in Sect. 6.5.2

[18] Note that this involves a form of *data snooping*, but without the theoretical justification for methods of multiple comparisons such as Scheffé's.

(Eq. (6.27)). For us the sets A_i will all equal a field F, namely the finite field $GF(s)$. This means that each projection map P_I is a linear transformation from F^k to F^h where $h = |I|$.

Our example indicates that when projecting a given fraction onto a subset I of factors, the defining words involving only the factors in I will play a central role. These correspond to the elements $\mathbf{a}$ in the defining subspace E of the fraction such that $\mathbf{a}_{I^c} = \mathbf{0}$. The set

$$E_0 = \{\mathbf{a} \in E \colon \mathbf{a}_{I^c} = \mathbf{0}\} \tag{6.63}$$

is a subspace of E, as is easily checked. (We should really write something like $E_0(I)$ as it actually depends on I, but we are suppressing this in our notation for ease of reading.) Note that we have defined E_0 so that its elements involve *some or all* of the factors in I. This subspace may be described another way: the fact that $\mathbf{a}_{I^c} = \mathbf{0}$ means that $\mathbf{a} \in N(P_{I^c})$, the nullspace of P_{I^c}, so that

$$E_0 = E \cap N(P_{I^c}). \tag{6.64}$$

This is a very useful characterization.

Lemma 6.79 *Let F be a field, and let $E \subset F^k$ be a subspace of dimension r. Let $I \subset \{1, \ldots, k\}$, and let $h = |I|$ and $d = \dim E_0$ where E_0 is given by (6.63).*

If $d = 0$, then for any basis $\mathbf{a}_1, \ldots, \mathbf{a}_r$ of E the vectors $\mathbf{a}_{1,I^c}, \ldots, \mathbf{a}_{r,I^c}$ are linearly independent.

If $d > 0$ then there is a basis $\mathbf{a}_1, \ldots, \mathbf{a}_d, \ldots, \mathbf{a}_r$ of E such that

a. $\mathbf{a}_1, \ldots, \mathbf{a}_d$ is a basis of E_0
b. $\mathbf{a}_{1,I^c} = \cdots = \mathbf{a}_{d,I^c} = \mathbf{0}$,
c. $\mathbf{a}_{1,I}, \ldots, \mathbf{a}_{d,I}$ are linearly independent, and
d. $\mathbf{a}_{d+1,I^c}, \ldots, \mathbf{a}_{r,I^c}$ are linearly independent.

In general we have $d \leq h$ and $r - d \leq k - h$.

Proof Let Q be the restriction of P_{I^c} to E. Note that equation (6.64) means that $E_0 = N(Q)$.

If $d = 0$ then $N(Q) = \{\mathbf{0}\}$, and so Q is one-to-one on E. Thus, given any basis $\mathbf{a}_1, \ldots, \mathbf{a}_r$ of E, the images $\mathbf{a}_{1,I^c}, \ldots, \mathbf{a}_{r,I^c}$ are linearly independent.

If $d > 0$, let $\mathbf{a}_1, \ldots, \mathbf{a}_d$ be a basis of E_0. These vectors of course satisfy (b), as do all elements of E_0. Condition (c) follows from this and the independence of $\mathbf{a}_1, \ldots, \mathbf{a}_d$. Extend this to a basis $\mathbf{a}_1, \ldots, \mathbf{a}_r$ of E, and let $E_1 = \langle \mathbf{a}_{d+1}, \ldots, \mathbf{a}_r \rangle$. Then

$$E = E_0 \oplus E_1 \quad \text{(direct sum)}.$$

Now Q is one-to-one on E_1 (easy proof). Therefore, since $\mathbf{a}_{d+1}, \ldots, \mathbf{a}_r$ are linearly independent, so are their images under Q. But this is statement (d).

Lastly, let $\mathbf{e}_1, \ldots, \mathbf{e}_k$ be the standard basis of F^k ($\mathbf{e}_i$ has 1 in the ith coordinate and zeros elsewhere). Then clearly E_0 is contained in the span of $\{\mathbf{e}_i : i \in I\}$, so $d \leq h$. Similarly, the vectors $\mathbf{a}_{d+1,I^c}, \ldots, \mathbf{a}_{r,I^c}$ are contained in the span of $\{\mathbf{e}_i : i \in I^c\}$, so by (d) we have $r - d \leq k - h$. □

With this lemma in hand, we turn to our main result. In order to visualize the repetition of elements in a projection of an s^{k-r} fraction S, we display S as a $k \times N$ *orthogonal array* O, where $N = s^{k-r}$. The columns of O are the elements of S. (In Example 6.78 we transposed O for convenience.) Recall that when we project the array on a set $I \subset \{1, \ldots, k\}$ of rows (factors), we delete the rows not indexed by I. We will denote the resulting $h \times N$ sub-array by O_I (where $h = |I|$).

Theorem 6.80 *Suppose S is a regular s^{k-r} fraction with defining subspace E. Let O be the $k \times s^{k-r}$ orthogonal array displaying S. Let $\emptyset \neq I \subset \{1, \ldots, k\}$ with $h = |I|$, and let $d = \dim E_0$ where E_0 is given by (6.63).*

a. If $d = 0$ then O_I consists of s^{k-h-r} copies of the full factorial (that is, $(GF(s))^h$) on the factors in I.
b. If $d > 0$ then O_I consists of $s^{k-h-(r-d)}$ copies of a regular fraction P of size s^{h-d}. The defining subspace of P is precisely E_0.

Because of this theorem, it is reasonable to refer to E_0 as the *defining subspace of the projection*, with the understanding that it may contain no defining vectors at all ($d = 0$).

Proof For each $\mathbf{t} \in S$—that is, each column $\mathbf{t}$ in O—the corresponding column of O_I is an $h \times 1$ vector $\mathbf{t}_I$, and the deleted components form a vector $\mathbf{t}_{I^c}$. While the vectors $\mathbf{t} \in S$ are distinct, we understand that the vectors $\mathbf{t}_I$ need not be, and similarly for the vectors $\mathbf{t}_{I^c}$.

Proof of (a): Let S be the solution set of a system

$$\begin{aligned} \mathbf{a}_1'\mathbf{t} &= b_1 \\ &\vdots \\ \mathbf{a}_r'\mathbf{t} &= b_r \end{aligned} \tag{6.65}$$

where $\mathbf{a}_1, \ldots, \mathbf{a}_r$ is a basis of E. Let us rewrite this in the form

$$\begin{aligned} \mathbf{a}_{1,I^c}'\mathbf{t}_{I^c} &= b_1 - \mathbf{a}_{1,I}'\mathbf{t}_I \\ &\vdots \\ \mathbf{a}_{r,I^c}'\mathbf{t}_{I^c} &= b_r - \mathbf{a}_{r,I}'\mathbf{t}_I \end{aligned} \tag{6.66}$$

where each $\mathbf{a}$ is partitioned into $\mathbf{a}_I$ and $\mathbf{a}_{I^c}$, the same as $\mathbf{t}$. For each fixed value of $\mathbf{t}_I \in (GF(s))^h$ on the right-hand side of (6.66) we have a system of r equations in the unknown $\mathbf{t}_{I^c}$—that is, in $k - h$ variables. Moreover, the vectors $\mathbf{a}_{i,I^c}$ are linearly independent because of Lemma 6.79, and so by Lemma 5.43(d) the system has s^{k-h-r} solutions $\mathbf{t}_{I^c}$. Thus each h-tuple $\mathbf{t}_I$ in O_I occurs s^{k-h-r} times.

Proof of (b): Let $\mathbf{a}_1, \ldots, \mathbf{a}_r$ be a basis of defining vectors of S satisfying (a)–(d) of Lemma 6.79. The system (6.65) now takes the form

$$\begin{aligned} \mathbf{a}'_{1,I}\mathbf{t}_I &= b_1 \\ &\vdots \\ \mathbf{a}'_{d,I}\mathbf{t}_I &= b_d \end{aligned} \tag{6.67}$$

$$\begin{aligned} \mathbf{a}'_{d+1,I^c}\mathbf{t}_{I^c} &= b_{d+1} - \mathbf{a}'_{d+1,I}\mathbf{t}_I \\ &\vdots \\ \mathbf{a}'_{r,I^c}\mathbf{t}_{I^c} &= b_r - \mathbf{a}'_{r,I}\mathbf{t}_I \end{aligned} \tag{6.68}$$

In (6.67) (the first d equations), the vectors $\mathbf{a}_{1,I}, \ldots, \mathbf{a}_{d,I}$ are linearly independent, and $\mathbf{t}_I$ is $h \times 1$, so by Lemma 5.43(d) the system has $h-d$ distinct solutions $\mathbf{t}_I$. These solutions to the system form a regular s^{h-d} design P, say, with defining subspace E_0. The strength of P is at least t since the minimum Hamming weight (= minimum wordlength) of a vector in E_0 is no less than that of E.

If we fix any one solution $\mathbf{t}_I$ of (6.67), system (6.68) contains $r-d$ equations in the unknown $(k-h)$-component vector $\mathbf{t}_{I^c}$, where the coefficient vectors $\mathbf{a}_{i,I^c}$ are independent. This system therefore has $s^{k-h-(r-d)}$ solutions $\mathbf{t}_{I^c}$. Thus each vector $\mathbf{t}_I$ occurs $s^{k-h-(r-d)}$ times as a column in O_I. □

Just as the defining subspace E of a fraction corresponds to its defining subgroup H, the subspace $E_0(= E_0(I))$ corresponds to the subgroup

$$H_0(= H_0(I)) = \{A_1^{a_1} \cdots A_k^{a_k} \in H\colon\ a_i = 0 \text{ for all } i \notin I\} \tag{6.69}$$

consisting of those defining words only involving the factors indexed by I (together with the identity). A basis of E_0 corresponds to a set of *independent generators*[19] of H_0. It is thus natural to refer to H_0 as the *defining subgroup of the projection*. We may restate Theorem 6.80 in the following way:

Corollary 6.81 *Suppose S is a regular s^{k-r} fraction with defining group H. Let O be the $k \times s^{k-r}$ orthogonal array displaying S. Let $\emptyset \neq I \subset \{1, \ldots, k\}$ with $h = |I|$, and let H_0 be the defining subgroup (6.69) of the projection.*

---

[19] Independence of elements of the effects group is defined in equation (5.42). The notion of a group generator is given in the Appendix (page 297).

a. *If $H_0 = \{identity\}$—that is, if there are no defining words that depend only on the factors in I—then O_I consists of s^{k-h-r} copies of the full factorial $(GF(s))^h$ on the factors in I.*
b. *If H_0 is generated by d independent group elements, then O_I consists of $s^{k-h-(r-d)}$ copies of a regular fraction P of size s^{h-d}. The defining group of P is precisely H_0.*

Example 6.82 Consider the 3^{6-3} design generated by ABD, ACE and BCF. Here $k = 6$ and $r = 3$. The reader can verify that the defining group consists of

$$ABD, ACE, BCF, A^2BCDE, AB^2CDF, ABC^2EF,$$
$$BC^2DE^2, AC^2DF^2, AB^2EF^2,$$
$$A^2B^2C^2DEF, B^2DEF^2, A^2DE, CDE^2F^2$$

and their squares, together with the identity,[20] so that the design has resolution 3 (strength $t = 2$).

Suppose we project this fraction on factors A through E, so that $h = 5$. The defining words containing only those letters are ABD, ACE, A^2BCDE, BC^2DE^2 and A^2DE and their squares. These may be generated by the independent words ABD, ACE and A^2DE (or AD^2E^2), so the projection's defining subgroup H_0 has $d = 3$ generators. The projection thus consists of $3^{6-5-(3-3)} = 3$ copies of the 3^{5-3} design on factors A through E, with defining words ABD, ACE and AD^2E^2. We see that this design has resolution 3 (= strength 2).

The original design has no defining words involving only factors A, B and C, so that if we project on these three factors ($h = 3$) we get $3^{6-3-3} = 1$ copy of the full factorial on these three factors.

We return to an earlier result (page 257), which is now an easy corollary:

Proof of Theorem 6.52 Let S be a regular fraction of maximum resolution R. We claim that S has maximum strength $R - 1$. As we noted earlier, S clearly cannot have strength R since then it would have resolution $R + 1$, by Theorem 6.51, so we just need to show that it has strength $R - 1$.

By Corollary 6.26, S has no defining words of length less than R. Thus Corollary 6.81 implies that for any $I \subset \{1, \ldots, k\}$ with $|I| = R - 1$, the subgroup $H_0(I)$ is trivial, so that the projection of S on any $R - 1$ factors must consist of copies of the complete factorial design on those factors. But this is precisely the definition of strength $R - 1$. □

Remark 6.83 A proof of Theorem 6.52 along the same lines, but for principal fractions, can be found in [136, pages 209–210].

[20] In Example 6.82, if we put $X = ABD$, $Y = ACE$, $Z = BCF$, then this list consists of X, Y, Z, XY, XZ, YZ, XY^2, XZ^2, YZ^2, XYZ, XY^2Z, XYZ^2, and XY^2Z^2.

The result stated in Corollary 6.26 appears to be widely known—see, for example, [36, page 159] or [97, page 11]. Oddly, there does not appear to be a proof in the published literature.

The projection on R factors of a regular fraction of resolution R is easy to see: If the R factors appear in a defining word X of length R (there must be one), then the projection consists of copies of a regular s^{R-1} fraction whose sole defining word is X. Note that there are no smaller defining words based on a subset of those factors, since R is the minimum wordlength defining the parent fraction.

There do not seem to be many results for projections on $h > R$ factors. When $s = 2$, H. Chen [34, Lemma 1] observed the following:

Proposition 6.84 *Consider projecting a 2^{k-r} fraction of maximum resolution R on h factors. If*

$$R + 1 \leq h \leq R + [(R-1)/2], \tag{6.70}$$

then the defining subspace E_0 of the projection has dimension 0 or 1. Equivalently, the defining subgroup H_0 either is trivial or has one generator. (As usual, $[\cdot]$ is the greatest integer function.)

Of course, this means that any such projection consists of copies either of a complete 2^h factorial or of a 2^{h-1} fraction. Chen [34, Theorem 1] gives a count of the number of projections of each type.

Proof of Proposition 6.84 If $\dim E_0 = 0$, we are done, so assume there is a nonzero vector $\mathbf{a} \in E_0$. We claim that if there is another nonzero $\mathbf{b} \in E_0$ such that $\mathbf{a}$ and $\mathbf{b}$ are independent, then (6.70) implies that $\ell(\mathbf{a} + \mathbf{b}) < R$, where ℓ is the Hamming length (= wordlength). Since $\mathbf{a} + \mathbf{b}$ is a defining vector of the parent fraction, this contradicts the fact that R is the minimum wordlength of the fraction.

Let I be the set of factors on which we are projecting. Vectors $\mathbf{a} \in E_0$ are such that $\mathbf{a}_{I^c} = \mathbf{0}$, so we may ignore the components of $\mathbf{a}$ and $\mathbf{b}$ corresponding to the factors in I^c, and assume that both vectors are in $(\mathbb{Z}/2)^h$. Since $1 + 1 = 0 \pmod 2$, we maximize $\ell(\mathbf{a} + \mathbf{b})$ (the worst case) by minimizing their "overlap", that is, the number of component positions in which both have a 1.

Solving the right-hand side of (6.70) for R, we find that

$$\begin{aligned} R \geq & (2/3)h + (1/3), \quad R \text{ odd}, \\ & (2/3)h + (2/3), \quad R \text{ even}, \end{aligned} \tag{6.71}$$

so that the bound (6.71) holds in all cases. Let $\ell_1 = \ell(\mathbf{a})$ and $\ell_2 = \ell(\mathbf{b})$. Then $\ell_i \geq R$, so

$$\ell_i \geq (2/3)h + (1/3).$$

If $h = 3m$ for some m, then $\ell_i \geq 2m + (1/3)$, so $\ell_i \geq 2m + 1$, and we minimize the overlap of $\mathbf{a}$ and $\mathbf{b}$ by assuming $\ell_1 = \ell_2 = 2m + 1$. Then the number of components in the overlap is $m + 2$, and so

$$\begin{aligned}\ell_1 + \ell_2 &= 2(2m + 1 - (m + 2)) \\ &= 2m - 2 \\ &= (2/3)h - 2 < (2/3)h + (1/3) \leq R,\end{aligned}$$

a contradiction. The cases $h = 3m + 1$ and $h = 3m + 2$ are proved similarly and are left as an exercise. □

6.9.1 In Non-regular Designs

In projecting a fractional design onto a subset of factors, the interest is in the structure of the projection. In the case of regular designs, as we have seen, the projected design is a set of replicates, either of a complete factorial or of a regular fraction. We may say that the projected design has been *decomposed* into the juxtaposition of several copies of a smaller array.

In this way the question of projection leads to the analysis of the structure of an orthogonal array of strength t as a juxtaposition of several smaller ones of that strength, where the number of factors is greater than t. Perhaps the first such result is that of Seiden and Zemach [129, Proposition 2.5], who showed that every symmetric orthogonal array having $t + 1$ factors and $s = 2$ symbols is a juxtaposition of arrays of size 2^t. Such arrays are the smallest possible of strength t, having *index* $\lambda = 1$. Cheng [35] utilized this fact to show that every array on $s = 2$ symbols with $t + 1$ factors is the juxtaposition of half-replicates of a 2^{t+1} factorial design and copies of the full 2^{t+1} design.

When $s > 2$, the question of decomposition of arrays having $t + 1$ factors is far more complicated. Diestelkamp [46] proved that *simple* arrays with $s = 3$ symbols decompose into arrays of index $\lambda = 1$, but gave an example of an indecomposable array of index $\lambda = 2$. Verification of that example, and an analysis of decomposable arrays with $s = 3$ symbols, are discussed in [48]. Note that symmetric arrays of index 1 are guaranteed to be regular only when $s = 2$ or 3 [48, 71].

In [28] Box and Tyssedal defined an orthogonal array as having *projectivity* P if every projection on P factors contains a complete s^P factorial design. (Their original definition assumed $s = 2$.) A regular fraction of resolution R has projectivity $R - 1$ (its strength), but cannot have projectivity R: for it must have a defining word of length R, and by Theorem 6.80 the projection on the factors comprising that word must consist of copies of a fractional design. By contrast, Box and Tyssedal showed that there are non-regular designs of resolution 3 and projectivity 3. Similar results were obtained around the same time by Lin and

Draper [92], who studied projections of Plackett-Burman designs. Further results and discussion may be found in [31] and [36], primarily for 2-level designs. Projection properties of orthogonal arrays continue to be a major area of research.

6.10 Exercises

Section 6.1

6.1. Prove Proposition 6.6(a, b). (For (a), identify the constant b.)

6.2. Prove Lemma 6.7(b).

6.3. Regarding Example 6.19:

(i) Find the aliases of C and D. Are any of the five main effects aliased with each other?

(ii) How many alias sets should there be? Find a representative of each. (You may find it easier to consider linear independence in $(\mathbb{Z}/3)^5$.)

(iii) Suppose the fraction was constructed using the principal block of the 3^5 factorial design. List three of the treatment combinations in this fraction. How many should there be in all?

6.4. Consider a regular 4^{3-1} design generated by ABC. Find the alias sets, expressing each effect in reduced (i.e., monic) form. Which effects are lost in the fraction? (The arithmetic of $GF(4)$ is given in Example A.17.)

Section 6.2

6.5. Show that the Hamming length in $(GF(s))^k$ satisfies the triangle inequality.

6.6. Prove Theorem 6.24(c). (A key step is to show that one can choose distinct F_1 and F_2 of length $R/2$ so that $\ell(F_1 F_2{}^{-1}) < R$.)

6.7. Find all the alias sets for the 2^{6-3} fraction in Example 6.27.

6.8. Prove Corollary 6.29. (Use parts (a) and (c) of Theorem 6.24. Keep in mind the correspondence of effects F with elements $\mathbf{a} \in (GF(s))^k$.)

Section 6.3

6.9. Construct the principal 3^{4-2} fraction having defining words ABC^2 and AB^2D^2 two ways:

(i) using the method of Example 6.32.

(ii) using the method of Remark 6.33.

Compare the two results (they should give the same 9 cells).

Section 6.4

6.10. Create a table of contrast columns for a 2^3 factorial design, associating -1 with level 0 and $+1$ with level 1 of each factor. Let $S = \{001, 010, 100, 111\}$ be the non-principal fraction defined by $I = ABC$. Show that the sum of the contrasts belonging to any aliased pair (such as A and BC) is a contrast whose support is S, and and whose restriction to S belongs to the effects in that pair.

6.11. Prove Theorem 6.35.

6.12. Let S be a principal fraction as in Theorem 6.35, and let $\ell'_0, \ldots, \ell'_{s-1}$ be another set of numbers that sum to zero. For each $\mathbf{a} \in \mathbf{a}_0 + E$ define another contrast function $d_\mathbf{a}$ by (6.26) using the numbers ℓ'. Show that if $c_{\mathbf{a}_0}$ and $d_{\mathbf{a}_0}$ are linearly independent then so are $c_\mathbf{a}$ and $d_\mathbf{a}$. Thus in particular, a basis of $U_{\mathcal{B}(L_{\mathbf{a}_0})}$ defines a basis of $U_{\mathcal{B}(L_\mathbf{a})}$.

6.13. State and prove versions of Lemma 6.34 and Theorem 6.35 for non-principal regular fractions.

Section 6.5

6.14. Prove Proposition 6.37.

6.15. An orthogonal array with N runs, k factors, s symbols (levels) and strength t is said to be an $OA(N, k, s, t)$.

(i) Show that the juxtaposition of an $OA(N_1, k, s, t_1)$ and an $OA(N_2, k, s, t_2)$ is an $OA(N, s, k, t)$ where $N = N_1 + N_2$ and $t \geq \min(t_1, t_2)$.
(ii) Show how to create an $OA(54, 4, 3, 3)$.

6.16. Prove Corollary 6.45.

6.17. By taking dimensions in Corollary 6.47(a), write out the Rao inequalities and justify your statements.

Section 6.7

6.18. With respect to the nonregular fraction $\{000, 001, 010, 100\}$ of Example 6.58:

(i) Assuming interactions absent, derive (6.40).
(ii) Substituting these relations in (6.31)–(6.33), verify that these contrasts reduce to (6.41).
(iii) Show that the fraction $\{000, 001, 010, 100\}$ doesn't have Resolution II, according to Definition 6.25. (For example, show that it doesn't have strength 1.)

6.19. Show that we may estimate ψ_{ABC} (Eq. (6.38)) in the principal fraction of Examples 6.54 and 6.57 by assuming that the sum (or average) of the eight cell means is zero. (Statisticians are usually unwilling to make such a "low-order" assumption when higher-order effects are allowed to be present.)

6.20. For the Plackett-Burman design in Example 6.53, show that every column of the alias matrix $\mathbf{A}$ contains three zeros. In particular, show that each two-factor interaction is unaliased with the two corresponding main effects.

Section 6.8

6.21. Show that design (c) has minimum aberration among all regular 2^{7-2} designs. (Consider, and eliminate, possible wordlength patterns.)

6.22. Prove Lemma 6.63(c). (Fix an order of the defining words, and let $\delta_{wj} = 1$ if the wth word contains the letter A_j, and = 0 otherwise, for $w = 1, \ldots, s^r - 1$. Compute $\sum_w \sum_j \delta_{wj}$ and $\sum_j \sum_w \delta_{wj}$.)

6.23. Prove the claim indicated in the proof of Proposition 6.66. (Of the independent defining vectors $\mathbf{a}_1, \ldots, \mathbf{a}_r$ let r_1 be the number of them having a nonzero entry in the jth coordinate. By assumption, $r_1 \geq 1$; without loss of generality we may assume that these vectors are $\mathbf{a}_1, \ldots, \mathbf{a}_{r_1}$. Quote any result from Section 5.6.1 that is helpful.)

6.24. Show that the vector $\mathbf{c_a}$ defined by Eq. (6.60) is a contrast vector in the full $s_1 \times \cdots \times s_k$ factorial design. (Hint: The sum can be iterated.)

6.25. Find the J-characteristics and generalized wordlength patterns of the following non-regular fractions.

(i) $\begin{bmatrix} 0 & 0 & 0 & 1 \\ 0 & 0 & 1 & 0 \\ 0 & 1 & 0 & 0 \end{bmatrix}$, 1/2 of a 2^3 factorial experiment.

(ii) $\begin{bmatrix} 0 & 0 & 0 & 0 & 1 & 1 & 1 & 1 & a & a & a & a & b & b & b & b \\ 0 & 1 & a & b & 0 & 1 & a & b & 0 & 1 & a & b & 0 & 1 & a & b \\ 0 & 1 & a & b & a & 0 & b & 1 & 1 & b & 0 & a & b & a & 1 & 0 \end{bmatrix}$, 1/4 of a 4^3 factorial experiment. (This is taken from [48, Theorem 3.8], where it is shown to be non-regular. One can easily check that it has strength 2.)

Section 6.9

6.26. Consider the 3^{6-3}_{III} design in Example 6.82.

(i) The projection onto factors A, B, C and E, results in a fraction. How many copies? Describe the fraction as 3^{h-d}, give d independent defining words, and determine its resolution.
(ii) What projections onto four factors, if any, give (copies of) a full factorial design?
(iii) Of the six possible projections onto five factors, which have resolution 5? What is the resolution of the others?

6.27. Complete the proof of Proposition 6.84.

6.2 [illegible] in order of the [illegible] words, and let [illegible] one with [illegible] contains the letter A [illegible] = 0 otherwise, for [illegible]
(Compute [illegible])

6.3 [illegible] indicated in the proof of the converse to [illegible] [illegible] vectors [illegible] the number of [illegible] [illegible] [illegible] without [illegible] [illegible]

6.4 [illegible] defined [illegible] [illegible] [illegible] design [illegible] and [illegible] consists of the following [illegible]

[illegible]

[illegible] with [illegible] 2.

Solutions

6.6 [illegible]

(a) [illegible] [illegible] delete [illegible] defining [illegible]

(b) What [illegible] (compare [illegible]) design?

(c) [illegible] possible [illegible] [illegible] solution [illegible]

6.7 Complete [illegible]

Appendix A
Mathematical Background

Throughout we use $|E|$ to denote the cardinality of the set E. We use $\mathbb{Z}$, $\mathbb{Q}$, $\mathbb{R}$ and $\mathbb{C}$ to denote the integers, the rational numbers, the real numbers, and the complex numbers, respectively.

A.1 Functions

We write $f{:}A \to B$ to denote a function defined on the set A with values in the set B. We use the terms *function* and *map* interchangeably. If $f(a) = b$, we also write $f{:}a \mapsto b$. The set A is called the *domain* of f, while the *range* of f is the set

$$\text{range}(f) = \{b \in B{:}b = f(a) \text{ for some } a \in A\}.$$

Of course, range$(f) \subseteq B$. If range$(f) = B$, we say that f maps A *onto* B, or that f is *surjective*. If $C \subset A$, then the *image* of C under the function is the set $\{b \in B{:}b = f(a) \text{ for some } a \in C\}$.

If, for any $a_1, a_2 \in A$, $f(a_1) = f(a_2)$ implies $a_1 = a_2$, then we say that f is a *one-to-one* function, or is *injective*.

If f maps A one-to-one onto B, then it has an *inverse function* $f^{-1}{:}B \to A$, where $f^{-1}(b) = a$ iff $f(a) = b$. In this case we say that f is *invertible*.

If $f{:}A \to B$ and $g{:}B \to C$, then their *composite* is the function $g \circ f{:}A \to C$ such that $g \circ f(a) = g(f(a))$. The *identity function* $id_A{:}A \to A$ is the function $id_A(a) = a$ for all $a \in A$. If $f{:}A \to B$ is invertible, then $f^{-1} \circ f = id_A$ and $f \circ f^{-1} = id_B$.

J. H. Beder, *Linear Models and Design*,
https://doi.org/10.1007/978-3-031-08176-7

A.2 Relations

The *power set* of a set S is the set of all subsets of S.

A *relation* on a set S is a subset $R \subset S \times S$. We write xRy if $(x, y) \in R$. Properties that we will be interested in are:

Reflexivity: xRx for all $x \in S$.
Symmetry: xRy implies yRx.
Antisymmetry: xRy and yRx implies $x = y$.
Transitivity: xRy and yRz implies xRz.

A.2.1 *Partially Ordered Sets and Lattices*

A *partial order* on a set S is a relation that is reflexive, antisymmetric, and transitive. The most basic examples of partial orders are the relation $\leq$ on $\mathbb{R}$ and the subset relation $\subset$ (or $\subseteq$) on the power set of a given set. Because of the former, the symbol $\leq$ is adopted generically for partial orders.

The order is called "partial" because there may be elements which are *unrelated*, that is, elements x and y for which neither $x \leq y$ nor $y \leq x$. A partially ordered set is called a *poset*. A poset with no unrelated elements is said to be *totally* (or *linearly*) *ordered*. Thus a total order is a partial order satisfying the additional condition that for any x and y, $x \leq y$ or $y \leq x$. A totally ordered subset of a poset is called a *chain*.

Example A.1 Consider a Cartesian product $S = A_1 \times \cdots \times A_k$ where $A_i \subset \mathbb{R}$. Its elements are k-tuples $\mathbf{x} = (x_1, \ldots, x_k)$, with $x_i \in A_i$. The relation

$$\mathbf{x} \leq \mathbf{y} \quad \text{iff} \quad x_i \leq y_i \text{ for all } i$$

defines a partial order on S.

We can define a total order on S by writing

$$\mathbf{x} < \mathbf{y} \quad \text{iff} \quad x_i < y_i \text{ for the first } i \text{ at which they differ.}$$

This is the *lexicographic order* on S, so named because of its relation to the alphabetical order of words in a dictionary.

If S is a poset and $A \subset S$, an *upper bound* for A is an element $y \in S$ such that $x \leq y$ for all $x \in A$. The element y is a *least upper bound (lub)* or *supremum* of A if it is an upper bound and if $y \leq z$ for any other upper bound z. *Lower bound* and *greatest lower bound (glb)* or *infimum* are defined analogously. Antisymmetry implies that lubs and glbs are unique.

If a poset S itself has a least upper bound, we call that element the *top element*. Similarly, the greatest lower bound of S, if it exists, is called its *bottom element*. We will use $\hat{1}$ and $\hat{0}$, respectively, for the top and bottom elements.[1] A poset having $\hat{1}$ and $\hat{0}$ is said to be *bounded*.

The lub and glb of x and y are denoted $x \vee y$ and $x \wedge y$. The operations $\vee$ and $\wedge$ are known as the *join* and the *meet*.

We say that z *covers* y if $y \leq z$ and there is no element between them. A *Hasse diagram* of a poset S is a graph whose vertices are the elements of S, such that there is an ascending edge from y to z if z covers y, and no edge between unrelated elements. The four-element poset consisting of $x, y, x \vee y$ and $x \wedge y$ has a Hasse diagram pictured below.

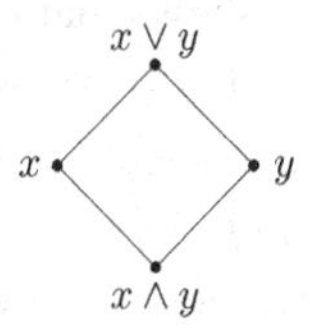

The *dual of a statement* about a poset is a statement which replaces $\leq$ by $\geq$, $\vee$ by $\wedge$, and $\wedge$ by $\vee$.

A *lattice* is a poset in which every finite subset has a least upper bound and a greatest lower bound. (The four-element poset pictured above is obviously a lattice, known in the literature as M_2 [40, p. 30].) The lattice L is *distributive* if

$$\text{for all } x, y, z \in L, x \wedge (y \vee z) = (x \wedge y) \vee (x \wedge z). \tag{A.1}$$

This is known, of course, as a *distributive law*. It is not hard to show that if the distributive law holds in L, then so does its dual [40, Lemma 6.3]. The classical example of a (bounded) distributive lattice is the power set of a set under the operations $\cup$ and $\cap$. (The power set has the stronger property that it contains the meet and join, not just of finite families of sets, but of *arbitrary* families. Such a lattice is said to be *complete*.)

For us, an important example of a lattice is the family of subspaces of a vector space under inclusion. We will describe its meet and join operations in Sect. A.4.1. It turns out that this type of lattice only satisfies the distributive law (A.1) under the assumption that $x \geq z$. Since then $x \wedge z = z$, the law may be restated as follows:

$$\text{For all } x, y, z \in L, \;\; x \geq z \Rightarrow x \wedge (y \vee z) = (x \wedge y) \vee z. \tag{A.2}$$

This is known as the *modular law*, and a lattice satisfying it is a *modular lattice*. By rearranging it and using commutativity, we get the dual law as well:

$$\text{For all } x, y, z \in L, \;\; z \leq x \Rightarrow z \vee (y \wedge x) = (z \vee y) \wedge x. \tag{A.3}$$

---

[1] Other common notations are $\bigvee S$ and $\bigwedge S$, or $\top$ and $\bot$.

(The modular law is said to be *self-dual.*) This law holds not only for vector spaces but more generally for modules over rings, hence its name. (See Theorem A.21 and Proposition A.27.)

It is useful to note that every lattice is half-distributive and thus half-modular, in the following sense [40, Lemma 6.1]:

Lemma A.2 *Let x, y and z be elements of a lattice L. Then:*

a. $x \wedge (y \vee z) \geq (x \wedge y) \vee (x \wedge z)$.
b. $x \geq z$ *implies* $x \wedge (y \vee z) \geq (x \wedge y) \vee z$.

Proof An application of transitivity shows that if $b \geq c$ then $a \wedge b \geq a \wedge c$. Thus $x \wedge (y \vee z) \geq (x \wedge y)$ and $\geq x \wedge z$. This gives the first part, and the second follows easily. □

In a bounded lattice L, the *complement* of $x \in L$ is an element y such that $x \vee y = \hat{1}$ and $x \wedge y = \hat{0}$. A lattice in which every element has a complement is said to be *complemented*. If each element x has a unique complement, we denote it by x'. The defining properties of complementation are thus

- $x \vee x' = \hat{1}$ and $x \wedge x' = \hat{0}$.

If in addition we have

- $x'' = x$ ($'$ is an *involution*)
- $x \leq y$ implies $x' \geq y'$

then we call the operation $'$ *orthocomplementation*. The example from which this gets its name is the orthocomplement of a subspace of a vector space. In the power set of a set, this operation is the usual set complementation. An *ortholattice* is a lattice having an orthocomplementation operation.

Lemma A.3 *For all x and y in an ortholattice L, we have the* De Morgan laws

$$\begin{aligned} (x \wedge y)' &= x' \vee y', \\ (x \vee y)' &= x' \wedge y'. \end{aligned} \tag{A.4}$$

Proof $z = (x \wedge y)'$

$$\begin{aligned} &\iff z' = x \wedge y \\ &\iff z' = \text{ the largest element of } L \text{ such that } z' \leq x \text{ and } z' \leq y \\ &\iff z = \text{ the smallest element of } L \text{ such that } z \geq x' \text{ and } z \geq y' \\ &\iff z = x' \vee y'. \end{aligned}$$

The second law is proved similarly. □

A.2.2 *Equivalence Relations and Partitions*

An *equivalence relation* on a set S is a relation that is reflexive, symmetric, and transitive. There are numerous ways of denoting the equivalence of x and y, two generic notations being $x \sim y$ and $x \equiv y$.

Let $\sim$ be an equivalence relation on S, and let $x \in S$. The *equivalence class* of x is the set $\{y \in S{:}x \sim y\}$. Let C_x denote the equivalence class of x. Then $x \in C_x$, and $C_x = C_y$ iff $x \sim y$.

A *partition* of a set S is a family of pairwise disjoint subsets whose union is S. We will refer to these subsets as *blocks*, and denote the family by script letters $\mathcal{A}, \mathcal{B}, \ldots$. In general we deal with finite partitions, that is, partitions into finitely many blocks (and in fact with finite sets, which can only have finite partitions). Thus $\mathcal{B} = \{B_1, \ldots, B_k\}$ is a partition of S iff $B_i \cap B_j =$ for $i \neq j$ and $\cup_{i=1}^{k} B_i = S$. We will denote by Part(S) the set of partitions of S.

A common way for partitions to arise is through functions. Let $f{:}S \to T$ be a function. The sets $f^{-1}(y) = \{x \in S{:}f(x) = y\}$ are the *contours*, *level sets* or *level curves* of f. Clearly every $x \in S$ belongs to some contour. Moreover, if $x \in f^{-1}(y_1) \cap f^{-1}(y_2)$ then $f(x) = y_1$ and $f(x) = y_2$, so $y_1 = y_2$, and so contours that are not disjoint must be equal. We thus have:

Lemma A.4 *The level curves of a function f form a partition of its domain.*

Partitions also arise from equivalence relations—and vice versa. Given a partition $\mathcal{A}$ of S, we define the relation R on S by saying that

$$xRy \text{ if and only if } x \text{ and } y \text{ belong to the same block of } \mathcal{A}.$$

The relationship between partitions and equivalence relations is summarized in the following result.

Theorem A.5 *Let S be a set.*

a. *If $\sim$ is an equivalence relation on S, then the equivalence classes of $\sim$ are a partition of S. The relation determined by this partition is precisely $\sim$.*
b. *If $\mathcal{A}$ is a partition of S, then the relation R determined by $\mathcal{A}$ is an equivalence relation on S. Its equivalence classes are precisely the blocks of $\mathcal{A}$.*

We say that the partition $\mathcal{D}$ is a *refinement* of $\mathcal{C}$, and that $\mathcal{C}$ is *coarser than* $\mathcal{D}$, if the blocks of $\mathcal{C}$ are unions of blocks of $\mathcal{D}$, and we will write $\mathcal{C} \leq \mathcal{D}$. Alternatively, a useful way of saying this is the following:

Lemma A.6 *Let $\mathcal{C}$ and $\mathcal{D}$ be partitions of S. Then $\mathcal{C} \leq \mathcal{D}$ iff every block of $\mathcal{D}$ is contained in a block of $\mathcal{C}$.*

It is easy to see from this that the relation of refinement is a partial order on Part(S). To show antisymmetry, for example, suppose $\mathcal{C} \leq \mathcal{D} \leq \mathcal{C}$, and let C be a block of $\mathcal{C}$. Then there are blocks $D \in \mathcal{D}$ and $C' \in \mathcal{C}$ such that $C \supset D \supset C'$. But since $\mathcal{C}$ is a partition, $C = C'$, so $D = C$. Thus $\mathcal{C}$ and $\mathcal{D}$ contain the same blocks, and so $\mathcal{C} = \mathcal{D}$. The proofs that $\leq$ is reflexive and transitive follow in a similar manner.

Clearly the finest partition of S the set of singleton subsets, $\{\{x\}:x \in S\}$, and the coarsest is the *trivial partition*, $\{S\}$. Thus $\mathrm{Part}(S)$ is a bounded poset.

In fact, we may define the *meet* and *join* of two partitions of S. We define the blocks of the meet by saying that x and y are in the same block of $\mathcal{C} \wedge \mathcal{D}$ if there is a sequence $x = x_1, x_2, \ldots, x_n = y$ in S such that x_i and x_{i+1} are in the same block of either $\mathcal{C}$ or $\mathcal{D}$. The join is simpler:

$$\mathcal{C} \vee \mathcal{D} = \{C \cap D : C \in \mathcal{C}, D \in \mathcal{D}\}.$$

Theorem A.7 *The relation $\leq$ and the operations $\vee$ and $\wedge$ make* $\mathrm{Part}(S)$ *a bounded lattice. The top element is the finest partition and the bottom element is the coarsest one.*

Proof We must show that $\mathcal{C} \vee \mathcal{D}$ is the least upper bound of $\mathcal{C}$ and $\mathcal{D}$, and that $\mathcal{C} \wedge \mathcal{D}$ is their greatest lower bound. We consider the latter.

First, $\mathcal{C} \wedge \mathcal{D} \leq \mathcal{C}$. To show this we must show that every block of $\mathcal{C}$ is contained in a block of $\mathcal{C} \wedge \mathcal{D}$. But if $x, y \in C \in \mathcal{C}$, then x and y are trivially in the same block of $\mathcal{C} \wedge \mathcal{D}$ (take $x_1 = x$ and $x_2 = y$). Similarly we have $\mathcal{C} \wedge \mathcal{D} \leq \mathcal{D}$.

Second, let $\mathcal{E} \leq \mathcal{C}$ and $\mathcal{E} \leq \mathcal{D}$. We must show that $\mathcal{E} \leq \mathcal{C} \wedge \mathcal{D}$. To do this, let $B \in \mathcal{C} \wedge \mathcal{D}$. We must show that B is contained in a block of $\mathcal{E}$. Let $x, y \in B$. By assumption, there is a sequence $x = x_1, \ldots, x_n = y$ such that x_i and x_{i+1} are in the same block of $\mathcal{C}$ or in the same block of $\mathcal{D}$. Let this block be B_i. If $B_i \in \mathcal{C}$, then since $\mathcal{E} \leq \mathcal{C}$ it follows that $B_i \subset E_i$ for some block $E_i \in \mathcal{E}$. Since $\mathcal{E} \leq \mathcal{D}$, the same holds if $B_i \in \mathcal{D}$. Thus $\mathcal{E}$ contains a sequence of blocks $E_1, \ldots, E_n$, and x_i and x_{i+1} belong to E_i. But x_{i+1} (along with x_{i+2}) also belongs to E_{i+1}, so that $E_i \cap E_{i+1} \neq \emptyset$, and since distinct blocks of $\mathcal{E}$ are disjoint we must have $E_i = E_{i+1}$. Thus $E_1 = \cdots = E_n = E$, say, and $x, y \in E$. Therefore $B \subset E$, so E is the block of $\mathcal{E}$ that we sought.

This shows that $\mathcal{C} \wedge \mathcal{D}$ is indeed the greatest lower bound of $\mathcal{C}$ and $\mathcal{D}$. The proof that $\mathcal{C} \vee \mathcal{D}$ is their least upper bound follows similar lines (and is somewhat easier). □

We refer to $\mathrm{Part}(S)$ as the *partition lattice* of S.

The join and meet of a finite family $\mathcal{C}_1, \ldots, \mathcal{C}_k$ of partitions is defined inductively. The join will be denoted by $\bigvee_{i=1}^{k} \mathcal{C}_i$, or $\bigvee_{i \in I} \mathcal{C}_i$ for an index set I. The meet may be denoted similarly. The empty join $\bigvee_{i \in \emptyset} \mathcal{C}_i$ is the partition $\{S\}$.

Remark A.8 Because of Theorem A.5, the lattice $\mathrm{Part}(S)$ is isomorphic (in the obvious sense) to the lattice of equivalence relations on S, and it is in that form that it was first studied by Ore [104]. Partition lattices are discussed by Aigner [2], Anderson [4], Bailey [8], Crawley and Dilworth [38], Doubilet [50], Grätzer [64], Pudlák and Tůma [107], Stanley [135], Andrews [6], and Tjur [141]. It should be emphasized that, except for the last two, all authors use the *reverse* of our partial ordering (and thus interchange $\vee$ and $\wedge$). This is natural when dealing with equivalence relations, since a "larger" equivalence relation contains more ordered pairs and thus corresponds to a coarser partition. However, there are many reasons that the opposite is more natural. For example, if we put "fine" above "coarse", as we have done, then

- the rank of a partition $\mathcal{C}$ on a set of size n would then simply be $|\mathcal{C}|$, rather than $n - |\mathcal{C}|$ [4, p. 19].
- if one considers the algebra of sets[2] generated by a partition, say $A(\mathcal{C})$, then we have $A(\mathcal{C}) \subset A(\mathcal{D})$ iff $\mathcal{C} \leq \mathcal{D}$.

There is a related reason for our choice, which we elaborate in Sect. 5.2.

A.3 Algebra

A *group* G is a set with an associative binary operation, say $\cdot$, such that

- the operation has an *identity element* e such that $x \cdot e = x = e \cdot x$, and
- every element has an inverse: for each $x \in G$ there is a $y \in G$ such that $x \cdot y = e = y \cdot x$.

It is easy to see that the identity element and inverses are unique. When the operation is written as multiplication (as above), the inverse of x is written x^{-1}, and the identity element is often denoted e. If it is written as addition, the identity is often written 0 and the inverse of x is denoted $-x$.

The *order* of an element g is the smallest positive integer n such that $g^n = e$ if the group is multiplicative, or $ng = 0$ if the group is additive. If there is no such n, we say that g has infinite order. If the group G is finite, then every element has finite order. Indeed, if $n = |G|$ then $g^n = e$ for every $g \in G$ (the order of g may be smaller than n).

If the (multiplicative) group G consists of powers of a given element g, then G is said to be *cyclic* and g is a *generator* of G. If the operation is addition, then G consists of the multiples of a generator. More generally, a set $S \subset G$ is said to *generate* the (multiplicative) group G if every element of G can be written as finite products of elements of S and their inverses.

Example A.9 The numbers $0, 1, \ldots, n-1$ form a group, denoted $\mathbb{Z}/n$, under addition modulo n.[3] The group is cyclic, generated by the elements k that are relatively prime to n. If n is prime, all the nonzero elements of $\mathbb{Z}/n$ are generators.

A *subgroup* of a group G is a subset $H \subset G$ that is closed under products and inverses: $a, b \in H$ implies that $ab \in H$ and $a^{-1} \in H$.

---

[2] The algebra (or field) of sets generated by the family $\mathcal{F}$ is the smallest family of sets containing $\mathcal{F}$ that is closed under complements and finite unions and intersections.

[3] It is assumed that the reader is familiar with modular arithmetic.

Groups G and G' are *isomorphic* if there is a one-to-one map ϕ of G onto G' such that $\phi(gh) = \phi(g)\phi(h)$ for all $gh \in G$. Isomorphic groups thus have the same multiplication table.

The group G is *commutative* or *abelian* if the binary operation is commutative. All cyclic groups are commutative.

A *subgroup* of G is a subset H that is closed under the binary operation of G. Given a subgroup H, one may define an equivalence relation $\equiv$ on G by saying that

$$g_1 \equiv g_2 \mod H \quad \text{iff} \quad {g_1}^{-1}g_2 \in H$$

(writing the group operation as multiplication). Equivalently,

$$g_1 \equiv g_2 \mod H \quad \text{iff} \quad g_2 = g_1 h$$

for some $h \in H$. The equivalence classes are thus the sets

$$gH = \{gh{:}h \in H\},$$

called *(left) cosets of* H. (Right cosets Hg are defined by a corresponding equivalence relation. In an abelian group, of course, $gH = Hg$.) If the group is written additively, as is common for abelian groups, then the left cosets are $g + H = \{g + h{:}h \in H\}$, and similarly for right cosets.

By a *ring* we shall mean a set R having two binary operations, + and $\cdot$, and two distinguished elements, denoted 0 and 1, such that

- $(R, +, 0)$ is a commutative group,
- the multiplication operation $\cdot$ is associative and 1 is its identity element, and
- multiplication is distributive over addition.

It follows that $0 \cdot x = 0 = x \cdot 0$ for all $x \in R$. A ring is

- *commutative* if multiplication is.
- an *integral domain* if it has no zero divisors—i.e., if $ab = 0$ implies $a = 0$ or $b = 0$.
- a *field* if it is an integral domain, if multiplication is commutative, and if every nonzero element has a multiplicative inverse.

Example A.10 The set $\mathbb{Z}/n$ is a ring under addition and multiplication modulo n. It is a field if n is prime, while it has zero-divisors if n is composite. Rings of this type are called *residue rings*.

The *characteristic* of a ring R, denoted char(R), is the smallest integer n for which $na = 0$ for all $a \in R$. If no such n exists, R has characteristic zero. If $\mathbb{Q}$ denotes the field of rational numbers, then char$(\mathbb{Q}) = 0$.

Proposition A.11 *If R is an integral domain, and in particular a field, and if* char(R) *is positive, then it is a prime.*

If char$(R) = 0$ *then R contains a copy of* $\mathbb{Q}$. *If* char$(R) = p > 0$ *then R contains a copy of* $\mathbb{Z}/p$.

We will use the notation

$$R[x] = \text{the set of polynomials in the variable } x \text{ with coefficients in the ring } R.$$

The number $\alpha \in \mathbb{C}$ is *algebraic over* $\mathbb{Q}$ if there is a polynomial $f(x) \in \mathbb{Q}[x]$ such that $f(\alpha) = 0$. A polynomial is *monic* if the leading coefficient is 1.

We will assume the following facts. Proofs may be found in standard texts such as [86].

Theorem A.12 *Let* $\alpha \in \mathbb{C}$ *be algebraic over* $\mathbb{Q}$. *Then there is a unique monic polynomial* $m(x) \in \mathbb{Q}[x]$ *of minimal degree such that* $m(\alpha) = 0$. *It is irreducible over* $\mathbb{Q}$. *If* $f(x) \in \mathbb{Q}[x]$ *is such that* $f(\alpha) = 0$, *then* $f(x) = m(x)q(x)$ *for some* $q(x) \in Q[x]$.

The polynomial $m(x)$ in Theorem A.12 is called the *minimal polynomial* of α over $\mathbb{Q}$.

Theorem A.13 (Fundamental Theorem of Algebra) *A polynomial* $f(x) \in \mathbb{C}[x]$ *may be factored completely as*

$$f(x) = c(x - \lambda_1) \cdots (x - \lambda_k)$$

for some $c, \lambda_1, \ldots, \lambda_k \in \mathbb{C}$, *where k is the degree of f.*

An *nth root of unity* is a number $\omega \in \mathbb{C}$ such that $\omega^n = 1$. Since these are the roots of the equation $x^n - 1 = 0$, the Fundamental Theorem says that there are precisely n of them. They are the numbers $\omega_k = e^{2\pi i k/n}$, $k = 0, \ldots, n-1$. These numbers are equispaced around the unit circle in the complex plane.

Example A.14 The number $\omega = e^{2\pi i/n}$ is a primitive nth root of unity. The nth roots of unity are $1, \omega, \omega^2, \ldots, \omega^{n-1}$.

The primitive square root of unity is -1. The primitive cube roots of unity are $(-1 \pm i\sqrt{3})/2$. The primitive 4th root of unity is i.

Proposition A.15 *Let p be a prime. If* ω *is a pth root of unity, then the minimal polynomial of* ω *over* $\mathbb{Q}$ *is* $\Phi_p(x) = 1 + x + \cdots + x^{p-1}$.

The nth roots of unity satisfy $\omega^a\omega^b = \omega^{a+b}$. In fact, they form a cyclic group, say U_n, under multiplication, generated by ω_k where k is relatively prime to n. In particular, when n is prime all the roots are primitive except the number 1. If this sounds familiar, it is due to the following fact:

Proposition A.16 *Let* ω *be a primitive nth root of unity. The map* $k \mapsto \omega^k$ *defines an isomorphism from* $\mathbb{Z}/n$ *(under addition) to* U_n *(under multiplication).*

For each prime p and each positive integer r there is a unique (up to isomorphism) finite field having $s = p^r$ elements. We will denote it $GF(s)$ (= the Galois field of order s). We note that $GF(p) = \mathbb{Z}/p$, the integers modulo the prime p, that $GF(p) \subset GF(p^2) \subset \cdots$, and that each of these fields has characteristic p. In general, $GF(s) \neq \mathbb{Z}/s$; in fact, $\mathbb{Z}/n$ is a field if and only if n is prime.

Example A.17 The smallest finite field not of the form $\mathbb{Z}/n$ is $GF(4)$. It contains $\mathbb{Z}/2$ as a subfield, and in fact it is generated by the roots of

$$x^2 + x + 1 = 0 \tag{A.5}$$

The left hand side is an irreducible polynomial in $(\mathbb{Z}/2)[x]$ as the equation has no roots in $\mathbb{Z}/2$; we may denote the two roots by a and b. From the arithmetic of $\mathbb{Z}/2$ and the relation (A.5), we get these tables for the arithmetic of $GF(4)$:

+	0	1	a	b
0	0	1	a	b
1	1	0	b	a
a	a	b	0	1
b	b	a	1	0

×	0	1	a	b
0	0	0	0	0
1	0	1	a	b
a	0	a	b	1
b	0	b	1	a

Since the nonzero elements of $GF(s)$ form a group with $s - 1$ elements, we have this result:

Proposition A.18 *If $0 \neq x \in GF(s)$ then $x^{s-1} = 1$. Every element of $GF(s)$ is a root of the equation $x^s - x = 0$. We have $x^s - x = \prod_{a \in GF(s)}(x - a)$.*

A standard source for this subject is [90]. General algebra texts such as [86] treat the basic theory.

A.4 Linear Algebra

Let K be a field. A *vector space V over K* is a commutative group, usually written additively, with an operation $K \times V \to V$ called *scalar multiplication*, written av for $a \in K$ and $v \in V$, such that for all $a, b \in K$ and $v, w \in V$ we have

- $a(v + w) = av + aw$
- $(a + b)v = av + bv$
- $a(bv) = (ab)v$
- $1v = v$, where 1 is the multiplicative identity of K.

The elements of K are called *scalars*. Our main interest will be in *real* vector spaces, that is, vector spaces over the field $\mathbb{R}$. Occasionally we will need to use the complex field $\mathbb{C}$ or a finite field $GF(s)$. In general we will use 0 to denote both the zero vector in V and the zero element in K. Context will clarify which is meant.

If K is a field, then the Cartesian product K^n, consisting of n-tuples of elements of K, is a vector space over K. Vectors in K^n will often be denoted in boldface.

An *algebra* over K is a vector space over K equipped with a bilinear vector product. That is, for vectors u and v there is a *vector* uv; this product is distributive over addition, and for any scalar $a \in K$ we have $(au)v = a(uv) = u(av)$. Distributivity is assumed to be two-sided: $u(v + w) = uv + uw$ and $(v + w)u = vu + wu$. Multiplication may or may not be associative or commutative or have an identity element.

The vector space K^n becomes an algebra under componentwise multiplication of vectors. This product is associative and commutative and has a multiplicative identity, namely $\mathbf{1}$, the vector of ones.

A.4.1 Subspaces and Bases

Definition A.19 Let V be a vector space.

a. A *subspace* of V is a subset that is closed under addition and scalar multiplication.
b. If W_1 and W_2 are subspaces of V, then their *sum* is defined to be

$$W_1 + W_2 = \{w_1 + w_2 : w_i \in W_i\}.$$

Proposition A.20 *If W_1 and W_2 are subspaces of the vector space V, then so are $W_1 + W_2$ and $W_1 \cap W_2$. $W_1 + W_2$ is the smallest subspace containing both W_1 and W_2, and $W_1 \cap W_2$ is the largest subspace contained in both.*

Proof The fact that $W_1 + W_2$ and $W_1 \cap W_2$ are closed under addition and scalar multiplication is straightforward. $W_1 + W_2$, contains W_1 as every $w \in W_1$ may be written $w + 0$, and similarly it contains W_2. Any subspace W containing both W_1 and W_2, being closed under addition, must contain all sums $w_1 + w_2$, $w_i \in W_i$, and so contains $W_1 + W_2$. The corresponding property of $W_1 \cap W_2$ is proved similarly. □

If we order the subspaces of V by inclusion, then $W_1 \cap W_2$ *and* $W_1 + W_2$ *are the meet and join of the subspaces* W_1 *and* W_2.

Theorem A.21 *Let L be the set of subspaces of a vector space V (including V and $\{0\}$), ordered by inclusion ($W_1 \leq W_2$ means $W_1 \subset W_2$). Then L is a bounded lattice, and satisfies the modular law*

$$W_1 \supset W_3 \Rightarrow W_1 \cap (W_2 + W_3) = (W_1 \cap W_2) + W_3. \tag{A.6}$$

Proof That L is a lattice is a restatement of Proposition A.20. It is obviously bounded, with $\hat{1} = V$ and $\hat{0} = \{0\}$. Let $W_1 \supset W_3$. By Lemma A.2 or directly we may show that $W_1 \cap (W_2 + W_3) \supset (W_1 \cap W_2) + W_3$. For the reverse inclusion, let $x \in W_1 \cap (W_2 + W_3)$. Then $x \in W_1$ and also $x = y + z$ where $y \in W_2$ and $z \in W_3$. Since we assume $W_1 \supset W_3$, it follows that $z \in W_1$ and therefore that $y = x - z \in W_1$. Thus $y \in W_1 \cap W_2$, so that $x = y + z \in (W_1 \cap W_2) + W_3$. □

Thus the lattice of subspaces of a vector space is modular. We will see in a moment that it is not distributive in general.

Definition A.22 Let V be a vector space. A *linear combination* of the elements $v_1, \ldots, v_n \in V$ is an element of the form $\sum_i c_i v_i$, for scalars c_i. The elements v_i are *linearly independent* if $\sum_i c_i v_i = 0$ implies $c_1 = \cdots = c_n = 0$.

Let $S \subset V$ be a set of vectors. The *span* of S, denoted $\langle S \rangle$, is the set of linear combinations of elements of S. If $\langle S \rangle = V$, we say that the set S *spans* V. The set S is *linearly independent* if every finite subset of S is linearly independent.

The set S is a *(linear) basis* for V if S is a linearly independent set and S spans V.

Theorem A.23

a. $B \subset V$ is a basis of V iff B is a maximal linearly independent set.
b. Every vector space V has a basis.
c. Every spanning set of V contains a basis.
d. Every basis of V has the same number[4] of elements.

Definition A.24 The *dimension* of the vector space V, $\dim(V)$, is the number of elements in a basis of V.

Example A.25 If K is a field, then $V = K^n$ has a basis consisting of the vectors $(1, 0, \ldots, 0), (0, 1, 0, \ldots, 0), \ldots, (0, \ldots, 0, 1)$. Thus $\dim(V) = n$. This basis is often called the *standard basis* of K^n.

Theorem A.26 *If W is a subspace of V, then any basis of W may be extended to a basis of V.*

We saw above that the lattice L of subspaces of a vector space V is modular. It is easy to see that L is distributive if $\dim(V) = 1$. It turns out that is the only case:

Proposition A.27 *If $\dim(V) > 1$, then L is not distributive.*

Sketch of Proof Let W be a two-dimensional subspace of V, and choose W_1, W_2, and W_3 to be distinct one-dimensional subspaces of W (one can always do this). Then $W_1 \cap (W_2 + W_3) = W_1$ but $W_1 \cap W_2 = W_1 \cap W_3 = \{0\}$. □

Definition A.28 If W_1 and W_2 are subspaces of a vector space V, their sum $W_1 + W_2$ is said to be *direct* if $W_1 \cap W_2 = \{0\}$.

[4] We may understand "number" to mean "cardinality". With this understanding, Theorem A.23 applies to infinite-dimensional vectors spaces as well.

Theorem A.29 *Suppose $W = W_1 + W_2$, where W_i are subspaces of V. If the sum is direct, then*

a. every element of W has a unique expression of the form $w_1 + w_2$ with $w_i \in W_i$.
b. $\dim(W) = \dim(W_1) + \dim(W_2)$.

Proof (a) The zero vector has a unique expression, as $0 = w_1 + w_2$ implies that $w_2 = -w_1$ so that both w_1 and w_2 are in $W_1 \cap W_2$. It follows that if $w = w_1 + w_2 = w_1' + w_2'$ then $0 = (w_1 - w_1') + (w_2 - w_2')$ and so uniqueness follows. (b) If B_1 is a set of vectors forming a basis of W_1 and B_2 is a basis of W_2, then it follows from (a) that $B_1 \cup B_2$ is linearly independent, and it spans $W_1 + W_2$ by the definition of this sum. □

The direct sum is typically denoted $W_1 \oplus W_2$, though we will usually use the $\oplus$ notation for *orthogonal* sums, defined in Sect. A.4.3. When $W = W_1 \oplus W_2$, we say that W_2 is the *complement* of W_1 in W.

Note In succeeding sections, reference is made repeatedly to "scalars". As mentioned earlier, **scalars are always assumed to be elements of the field K over which the vector space is defined.**

A.4.2 Linear Transformations

Definition A.30 Let U and V be vector spaces over the same field K. A map $T{:}U \rightarrow V$ is a *linear transformation* if $T(cu) = cT(u)$ and $T(u_1 + u_2) = T(u_1) + T(u_2)$ for any scalar c and $u, u_1, u_2 \in U$. If T maps U one-to-one onto V, then T is said to be an *isomorphism* of vector spaces.

A linear transformation $T{:}U \rightarrow K$ (where K is viewed as a vector space over itself) is called a *linear functional on U*.

Theorem A.31 *Let $c_1, \ldots, c_n \in K$. The function $T{:}K^n \rightarrow K$ defined for each $\mathbf{u} = (u_1, \ldots, u_n)$ by*

$$T(\mathbf{u}) = c_1 u_1 + \cdots + c_n u_n \tag{A.7}$$

is a linear functional on K^n. Conversely, every linear functional on K^n has the form (A.7) for unique $c_1, \ldots, c_n \in K$.

Proof The linearity of T given by (A.7) is straightforward. Conversely, suppose T is a linear functional on K^n. Let $\mathbf{e}_1, \ldots, \mathbf{e}_n$ be the standard basis of K^n (Example A.25), and put $c_j = T(\mathbf{e}_j)$. The quantities c_j are uniquely determined by T, and it's easy to see that T satisfies (A.7). □

Definition A.32 Let $T:U \to V$ be a linear transformation. The *nullspace* or *kernel* of T is the set

$$N(T) = \{u \in U : T(u) = 0\}.$$

As with any function, the *range* of T is the set

$$R(T) = \{v \in V : v = T(u) \text{ for some } u \in U\}.$$

Proposition A.33 *If $T:U \to V$ is a linear transformation, then $N(T)$ is a subspace of U and $R(T)$ is a subspace of V.*

This proposition follows immediately from the linearity of T.

Theorem A.34 *Let $T:U \to V$ be a linear transformation, with* $\dim U < \infty$. *Then* $\dim U = \dim N(T) + \dim R(T)$.

Sketch of Proof The image of a basis of U must span $R(T)$, so $\dim R(T) < \infty$. Let $v_1, \ldots, v_r$ be a basis of $R(T)$, and choose u_i such that $T(u_i) = v_i$, $i \leq r$. Let $u_{r+1}, \ldots, u_{r+q}$ be a basis of $N(T)$. Then $u_1, \ldots, u_{r+q}$ span U. (If $u \in U$, put $T(u) = \sum_1^r c_i v_i$. Then $u - \sum_1^r c_i u_i \in N(T)$, so there are $c_{r+1} \ldots, c_{r+q}$ such that $u = \sum_1^{r+q} c_i u_i$.) It is straightforward to show that they are linearly independent and thus a basis of U. Therefore, $\dim U = r + q = \dim R(T) + \dim N(T)$. □

The zero map $0:U \to V$ that takes every $u \in U$ to the vector $0 \in V$ is trivially a linear transformation. **Caution**: Note that now 0 may denote a scalar, a vector, or a linear transformation.

Notation As with any function, we write $T(E)$ for the *image* of a set E under the map T, and $T^{-1}(F)$ as the *inverse image* of F. Thus we may write $R(T) = T(U)$ and $N(T) = T^{-1}(0)$. Of course, T^{-1} also denotes the inverse function of T if T is an isomorphism. If T^{-1} exists, we say that T is *invertible*; otherwise, *singular*.

We also introduce the following:

- $\mathcal{L}(U, V)$ = set of linear transformations from U to V;
- $\mathcal{L}(V) = \mathcal{L}(V, V)$.

In using this notation, we assume that the field of scalars is the same for U, V, and the elements of $\mathcal{L}(U, V)$. If we need to indicate the field of scalars explicitly, we will use a subscript (e.g., $\mathcal{L}_{\mathbb{R}}(V)$).

Theorem A.35 *If $T \in \mathcal{L}(U, V)$, then $N(T)$ is a subspace of U and $R(T)$ is a subspace of V.*

More generally, if U_0 is a subspace of U then $T(U_0)$ is a subspace of V, and if V_0 is a subspace of V then $T^{-1}(V_0)$ is a subspace of U.

Example A.36 Let K be a field, let $a_1, \ldots, a_n \in K$, and let $T(x_1, \ldots, x_n) = a_1x_1 + \cdots + a_nx_n$. Then the map $T : K^n \to K$ given by $y = T(x_1, \ldots, x_n)$ is linear. More generally, a system of equations

$$\begin{aligned} a_{11}x_1 + \cdots + a_{1n}x_n &= y_1 \\ \vdots \qquad\quad \vdots \quad &\quad \vdots \\ a_{m1}x_1 + \cdots + a_{mn}x_n &= y_m, \end{aligned} \tag{A.8}$$

defines a linear map $T : K^n \to K^m$ taking $\mathbf{x} = (x_1, \ldots, x_n)$ to $\mathbf{y} = (y_1, \ldots, y_m)$.

We may recast this in terms of matrices (matrix theory is reviewed in Sect. A.4.8 below). Let $\mathbf{T}$ be an $m \times n$ matrix of elements $a_{ij} \in K$, let $\mathbf{x}$ be an $n \times 1$ column vector, and define $\mathbf{y} = \mathbf{Tx}$, so that $\mathbf{y}$ is $m \times 1$. Then the map $\mathbf{x} \mapsto \mathbf{y}$ is a linear transformation T from K^n to K^m, as is easily verified. If we let $\mathbf{a}_1, \ldots, \mathbf{a}_n$ be the columns of $\mathbf{T}$ and $\mathbf{x} = (x_1, \ldots, x_n)'$, then $\mathbf{Tx} = x_1\mathbf{a}_1 + \cdots + x_n\mathbf{a}_n$, so that the columns of $\mathbf{T}$ span $R(T)$.

Theorem A.37 *Let $T \in \mathcal{L}(U, V)$.*

a. *T is one-to-one iff $N(T) = \{0\}$.*
b. *Let T be one-to-one. If $u_1, \ldots, u_n$ are linearly independent then so are $Tu_1, \ldots, Tu_n$.*
c. *If $\dim U = \dim V < \infty$, then T is one-to-one iff T is onto.*

Proof (c) If $u_1, \ldots, u_n$ is a basis of U and if T is one-to-one, then $Tu_1, \ldots Tu_n$ must be a basis of V, and it is easy to see that T is onto. If T is onto, then given a basis $v_1, \ldots, v_n$ of V, let u_i be such that $Tu_i = v_i$. Then $u_1, \ldots, u_n$ must be linearly independent and therefore a basis of U. □

Definition A.38 Let V be a vector space. An *affine set*, or a *flat*, is a coset of a subspace, that is, a set of the form $x + U = \{x + u{:}u \in U\}$ where $x \in V$ and U is a subspace of V. If $\dim(U) = r$, $x + U$ is called an *r-flat*. We say that $x + U$ is a *translation* of the subspace U by the vector x.

Part (b) of the following theorem says that an affine set can be viewed as the translation of U by any of its elements, a fact that is geometrically obvious in $\mathbb{R}^n$. Corollary A.66 below will pick out a particular translation representing the affine set when geometry (an inner product) is available.

Theorem A.39

a. *Let U be a subspace of V, and $x_1, x_2 \in V$. Then $x_1 + U = x_2 + U$ iff $x_1 - x_2 \in U$.*
b. *If $A = x + U$ is an affine set, then also $A = x' + U$ for any $x' \in A$.*
c. *Let $T \in \mathcal{L}(V, W)$ and $y \in W$. The solution set $T^{-1}(y) = \{x \in V{:}Tx = y\}$ is an affine set in V, namely $x_0 + N(T)$ where x_0 is a particular vector such that $Tx_0 = y$.*
d. *For every affine set $A \subset V$ there is a map $T \in \mathcal{L}(V, W)$ and a vector $y \in W$ such that A is the solution set of the equation $Tx = y$.*

Example A.40 Given $y_1, \ldots, y_m \in K$, the solution set of the linear system (A.8) is an affine set in K^n.

Theorem A.41 *Let $v_1, \ldots, v_n$ be a basis of V, and let T be a map from $\{v_1, \ldots, v_n\}$ to W. For any $v \in V$, define $T(v)$ as follows: If $v = \sum_j a_j v_j$, let $T(v) = \sum_j a_j T(v_j)$. Then $T \in \mathcal{L}(V, W)$, and if $S \in \mathcal{L}(V, W)$ and $S(v_i) = T(v_i)$, then $S = T$.*

We say that a linear transformation is *uniquely determined by its values on a basis*. The method of defining $T(v)$ in this theorem is referred to as *extending T to V by linearity*.

Theorem A.42 *Let T, T_1 and $T_2 \in \mathcal{L}(U, V)$ and $S \in \mathcal{L}(V, W)$, and let c be a scalar. Then the following are linear transformations:*

a. $cT{:}U \to V$ defined by $(cT)(u) = c \cdot T(u)$.
b. $T_1 + T_2{:}U \to V$ defined by $(T_1 + T_2)(u) = T_1(u) + T_2(u)$.
c. $ST{:}U \to W$ defined by $(ST)(u) = S(T(u))$.
d. $T^{-1}{:}V \to U$ if T is one-to-one and onto.

Theorem A.43 *$\mathcal{L}(U, V)$ is a vector space. If* $\dim V = n$ *and* $\dim W = m$*, then* $\dim \mathcal{L}(V, W) = mn$.

Sketch of Proof Theorem A.42(a,b) implies that $\mathcal{L}(U, V)$ is a vector space. As to its dimension, let $v_1, \ldots, v_n$ be a basis of V and $w_1, \ldots, w_m$ a basis of W. Define

$$E_{ij} v_j = w_i$$

$$E_{ij} v_k = 0 \text{ for } k \neq j$$

and extend E_{ij} to V by linearity. Clearly $E_{ij} \in \mathcal{L}(V, W)$, and there are mn such linear transformations. It is straightforward to check that they are a basis of $\mathcal{L}(V, W)$. □

The *identity map* $I{:}V \to V$ is in $\mathcal{L}(V)$, and if $T \in \mathcal{L}(V)$ then $T^n \in \mathcal{L}(V)$ for $n > 1$ (where $T^2 = TT$ and so on). Thus if V is a vector space over K and $f \in K[t]$, and if $T \in \mathcal{L}(V)$, then $f(T) \in \mathcal{L}(V)$, where $f(T)$ is defined by replacing t by T. (We we interpret the constant term a_0 of $f(T)$ as $a_0 I$.)

Definition A.44 If $T \in \mathcal{L}(V)$ and if $Tv = \lambda v$ for some scalar λ and nonzero $v \in V$, then we say that v is an *eigenvector* of T and λ is the corresponding *eigenvalue*. We say that v *belongs to* λ.

Note that the nonzero elements of the nullspace $N(T)$ are the eigenvectors belonging to the eigenvalue $\lambda = 0$. There are many approaches to the study of eigenvalues and eigenvectors. We will follow [85] and [86], with some modifications.

Theorem A.45 *Let $T \in \mathcal{L}(V)$, and let*

$$V_\lambda = \{v \in V : v \text{ belongs to } \lambda \text{ or } v = 0\}$$

if λ is an eigenvalue of T. Then:

a. *V_λ is a subspace of V.*
b. *If λ_1 and λ_2 are distinct eigenvalues of T then $V_{\lambda_1} \cap V_{\lambda_2} = \{0\}$.*
c. *If $\lambda_1, \ldots, \lambda_k$ are* distinct *eigenvalues of T and if v_i is an eigenvector belonging to λ_i, then $v_1, \ldots, v_k$ are linearly independent.*

Sketch of Proof The proof of (a) is straightforward. As to (b), if $v \in V_{\lambda_1} \cap V_{\lambda_2}$ then $(\lambda_1 - \lambda_2)v = 0$, so $v = 0$. Part (c) may be proved[5] by induction on k, using the distinctness of the eigenvalues and the fact that $T \sum_{i=1}^{k} c_i v_i - \lambda_k \sum_{i=1}^{k} c_i v_i = \sum_{i=1}^{k-1} c_i(\lambda_i - \lambda_k) v_i$. □

The subspace V_λ in this theorem is called the *eigenspace* of T belonging to λ. The dimension of V_λ is called the *geometric multiplicity* of λ. Since the sum of the eigenspaces of T is direct, we have the following:

Corollary A.46 *Let $T \in \mathcal{L}(V)$ have distinct eigenvalues $\lambda_1, \ldots, \lambda_k$, and let m_i be the geometric multiplicity of λ_i. Then*

$$\sum_{i=1}^{k} m_i \leq \dim(V). \tag{A.9}$$

In particular, T has at most $\dim(V)$ *distinct eigenvalues.*

A key question is whether a given linear transformation T has *any* eigenvalues. We answer this in two cases.

Definition A.47 A linear transformation $T : V \to V$ is *idempotent* if $T^2 = T$.

An idempotent linear transformation is also called a *projection*, or sometimes an *oblique projection* (to distinguish it from *orthogonal projections*, defined below).

Theorem A.48 *If $T : V \to V$ is idempotent, then its only eigenvalues are 0 and 1. We have*

$$V = V_0 \oplus V_1 \tag{A.10}$$

(direct sum), where V_0 and V_1 are the eigenspaces of 0 and 1.

Proof If λ is an eigenvalue of T with eigenvector v, then $\lambda^2 v = T(T(v)) = T(v) = \lambda v$, so $\lambda = 0$ or 1. Now $\dim V = \dim N(T) + \dim R(T)$ (Theorem A.34). Clearly

[5] Adapted from [85].

$V_0 = N(T)$, and it's not hard to see that $V_1 = R(T)$. Since $\dim V = \dim V_0 + \dim V_1$ and $V_0 \cap V_1 = \{0\}$, (A.10) follows. □

In the second case, we specialize the field of scalars to $\mathbb{C}$.

Theorem A.49 *Let V be a finite-dimensional vector space over $\mathbb{C}$, with* $\dim V \geq 1$, *and let $T \in \mathcal{L}_{\mathbb{C}}(V)$. Then T has a nonzero eigenvector.*

In this case, eigenvalues and eigenvectors may be complex. The proof of the theorem relies on the following result:

Lemma A.50 *Let V be a vector space of dimension n over the field K and let $T \in \mathcal{L}(V)$. Then there is a nonzero polynomial $f \in K[t]$ of degree at most n^2 with coefficients in K such that $f(T) = 0$ (the zero transformation).*

Proof By Theorem A.43, $\dim \mathcal{L}(V) = n^2$; call this N. The $N + 1$ powers $I, T, T^2, \ldots, T^N$ must be linearly dependent, so we have a relation

$$a_N T^N + \cdots + a_1 T + a_0 = 0$$

where not all a_i are 0, and we put $f(t) = a_n t^n + \cdots + a_1 t + a_0$. □

Proof of Theorem A.49 Let $f \in \mathbb{C}[t]$ such that $f(T) = 0$, as guaranteed by Lemma A.50. Assume f has degree k and leading coefficient a_k. Then

$$f(t) = a_k(t - \lambda_1) \cdots (t - \lambda_k)$$

for some $\lambda_i \in \mathbb{C}$. Thus

$$(T - \lambda_1 I) \cdots (T - \lambda_k I)$$

must be the zero linear transformation (it equals ${a_k}^{-1} f(T)$). But then the maps $T - \lambda_i I$ cannot all be one-to-one. Thus for some i there is a nonzero $v \in V$ such that

$$(T - \lambda_i I)(v) = 0.$$

But then $T(v) = \lambda_i v$, so v is a nonzero eigenvector. □

A.4.3 Inner Product Spaces

Definition A.51 An *inner product* on a (real) vector space V is a function assigning to each x and y in V a real number (x, y) satisfying these properties:

a. $(x, y) = (y, x)$;
b. $(x + y, z) = (x, z) + (y, z)$;

c. $(cx, y) = c(x, y)$ for any $c \in \mathbb{R}$;
d. $x \neq 0$ implies $(x, x) > 0$.

An *inner product space* is a vector space V together with an *inner product* (x, y). Property (a) is called *symmetry*. Properties (b) and (c) together are called *linearity*. Property(d) is called *positive-definiteness*.

It is immediate from symmetry that linearity holds for the right member of (x, y) as well, so that (x, y) is *bilinear*. Moreover, property (c) implies that $(0, y) = 0$, and so by symmetry $(x, 0) = 0$.

Remark A.52 We have defined a real inner product space. If V is a complex vector space, it may carry a *complex* (or *hermitian*) inner product $\langle \cdot, \cdot \rangle$, for which symmetry and linearity are modified:

a. $\langle x, y \rangle = \overline{\langle y, x \rangle}$;
b. $\langle x + y, z \rangle = \langle x, z \rangle + \langle y, z \rangle$;
c. $\langle cx, y \rangle = c\langle x, y \rangle$ for any $c \in \mathbb{C}$;
d. $x \neq 0$ implies $\langle x, x \rangle > 0$,

where $\bar{c}$ denotes the complex conjugate of the number c. Linearity still holds for the right member of $\langle x, y \rangle$ except that $\langle x, cy \rangle = \bar{c}\langle x, y \rangle$. Since $\langle x, y \rangle$ is not quite linear in the second variable, one sometimes says that it is *sesquilinear* (one and a half times linear). We will actually introduce a complex inner product briefly on the way to proving the Spectral Theorem (Theorem A.87).

Let $(\cdot, \cdot)$ be a inner product on V, and define a *norm*

$$\|v\| = \sqrt{(v, v)}.$$

It is easily verified that the norm has these properties:

- $\|cv\| = |c|\|v\|$ for any $c \in \mathbb{R}$ ($c \in \mathbb{C}$ in the complex case);
- $\|v\| = 0$ if and only if $v = 0$;
- $\|u + v\|^2 = \|u\|^2 + 2(u, v) + \|v\|^2$. We refer to this as "expanding $\|u + v\|^2$".

Somewhat more complicated to prove is

Lemma A.53

a. $|(u, v)| \leq \|u\|\|v\|$ (the Cauchy-Schwarz inequality[6]). *Equality holds iff u and v are linearly dependent.*[7]
b. $\|u + v\| \leq \|u\| + \|v\|$ (the triangle inequality). *Equality holds iff u or v is zero or $u = cv$ for some real $c > 0$.*
c. $|\|u\| - \|v\|| \leq \|u - v\|$.

[6] Note the spelling of Schwarz. The inequality is known by a variety of names, including Cauchy-Buniakowski-Schwarz.

[7] Linear dependence of u and v includes the case that one of them is 0.

Sketch of Proof For Cauchy-Schwarz, we note first that if $v = 0$ then both sides are zero. Assuming $v \neq 0$, we expand the right-hand side of

$$0 \leq \|u - cv\|^2$$

and set $c = (u, v)/\|v\|^2$. The triangle inequality follows from expanding $\|u + v\|^2$ and applying Cauchy-Schwarz. The third inequality comes from applying Cauchy-Schwarz to both $(u - v) + v$ and $(v - u) + u$. □

Example A.54 When $V = \mathbb{R}$, the triangle inequality is a statement about absolute values: $|x + y| \leq |x| + |y|$, with equality iff x and y have the same sign or at least one of them is zero.

When $V = \mathbb{C}$, we regard $\mathbb{C}$ as the plane $\mathbb{R}^2$ in the usual way, with the Euclidean distance function. Now $|z|$ is the usual modulus, and $|z + w| \leq |z| + |w|$, with equality iff either z or w is zero or $z = cw$ for some real $c > 0$.

Example A.55 Consider $V = \mathbb{R}^n$ as a vector space over $\mathbb{R}$, with elements viewed as column vectors. Then $(\mathbf{u}, \mathbf{v}) = \mathbf{u}'\mathbf{v} = \sum_i u_i v_i$, the usual dot product (so named from the notation $\mathbf{u} \cdot \mathbf{v}$), and $\|\mathbf{u}\| = (u_1^2 + \cdots + u_n^2)^{1/2}$, the Euclidean length. In this case, analytic geometry allows an alternate proof of the preceding properties. For example, since the vectors $\mathbf{u}$, $\mathbf{v}$, and $\mathbf{u} + \mathbf{v}$ form the sides of a triangle, the triangle inequality in this case simply asserts an obvious geometric fact about triangles. The cosine law tells us that the angle θ between $\mathbf{u}$ and $\mathbf{v}$ satisfies $\cos(\theta) = (\mathbf{u}, \mathbf{v})/\|\mathbf{u}\|\|\mathbf{v}\|$, from which the Cauchy-Schwarz inequality would follow directly.

A norm allows us to define a *distance function* or *metric* on V, the distance between vectors u and v given by

$$\|u - v\|. \tag{A.11}$$

The following properties are evident:

- $\|u - v\| \geq 0$, and $\|u - v\| = 0$ if and only if $u = v$;
- $\|u - v\| = \|v - u\|$; and
- $\|u - v\| \leq \|u - z\| + \|z - v\|$.

Definition A.56 We say that u and v are *orthogonal* or *perpendicular*, and write $u \perp v$, if $(u, v) = 0$. A set of vectors is *pairwise orthogonal* if any pair of vectors in the set is orthogonal.

If S and T are sets of vectors, we say that u is *orthogonal to* T ($u \perp T$) if $u \perp v$ for every $v \in T$, and that S and T are *orthogonal sets* ($S \perp T$) if $u \perp v$ for every $u \in S$ and $v \in T$.

Theorem A.57 *In an inner product space V:*

a. (Pythagorean Theorem) *If $u \perp v$ then $\|u+v\|^2 = \|u\|^2 + \|v^2\|$. If $u_1, \ldots, u_n$ are pairwise orthogonal, then $\|u_1 + \cdots + u_n\|^2 = \|u_1\|^2 + \cdots + \|u_n\|^2$.*
b. If $u_1, \ldots, u_n$ are nonzero and pairwise orthogonal then they are linearly independent.
c. $v \perp S$ iff $v \perp \langle S \rangle$.[8]
d. If $v \in W$ and $v \perp W$ then $v = 0$.
e. If W_1 and W_2 are orthogonal subspaces of V then the sum $W_1 + W_2$ is direct.

Proof

(a) For the first statement, expand $\|u+v\|^2$. For the second, do the same or use induction.
(b) Assume that $\sum_i c_i u_i = 0$ (a finite sum) and compute $(u_k, \sum_i c_i u_i)$ for each k to see that $c_k = 0$.
(c) Each $u \in U$ is a finite sum $u = \sum_i c_i u_i$ for some $u_i \in S$, so $(v, u) = \sum_i c_i (v, u_i)$. Thus $v \perp S$ implies $v \perp U$. The converse is trivial.
(d) $\|v\|^2 = (v, v) = 0$, so $v = 0$.
(e) Immediate from (d).

□

Definition A.58 If W_1 and W_2 are orthogonal subspaces of a vector space V, their sum said to be an *orthogonal sum*, and is denoted $W_1 \oplus W_2$.

Definition A.59 Let V be an inner product space and let W be a subspace. The *orthogonal complement of W in V*, or the *orthogonal difference between V and W*, is

$$V \ominus W = \{v \in V : v \perp W\}.$$

If the space V is understood, we write this as $W^\perp$. Similarly, if $w \in V$, we define $v^\perp = \{v \in V : v \perp w\}$. If $S \subset V$, then $S^\perp = \{v \in V : v \perp w \text{ for every } w \in S\}$.

If we have $W_1 \subset W_2 \subset V$, it is useful to note that

$$W_2 \ominus W_1 = W_2 \cap W^{\perp}{}_1. \tag{A.12}$$

Caution When writing $W^\perp$ one must be careful to identify the ambient space in which W sits. If $W_1 \subset W_2$, the notation $W^{\perp}{}_1$ may mean $W_2 \ominus W_1$, but it may also mean something else if both spaces sit inside some fixed larger space. That larger space will often be some Euclidean space $\mathbb{R}^n$.

[8] Recall that $\langle S \rangle$ is the span of S.

Proposition A.60 *Let V be an inner product space. Let $v \in V$, let $S \subset V$ be a subset, and let W_1 and W_2 be subspaces with $W_1 \subset W_2$. Then the following are subspaces:*

a. $S^{\perp}$.
b. $v^{\perp}$.
c. $W_2 \ominus W_1$.

Proof It is easy to see that $S^{\perp}$ is closed under addition and scalar multiplication. Statement (b) is a special case of (a) when $S = \{v\}$. From (a), $W^{\perp}{}_1$ is a subspace, and so (c) follows from Eq. (A.12) and Proposition A.20. □

Definition A.61 Vectors u and v are *orthonormal* if they are orthogonal and have length (norm) 1. An *orthonormal set* is a set of vectors that are pairwise orthonormal.

Orthonormal sets have a convenient feature that allows us to "read off" the coefficients of linear combinations:

Lemma A.62 *Let $u_1, \ldots, u_k$ be pairwise orthogonal in V, let $c_i \in \mathbb{R}$, and put $v = \sum_i c_i u_i$. Then $c_k = (v, u_k)/(u_k, u_k)$ for each k. If in particular $\{u_1, \ldots, u_k\}$ is an orthonormal set, then $c_k = (v, u_k)$.*

Proof Compute (v, u_k). □

Theorem A.63 *V contains a maximal orthonormal set. If $\dim(V) = n < \infty$, a maximal orthonormal set is a basis for V, and in particular has n elements.*

The word *basis* here is used in its usual sense (Definition A.22). Note that an orthonormal set cannot contain the zero vector.
Sketch of Proof In the finite-dimensional case, the first statement is obvious since orthogonal sets cannot contain more than n elements. In the infinite-dimensional case it follows from Zorn's Lemma or the Hausdorff Maximality Theorem.

Assume $\dim(V) = n < \infty$. Since an orthogonal set must be linearly independent, we must show that a *maximal* orthogonal set spans V. Let $u_1, \ldots, u_k$ be such a set. Suppose $v \in V$, and put $u = \sum_{i=1}^{k} (v, u_i) u_i$. We claim that $v = u$. (This will show incidentally that $k = n$.) A quick calculation shows that $v - u \perp u_i$ for each i. Were $v \neq u$,

$$\{u_1, \ldots, u_k, v - u\}$$

would be orthogonal, but this would contradict the maximality of $\{u_1, \ldots, u_k\}$. Thus $v = u$, as claimed.

Finally, given a maximal orthogonal set, we create a maximal orthonormal set by dividing each vector by its length. □

We call a maximal orthogonal resp. orthonormal set an *orthogonal* resp. *orthonormal basis*.

Theorem A.63 does not give a simple way to *construct* an orthogonal basis. One constructive method, known as the *Gram-Schmidt process*, will be discussed below.

Theorem A.64 (The Minimization Theorem) *Let W be a nonempty finite-dimensional subspace of an inner-product space V. For every $v \in V$ there is a unique $\hat{v} \in W$ that is closest to v, that is, such that $\|v - \hat{v}\| = \min_{w \in W} \|v - w\|$. If $u_1, \ldots u_k$ is an orthogonal basis of W, then $\hat{v}$ is given by*

$$\hat{v} = \sum_{i=1}^{k} \frac{(v, u_i)}{(u_i, u_i)} u_i. \tag{A.13}$$

Furthermore, we have $v - \hat{v} \perp W$.

If $v' \in W$ and $v - v' \perp W$, then $v' = \hat{v}$.

Theorem A.64 gives us two ways to find $\hat{v}$. Expression (A.13) requires first finding an orthonormal basis of W, and is thus not the most convenient. It is easier to exploit the necessary and sufficient condition that $v - \hat{v} \perp W$. Based on our experience with $\mathbb{R}^2$ and $\mathbb{R}^3$, this is known informally as *dropping a perpendicular* (that is, from v to W), and is the basis of the method of *least squares.*

Proof Fix an orthonormal basis $u_1, \ldots u_k$ of W. An arbitrary element $w \in W$ may be written in one and only one way as $w = \sum_{i=1}^{k} c_i u_i$ for constants $c_1, \ldots, c_k$, and so we must find the constants c_i to minimize $\|v - w\|$. Expanding $\|v - \sum_{i=1}^{k} c_i u_i\|^2$, applying Theorem A.57(a) to $\|\sum_{i=1}^{k} c_i u_i\|^2$, and completing the square term by term, we have

$$\|v - \sum_{i=1}^{k} c_i u_i\|^2 = \|v\|^2 + \sum_{i=1}^{k} \|u_i\|^2 \left(c_i - \frac{(v, u_i)}{\|u_i\|^2} \right)^2 - \sum_{i=1}^{k} \frac{(v, u_i)^2}{\|u_i\|^2}, \tag{A.14}$$

and the only way to minimize this over all choices of c_i is by letting $c_i = (v, u_i)/\|u_i\|^2$, which gives the expression (A.13). Direct computation shows that $(v - \hat{v}, u_i) = 0$ for all i, and so Theorem A.57(c) implies that $v - \hat{v} \perp W$.

Finally, if $v' \in W$ and $v - v' \perp W$, then for any $w \in W$ we have

$$\begin{aligned} \|v - w\|^2 &= \|v - v' + v' - w\|^2 \\ &= \|v - v'\|^2 + 2(v - v', v' - w) + \|v' - w\|^2. \end{aligned}$$

The middle term vanishes since $v' - w \in W$ and $v' - w \perp W$, and so $\|v - w\|$ is minimized when $w = v'$. But then $v' = \hat{v}$. □

Definition A.65 Given an inner-product space V, a finite-dimensional subspace W, and a vector $v \in V$, the vector $\hat{v} \in W$ closest to v is called the *orthogonal projection of v onto W*.

Corollary A.66 *Let V be an inner product space. A non-empty k-flat $A \subset V$ contains one and only one element $\hat{v}$ of minimum norm. If A is a translate of the subspace W, then $\hat{v}$ is the unique element of A orthogonal to W, and we have $A = \hat{v} + W$.*

In particular, if T is a linear transformation defined on V, then for each $y \in R(T)$ the solution set of $Tx = y$ can be written $x_0 + N(T)$ where x_0 is the unique solution orthogonal to $N(T)$.

Proof Let the k-flat be $A = v_0 + W$ where W is a subspace of V. Finding the shortest element of A means finding the element $v_0 + w \in A$ closest to 0, i.e., minimizing $\|v_0 + w\|$ over all $w \in W$. But $\|v_0 + w\| = \|w - (-v_0)\|$, so we are finding the vector $\hat{w} \in W$ closest to $-v_0$. That is, $\hat{w} = P(-v_0)$ where P is the orthogonal projection of V on W, and $v_0 - \hat{w} \perp W$. The vector $\hat{v} = v_0 - \hat{w}$ satisfies the conclusions of the corollary. The fact that $A = \hat{v} + W$ and the statement about the solution set of $Tx = y$ follow from Theorem A.39(b) and (c). □

Thus, in an inner product space, an *affine set arises by translating a subspace in the direction perpendicular to the subspace.*

Remark A.67 Letting $c_i = (v, u_i)$ in (A.14) gives $\|v\|^2 \geq \sum_{i=1}^{k}(v, u_i)^2$, which is known as *Bessel's inequality.*

The first statement of Theorem A.64 is actually true more generally if W is simply a nonempty *closed* and *convex* subset of V. See [19, Sec. III.5, Theorem 1], for example. This would allow us to avoid the use of orthonormal bases at this point. The theorem holds in the infinite-dimensional case if we replace $\dim(W) < \infty$ with the assumption that W is closed.

Similarly, the minimization part of Corollary A.66 holds for any nonempty closed and convex set in an inner product space.

The *Gram-Schmidt* process allows us to transform an ordinary (linear) basis into an orthogonal one. This depends, of course, on being able to construct a linear basis, but that is a simpler problem, and in many applications a linear basis is actually given. We state it in the finite-dimensional case:

Theorem A.68 (The Gram-Schmidt Process) *Let $\{v_1, \ldots, v_n\}$ be a basis of the inner-product space V. Let $W_k = \langle v_1, \ldots, v_k \rangle$ and $W_0 = (0)$, and let $\hat{v}_k =$ the orthogonal projection of v_k on W_{k-1}. Put*

$$u_k = v_k - \hat{v}_k.$$

Then $\{u_1, \ldots, u_k\}$ is an orthogonal basis of W_k, and in particular $\{u_1, \ldots, u_n\}$ is an orthogonal basis of V.

Proof We have $v_k \in W_k$ and $\hat{v}_k \in W_{k-1}$, so that on the one hand $u_k \in W_k$. On the other hand, the Minimization Theorem (Theorem A.64) implies that $u_k \perp W_{k-1}$ for each k. Thus $u_k \perp u_1, \ldots, u_{k-1}$. Since orthogonal sets are linearly independent, $\{u_1, \ldots, u_k\}$ is an orthogonal basis of W_k, and in particular $\{u_1, \ldots, u_n\}$ is an orthogonal basis of $V = W_n$. □

The Gram-Schmidt process is typically given by a set of explicit formulas:

$$\begin{aligned}
u_1 &= v_1 \\
u_2 &= v_2 - \frac{(v_2, u_1)}{(u_1, u_1)} u_1 \\
u_3 &= v_3 - \frac{(v_3, u_1)}{(u_1, u_1)} u_1 - \frac{(v_3, u_2)}{(u_2, u_2)} u_2 \\
&\vdots \\
u_n &= v_n - \frac{(v_n, u_1)}{(u_1, u_1)} u_1 - \frac{(v_n, u_2)}{(u_2, u_2)} u_2 - \cdots - \frac{(v_n, u_{n-1})}{(u_{n-1}, u_{n-1})} u_{n-1}.
\end{aligned} \tag{A.15}$$

These are a direct application of Eq. (A.13) in the Minimization Theorem. Formulas (A.15) are used inductively, defining u_k in terms of $u_1, \ldots, u_{k-1}$. However, Theorem A.68 allows one to define any u_k by projecting v_k orthogonally on W_{k-1}, using only the original vectors v_i.

Building on Theorem A.26, we have the following.

Corollary A.69 *If W is a subspace of V, then any orthonormal basis of W may be extended to one of V.*

Theorem A.70 *Let V be a finite-dimensional inner product space and let W, W_1 and W_2 be subspaces of V. Then*

a. $W \cap W^{\perp} = \{0\}$ *and* $W \oplus W^{\perp} = V$ *(orthogonal sum).*
b. $W^{\perp\perp} = W$ *($^{\perp}$ is an* involution*).*
c. $W_1 \subset W_2$ *iff* $W_1^{\perp} \supset W_2^{\perp}$.

That is, the subspaces of V form an ortholattice under the operations $+$, $\cap$, and $^{\perp}$.

Proof The fact that $W \cap W^{\perp} = \{0\}$ follows from Theorem A.57(d). Let $v \in V$ and let $\hat{v}$ be the orthogonal projection of v on W. Put $y = v - \hat{v}$; then $y \perp U$ (Theorem A.64) and $v = \hat{v} + y$, so $V = W + W^{\perp}$. Since $W \perp W^{\perp}$, their sum is orthogonal. This proves (a).

For (b), let $v = w + y$ be the decomposition of v with $w(= \hat{v}) \in W$ and $y \perp W$. Then $(v, y) = (w + y, y) = \|y\|^2$. But if in particular $v \in W^{\perp\perp}$, then $v \perp W^{\perp}$, and so $(v, y) = 0$. Thus $\|y\| = 0$, so $y = 0$ and $v = w \in W$. This shows that $W^{\perp\perp} \subset W$. The reverse inclusion is easy.

Finally, from $W_1 \subset W_2$ it easily follows that $W_1^{\perp} \supset W_2^{\perp}$. The opposite implication follows from applying part (b).

These are the three defining properties of an ortholattice (page 294). □

Corollary A.71 *Let V be a finite-dimensional inner product space and let W, W_1 and W_2 be subspaces of V, $W_1 \subset W_2$. Then*

$$W_2 = (W_2 \ominus W_1) \oplus W_1. \tag{A.16}$$

$$W^{\perp}{}_1 = (W_2 \ominus W_1) \oplus W^{\perp}{}_2. \tag{A.17}$$

$$\dim(W_2 \ominus W_1) = \dim(W_2) - \dim(W_1). \tag{A.18}$$

The direct sums above are orthogonal. In particular, we have

$$\dim(W^{\perp}) = \dim(V) - \dim(W). \tag{A.19}$$

Equations (A.16) and (A.17) may be visualized in the following diagram:

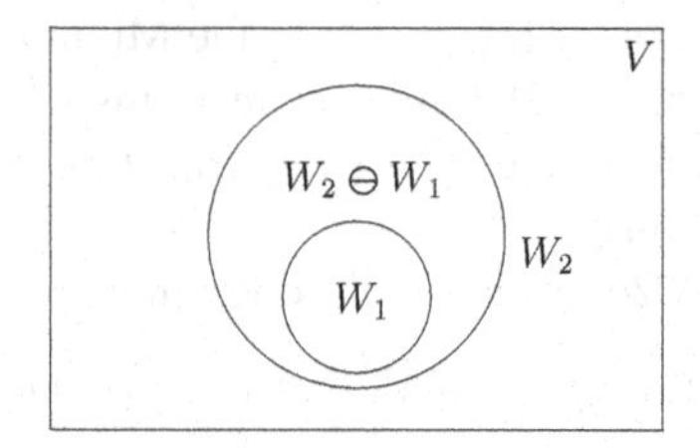

Proof Applying the modular law (A.6) to $(W_2 \cap W^{\perp}{}_1) + W_1$ and to $(W_2 \cap W^{\perp}{}_1) + W^{\perp}{}_2$ yields (A.16) and (A.17) (the sums are all orthogonal, as is easily checked). The dimension equations (A.18) and (A.19) follow by counting dimensions in (A.16) and in $V = W \oplus W^{\perp}$, using Theorem A.29(b). □

Corollary A.72 *Let V be a finite-dimensional inner product space. The lattice of subgroups of V satisfies the* De Morgan laws*:*

$$\begin{aligned} (W_1 \cap W_2)^{\perp} &= W^{\perp}{}_1 + W^{\perp}{}_2, \\ (W_1 + W_2)^{\perp} &= W^{\perp}{}_1 \cap W^{\perp}{}_2. \end{aligned} \tag{A.20}$$

This is just a re-writing of Eqs. (A.4).

A.4.4 The Transpose. Symmetric Maps

Definition A.73 Let V, V_1 and V_2 be *real* finite-dimensional inner product spaces. Let $T{:}V_1 \to V_2$ be a linear transformation. The map $T'{:}V_2 \to V_1$ such that

$$(Tu, v) = (u, T'v) \tag{A.21}$$

for all $u \in V_1$ and $v \in V_2$ is called the *transpose* of T.

If $T: V \to V$ and $T' = T$, we say that T is a *symmetric* linear transformation.

The terms "transpose" and "symmetric" come from the relationship of the matrices that represent T and T', which we discuss below. Existence and uniqueness of the transpose map are guaranteed by the following theorem:

Theorem A.74 *Let $T: V_1 \to V_2$ be a linear transformation of (real) finite-dimensional inner product spaces. Then T has a unique transpose.*

We will sketch the proof of this theorem. First, we note that if V is an inner product space, then for any $v \in V$ the map $L(u) = (u, v)$ is a linear functional. It turns out that all linear functionals arise this way:

Theorem A.75 *Let V be a finite-dimensional inner product space and let $L: V \to \mathbb{R}$ be a linear map. Then there exists a unique $v \in V$ such that $L(u) = (u, v)$ for all $u \in V$.*

We omit the proof of this theorem; see Remark A.76 below.

Sketch of Proof of Theorem A.74 Fix $v \in V_2$. The map $L(u) = (Tu, v)$ is easily seen to be a linear functional, so by Theorem A.75 there is a unique $u^* \in V_1$ such that $L(u) = (u, u^*)$ for all u. Define T' by $T'(v) = u^*$. Clearly T maps V_2 to V_1 and (A.21) holds, and we verify that T' is linear. □

Remark A.76 In these results (and in Definition A.73), "finite-dimensional" may be replaced by "complete"—that is, by the assumption that Cauchy sequences converge. It may be shown that finite-dimensional inner product spaces have this property. Complete inner product spaces are called *Hilbert spaces*. Theorem A.75 is variously known as the *Riesz* or *Fréchet-Riesz Representation Theorem.* A proof of that theorem in the finite-dimensional case may be found, e.g., in [85].

We note that the transpose of a map is also called its *adjoint*, the term that is used exclusively in the complex case.

Theorem A.77 *Let S and T be linear transformations from V_1 to V_2. Then*

$$(S + T)' = S' + T'.$$

Proof For all $v_1 \in V_1$ and $v_2 \in V_2$ we have

$$\begin{aligned}\langle v_1, (S+T)'v_2 \rangle &= \langle (S+T)v_1, v_2 \rangle = \langle Sv_1, v_2 \rangle + \langle Tv_1, v_2 \rangle \\ &= \langle v_1, S'v_2 \rangle + \langle v_1, T'v_2 \rangle = \langle v_1, (S' + T')v_2 \rangle.\end{aligned}$$

Thus $((S+T)' - (S' + T'))v_2$ is orthogonal to V_1, and so $= 0$ by Theorem A.57(d). Since this holds for all v_2, the result follows. □

Theorem A.78 *Let* $V_1 \overset{T}{\to} V_2 \overset{S}{\to} V_3$ *be linear transformations on finite-dimensional inner product spaces. Then:*

a. $T'' = T$.
b. $(ST)' = T'S'$.
c. The map $T'T$ *is symmetric.*

Outline of Proof We use Theorem A.57(d) to prove (a) and (b).

(a) Show that $\langle T''v_1, v_2 \rangle = \langle Tv_1, v_2 \rangle$ for all $v_i \in V_i$, and then apply the theorem to $T''v_1 - Tv_1$.
(b) Show that $\langle (ST)'v_3, v_1 \rangle = \langle T'S'v_3, v_1 \rangle$ for all $v_i \in V_i$, and then apply the theorem to $(ST)'v_3 - T'S'v_3$.
(c) $(T'T)' = T'T'' = T'T$.

□

Theorem A.79 *Let* $T: V_1 \to V_2$ *be a linear map of finite-dimensional inner product spaces. Then*

a. $N(T) = R(T')^\perp$.
b. $N(T)^\perp = R(T')$.
c. $N(T') = R(T)^\perp$.
d. $N(T')^\perp = R(T)$.

Proof For $v \in V_1$ and $w \in V_2$ we have $(Tv, w) = (v, T'w)$. Now to prove (a), suppose $v \in N(T)$ and $u \in R(T')$. Then $u = T'w$ for some $w \in V_2$, and $(v, u) = (v, T'w) = (Tv, w) = (0, w) = 0$, so $v \perp R(T')$. Thus $N(T) \subset R(T')^\perp$. Conversely, suppose $v \in R(T')^\perp$. Then $(v, T'w) = 0$ for all $w \in V_2$. But then $(Tv, w) = 0$ for all $w \in V_2$, so $Tv = 0$, i.e., $v \in N(T)$. Thus $N(T) \supset R(T')^\perp$, so we have (a).

Equation (b) follows by applying $^\perp$ to both sides of (a) and using Theorem A.70(b). The last two equations follow from the first two by interchanging the roles of T and T' and using the fact that $T'' = T$ (Theorem A.78). □

If T is defined on V, then so is $T'T$.

Corollary A.80 *Let* T *be a linear transformation defined on a finite-dimensional inner product space* V. *Then* $N(T'T) = N(T)$ *and* $R(T'T) = R(T)$.

Proof If $T'Tv = \mathbf{0}$ then $(T'Tv, v) = 0$. But $(T'Tv, v) = (Tv, Tv) = \|Tv\|^2$, so $Tv = 0$. Thus $N(T'T) \subset N(T)$. The reverse inclusion is obvious. The statement about ranges follows by applying $^\perp$ to both sides of $N(T'T) = N(T)$ and using Theorem A.79 and the symmetry of $T'T$. □

We end with a fact that will be useful in the next section. Its proof is an easy computation.

Lemma A.81 *Let* T *be symmetric. If* v *is an eigenvector of* T *and* $w \perp v$ *then* $Tw \perp v$.

A.4.5 Positive Maps

Definition A.82 Let V be an inner-product space (over $\mathbb{R}$) and $T \in \mathcal{L}(V)$. Then T is *positive* if $(Tv, v) \geq 0$ for all $v \in V$. It is *positive definite* if $(Tv, v) > 0$ for all $v \neq 0$.

Theorem A.83 *Let V be an inner-product space (over $\mathbb{R}$) and $T \in \mathcal{L}(V)$ be positive.*

a. If T is positive definite then it is invertible, in which case T^{-1} is positive definite.

b. The eigenvalues of T are non-negative, and are positive if T is positive-definite.

Proof (a) If $Tv = 0$ then $(Tv, v) = 0$, so $v = 0$. Thus $N(T) = \{0\}$, so T is one-to-one, and therefore onto (Theorem A.37). To show T^{-1} positive definite, let $v = Tw$ where w and v are nonzero. Then $(T^{-1}v, v) = (w, Tw) = (Tw, w) > 0$.

(b) If $Tv = \lambda v$, then $(Tv, v) = \lambda(v, v)$. Since $(Tv, v) \geq 0$ and $(v, v) \geq 0$, $\lambda \geq 0$. The positive definite case is proved similarly. □

Remark A.84 The converse of part (a) is false. For example, consider the invertible matrix

$$\mathbf{A} = \begin{pmatrix} 0 & 1 \\ -1 & 1 \end{pmatrix},$$

and define $T \in \mathcal{L}(\mathbb{R}^2)$ by $T\mathbf{u} = \mathbf{A}\mathbf{u}$, where the inner product on $\mathbb{R}^2$ is the usual dot product. Direct calculation shows that if $\mathbf{u} = (x, y)'$ then $(T\mathbf{u}, \mathbf{u}) = (\mathbf{A}\mathbf{u}) \cdot \mathbf{u} = y^2$, so T is positive but not definite.[9]

The converse holds if T is also symmetric. This follows from the Spectral Theorem (see Theorem A.88 below).

A linear transformation that is positive but not definite is sometimes called *semi-definite*.

A.4.6 The Spectral Theorem

This fundamental theorem guarantees that a symmetric linear transformation T on an inner-product space V yields an orthogonal basis consisting of eigenvectors. The theorem has a number of important by-products, as we shall see. The first step is to get a single nonzero eigenvector. Of course, its eigenvalue must be real.

---

[9] I thank Milan Lukic for this example.

We consider only the real case. Thus throughout this section V is a real vector space and $T \in \mathcal{L}(V)$ is symmetric.

Theorem A.49 showed that a linear transformation on a *complex* vector space has a nonzero eigenvector. Its eigenvalue is complex. The argument was fairly elementary, and in fact did not assume an inner product at all. In order to make use of this result, we will invoke a procedure known as *complexification*. That is, we will embed V in a complex inner-product space $\tilde{V}$, and construct from T a transformation $\tilde{T}$ on this new vector space that is linear over $\mathbb{C}$. This argument, which I have adapted from [86] (it probably comes from elsewhere), is probably the only unfamiliar technical step in the proof. The reader is welcome to consult other proofs of the spectral theorem, but some technicalities are inevitable. There is no free lunch.

We define $\tilde{V}$ informally[10] by

$$\tilde{V} = V + iV. \tag{A.22}$$

Its elements have the form $\tilde{v} = x + iy$, which may be added in the same way as complex numbers are added, although the real and imaginary parts are vectors in V rather than numbers. V is identified with the subspace $V + 0i \subset \tilde{V}$. Moreover,

$$x_1 + iy_1 = x_2 + iy_2 \quad \text{implies} \quad x_1 = x_2 \text{ and } y_1 = y_2.$$

We now make the following definitions:

- We define scalar multiplication in $\tilde{V}$ by formally multiplying $c \in \mathbb{C}$ by $\tilde{v}$ in the expected way: If $c = a + bi$, then

  $$c\tilde{v} = (a + bi)(x + iy) = (ax - by) + i(ay + bx).$$

  Note that the real and imaginary parts on the right are vectors in V. The verification that $\tilde{V}$ is a vector space over $\mathbb{C}$ is straightforward, although tedious.
- We define an inner product $\langle \cdot, \cdot \rangle$ on $\tilde{V}$ as follows:

  $$\begin{aligned}\langle \tilde{v}, \tilde{w} \rangle &= \langle v_1 + iv_2, w_1 + iw_2 \rangle \\ &= (v_1, w_1) + (v_2, w_2) + i((v_2, w_1) - (v_1, w_2)),\end{aligned}$$

  where $(\cdot, \cdot)$ is the inner product in V. (Imagine expanding $\langle \tilde{v}, \tilde{w} \rangle$ as expected except that $\langle x, iy \rangle = -i\langle x, y \rangle$.) One can verify that $\langle \cdot, \cdot \rangle$ is a hermitian inner product on $\tilde{V}$ (see Remark A.52 above).

[10] A formal definition of $\tilde{V}$ is as a direct sum $V + V$, that is, as the Cartesian product $V \times V$ with componentwise addition and with scalar multiplication given by $(a + bi)(x, y) = (ax - by, ay + bx)$. The informal definition (A.22) is easier to understand, and we will follow this approach.

- Finally, we define the map $\tilde{T}:\tilde{V} \to \tilde{V}$ from T in the obvious way:

$$\tilde{T}\tilde{v} = \tilde{T}(x + iy) = Tx + iTy.$$

It is again straightforward to verify that $\tilde{T}$ is $\mathbb{C}$-linear.

Lemma A.85 *The eigenvalues of $\tilde{T}$ are real.*

Proof[11] First we note that $\langle \tilde{T}\tilde{v}, \tilde{v} \rangle$ is real. For let $\tilde{v} = v_1 + iv_2$. Then

$$\begin{aligned}\langle \tilde{T}\tilde{v}, \tilde{v} \rangle &= (Tv_1, v_1) + (Tv_2, v_2) + i((Tv_2, v_1) - (Tv_1, v_2)) \\ &= (Tv_1, v_1) + (Tv_2, v_2),\end{aligned}$$

as $(Tv_2, v_1) = (v_1, Tv_2) = (Tv_1, v_2)$ by the symmetry of T. Now if $\tilde{v}$ is a nonzero eigenvector of $\tilde{T}$ with eigenvalue λ, then

$$\langle \tilde{T}\tilde{v}, \tilde{v} \rangle = \lambda \langle \tilde{v}, \tilde{v} \rangle,$$

and since both inner products are real, λ must be also. □

Because of this lemma, the eigenvalues of $\tilde{T}$ are potential eigenvalues of T. This is in fact the case, and is needed in the proof of the next result.

Proposition A.86 *If V is finite-dimensional, then T has a nonzero eigenvector.*

Proof By Theorem A.49, $\tilde{T}$ has a nonzero eigenvector $\tilde{v}$. Thus by Lemma A.85, $\tilde{T}\tilde{v} = \lambda\tilde{v}$ for some $\lambda \in \mathbb{R}$. Write $\tilde{v} = v_1 + iv_2$, $v_i \in V$. Then

$$Tv_1 + iTv_2 = \lambda v_1 + i\lambda v_2,$$

so $Tv_1 = \lambda v_1$ or $Tv_2 = \lambda v_2$. The result now follows since λ is real and at least one of v_1 and v_2 is nonzero. □

Theorem A.87 (Spectral Theorem) *If V is finite-dimensional and $T \in \mathcal{L}(V)$ is symmetric then V has an orthogonal basis consisting of eigenvectors of T.*

Proof By induction on $n = \dim(V)$. If $n = 1$, Proposition A.86 furnishes the orthogonal basis. Assume $n > 1$, and let v be an eigenvector of T, again furnished by the proposition. Put $W = v^{\perp}$; then $\dim W = n - 1$, and W inherits the inner product of V. Lemma A.81 shows that $T(w) \in W$ for all $w \in W$, so that $T \in \mathcal{L}(W)$, and T is symmetric as a map on W. The induction hypothesis now implies that W has an orthogonal basis of eigenvectors, and these are orthogonal to v, so that V has an orthogonal basis of eigenvectors. □

[11] An alternative proof of Lemma A.85 is to show that $\tilde{T}$ has hermitian symmetry.

From the Spectral Theorem we may immediately derive the converse of Theorem A.83(A.83) for positive symmetric maps, as mentioned above:

Theorem A.88 *Let V be a finite-dimensional inner-product space (over $\mathbb{R}$) and let $T \in \mathcal{L}(V)$ be positive and symmetric. If T is invertible then it is positive-definite.*

We also note that when T is symmetric the inequality (A.9) becomes an equality. For our purposes, though, the important applications of the Spectral Theorem are in the context of matrices, and will be described in Sect. A.4.8.

The approach we have followed does not give us an easy way to construct the basis given by the Spectral Theorem. For linear transformations on $\mathbb{R}^n$ there is a standard method, which we recall in Sect. A.4.8. For orthogonal projections the situation is simpler, as discussed in Sect. A.4.7.

A.4.7 Orthogonal Projections

Definition A.89 Let V be a finite-dimensional inner product space and W a subspace. The map $P: V \to V$ that associates to each $v \in V$ its orthogonal projection $\hat{v} \in W$ is the *orthogonal projection of V on W*.

Thus P is the identity map on V and the zero map on $V^\perp$; that is,

$$\begin{aligned} Pv &= v \text{ if } v \in V, \\ &= 0 \text{ if } v \in V^\perp. \end{aligned}$$

Theorem A.90 *Let V be an inner product space and W a finite-dimensional subspace. Let $P: V \to V$ be the orthogonal projection of V on W. Then*

a. P is a linear transformation.
b. $(Pv_1, v_2) = (v_1, Pv_2)$ for all $v_1, v_2 \in V$ (P is symmetric*).*
c. $P^2 = P$, that is, $P(Pv) = Pv$ for all $v \in V$ (P is idempotent*).*
d. $R(P) = W$ and $N(P) = W^\perp$.

Conversely, let $P: V \to V$ be linear, symmetric, and idempotent, and let $W = R(P)$. Then P is the orthogonal projection of V on W.

Corollary A.91 *If V is finite-dimensional and P is the orthogonal projection on the subspace W, then $I - P$ is the orthogonal projection on $W^\perp$.*

Proof $I - P$ is obviously linear, and it is easy to check that it is symmetric and idempotent, and that $R(I - P) = W^\perp$. □

Corollary A.92 *If P is a projection, then the eigenvalues of P equal 0 or 1. If P is the orthogonal projection of V on W, and if* $\dim V = n$*, then all the vectors in*

W are eigenvectors belonging to 1, and those belonging to $W^\perp$ are the eigenvectors belonging to 0.

Corollary A.93 *Let P_1 and P_2 be the orthogonal projections of V on W_1 and W_2, respectively. Then the following are equivalent:*

a. $W_1 \subset W_2$.
b. $P_2 P_1 = P_1$.
c. $P_1 P_2 = P_1$.
If these hold, then
d. $I - P_1$ *maps* W_2 *onto* $W_2 \ominus W_1$.

Proof Assume $W_1 \subset W_2$. Let $v \in V$ and $w = P_1 v$. Then $w \in W_1$, so $w \in W_2$, and so $P_2 w = w$. But then $P_1 v = w = P_2 w = P_2 P_1 v$. Since this holds for all $v \in V$, $P_2 P_1 = P_1$. Conversely, suppose $P_2 P_1 = P_1$, and let $w \in W_1$. Then $w = P_1 w = P_2 P_1 w \in R(P_2) = W_2$.

We have shown (a) $\iff$ (b). The equivalence of (b) and (c) follows by taking transposes.

As to the last statement, let $w \in W_2$. By (A.16), w may be written (uniquely) as $w = w_1 + w_2$ with $w_1 \in W_1$ and $w_2 \in W_2 \ominus W_1$. By Corollary A.91, $(I - P_1)w = w_2 \in W_2 \ominus W_1$. Thus $I - P_1$ maps W_2 into $W_2 \ominus W_1$. To show that this mapping is onto, we note that for any $w_2 \in W_2$ we have $(I - P_1)w_2 = w_2$. □

Theorem A.94 *If P, Q, and PQ are all orthogonal projections, then $R(PQ) = R(P) \cap R(Q)$.*

Proof First we note that $R(PQ) \subset R(P)$. But since PQ is symmetric, $QP = Q'P' = (PQ)' = PQ$. Thus we also have $R(PQ) = R(QP) \subset R(Q)$, so that $R(PQ) \subset R(P) \cap R(Q)$. Conversely, if $w \in R(P) \cap R(Q)$, then $Pw = w$ and $Qw = w$, so $PQw = Pw = w$, and so $w \in R(PQ)$. □

Remark A.95 Given projections P and Q, one can show that PQ is also a projection if and only if P and Q commute. We have adapted the above theorem and the following corollary from [68].

Corollary A.96 *Let V be a finite-dimensional inner product space and let W_1 and W_2 be subspaces such that $W_1 \subset W_2$. Let P_i be the orthogonal projection of V on W_i, $i = 1, 2$. Then $P_2 - P_1$ is the orthogonal projection of V on $W_2 \ominus W_1$.*

Proof From Theorem A.77 it is easy to see that $(P_2 - P_1)' = P_2 - P_1$, and since $P_1 P_2 = P_1 = P_2 P_1$ we see that $(P_2 - P_1)^2 = P_2 - P_1$, so that $P_2 - P_1$ is an orthogonal projection. On the other hand, $P_2 - P_1 = P_2(I - P_1)$ so by Theorem A.94 and Corollary A.91, $P_2 - P_1$ is the orthogonal projection on $W_2 \cap W^{\perp}{}_1 = W_2 \ominus W_1$.
□

Remark A.97 An inner product space V is an example of a *metric space*, where the metric is given by (A.11). Theorem A.90 and its corollaries hold without the assumption of finite dimension if we restrict ourselves to closed subspaces.

If V is *complete*, that is, if every Cauchy sequence in V converges to an element of V, then V is a *Hilbert space*.

A.4.8 Linear Algebra in $\mathbb{R}^n$. Matrices

We will view the elements of $\mathbb{R}^n$ as column vectors, or as $n \times 1$ matrices. The set $\mathbb{R}^n$ is vector space of dimension n, having the *standard basis* $\mathbf{e}_1, \ldots, \mathbf{e}_n$ where $\mathbf{e}_i$ is the vector with 1 in the ith position and 0 elsewhere.

Let $\mathbf{A} = (a_{ij})$ be $m \times n$. The span of the columns of $\mathbf{A}$ is called the *columnspace* of $\mathbf{A}$, and is a subspace of $\mathbb{R}^m$. The span of its rows is its *rowspace*, and is a subspace of $\mathbb{R}^n$. The *transpose* of $\mathbf{A}$ is the $n \times m$ matrix $\mathbf{A}' = (b_{ij})$ where $b_{ij} = a_{ji}$. If $\mathbf{A}$ is square ($m = n$), then it is *symmetric* if $\mathbf{A}' = \mathbf{A}$.

The most common inner product on $\mathbb{R}^n$ is

$$(\mathbf{u}, \mathbf{v}) = \mathbf{u}'\mathbf{v},$$

usually denoted $\mathbf{u} \cdot \mathbf{v}$ and called the *dot product*. Matrix multiplication is defined in the usual way: If $\mathbf{A}$ is $m \times n$ and $\mathbf{B}$ is a $n \times r$, and if $\mathbf{a}^i$ is the ith row of $\mathbf{A}$ and $\mathbf{b}_j$ is the jth column of $\mathbf{B}$, then $\mathbf{AB}$ is the $m \times r$ matrix whose ijth element is $\mathbf{a}^i \cdot \mathbf{b}_j$.

Theorem A.98 *Suppose* $\mathbf{A}$ *is* $m \times n$ *and* $\mathbf{B}$ *is* $n \times r$.

a. *For* $\mathbf{x} \in \mathbb{R}^n$, *define* $\mathbf{y} = \mathbf{Ax}$. *The correspondence* $A{:}\mathbf{x} \mapsto \mathbf{y}$ *is a linear transformation from* $\mathbb{R}^n$ *to* $\mathbb{R}^m$. *Conversely, if* $A{:}\mathbb{R}^n \to \mathbb{R}^m$ *is linear, then there is an* $m \times n$ *matrix* $\mathbf{A}$ *that represents*[12] *it in the sense that* $A(\mathbf{v}) = \mathbf{Av}$.
   The range $R(A)$ *is the columnspace of* $\mathbf{A}$.
b. *If* $B{:}\mathbb{R}^r \to \mathbb{R}^n$ *is the linear transformation defined by* $\mathbf{B}$, *then* $\mathbf{AB}$ *is the matrix of the linear transformation* $AB{:}\mathbb{R}^r \to \mathbb{R}^n$.
c. *The transposed matrix* $\mathbf{A}'$ *defines the linear transformation* A' *(the transpose map) from* $\mathbb{R}^m$ *to* $\mathbb{R}^n$. *The matrix* $\mathbf{A}$ *is symmetric if and only if the map* A *is symmetric.*

The proof is by direct computation. Due to Theorem A.98(a), we write $R(\mathbf{A})$ for the columnspace of $\mathbf{A}$. (**Caution**: R stands for *range*, not *rows*!) We will naturally use $N(\mathbf{A})$ for $N(A)$: $N(\mathbf{A}) = \{\mathbf{v}{:}\mathbf{Av} = \mathbf{0}\}$ = the *nullspace* of $\mathbf{A}$.

With the aid of Theorem A.98, **all the results we proved for linear transformations carry over naturally to matrices**. For example:

[12] In Theorem A.98(a), "represents" means "with respect to the standard basis."

Theorem A.99

a. $(\mathbf{A}')' = \mathbf{A}$.
b. $N(\mathbf{A}) = R(\mathbf{A}')^{\perp}$.
c. $N(\mathbf{A}'\mathbf{A}) = N(\mathbf{A})$.
d. $R(\mathbf{A}'\mathbf{A}) = R(\mathbf{A})$. *In particular,* $\text{rank}(\mathbf{A}'\mathbf{A}) = \text{rank}(\mathbf{A})$.

The reader may note that matrix proofs of these are sometimes simpler than the ones we have given. However, we have emphasized the role of linear transformations due to the usefulness of this perspective.

Theorem A.100 *Let A be the linear transformation defined by the $m \times n$ matrix $\mathbf{A}$.*

a. A is one-to-one iff the columns of $\mathbf{A}$ are linearly independent.
b. A is surjective ("onto") iff the columnspace of $\mathbf{A}$ is all of $\mathbb{R}^m$.

Definition A.101 The *rank* of $\mathbf{A}$ is the dimension of $R(\mathbf{A})$. The dimension of $N(\mathbf{A})$ is called[13] the *nullity* of $\mathbf{A}$.

Wardlaw [148] has given a remarkably short proof of the following classic fact:

Theorem A.102 $\text{Rank}(\mathbf{A}') = \text{rank}(\mathbf{A})$.

From Theorem A.34 we have:

Theorem A.103 (Rank-Plus-Nullity Theorem) *Let A be $m \times n$. Then* $n = \text{rank}(\mathbf{A}) + \dim N(\mathbf{A})$.

Square Matrices

An $n \times n$ matrix defines a linear transformation from $\mathbb{R}^n$ to $\mathbb{R}^n$. The identity map on $\mathbb{R}^n$ is given by an *identity matrix* $\mathbf{I}$, or $\mathbf{I}_n$ if we want to indicate the dimension, having 1's on the diagonal and 0's elsewhere.

To each square matrix $\mathbf{A}$ is associated two important constants: its trace $\text{tr}(\mathbf{A})$ and its determinant $\det(\mathbf{A})$. If $\mathbf{A} = [a_{ij}]$, then

$$\text{tr}(\mathbf{A}) = \sum_i a_{ii}.$$

That is, the trace is the sum of the diagonal elements of $\mathbf{A}$. Two useful properties of the trace are easy to verify:

- $\text{tr}(c\mathbf{A}) = c\,\text{tr}(\mathbf{A})$ for any constant c.
- $\text{tr}(\mathbf{AB}) = \text{tr}(\mathbf{BA})$.

The second property shows, for example, that $\text{tr}(\mathbf{ABC}) = \text{tr}(\mathbf{BCA})$.

[13] Less commonly.

We assume that the reader is familiar with the computation of the determinant and its basic properties, for example, $\det(\mathbf{I}) = 1$, $\det(\mathbf{AB}) = \det(\mathbf{A})\det(\mathbf{B})$, and $\det(\mathbf{A}') = \det(\mathbf{A})$.

Theorem A.104 *Let* $\mathbf{A}$ *be a square matrix. The following are equivalent:*

a. $\det(\mathbf{A}) \neq 0$.
b. $N(\mathbf{A}) \neq \mathbf{0}$.
c. There is a square matrix $\mathbf{B}$ *such that* $\mathbf{AB} = \mathbf{I} = \mathbf{BA}$.

A matrix $\mathbf{A}$ satisfying any of the conditions of Theorem A.104 is said to be *invertible* or *nonsingular*. As usual, we refer to the matrix $\mathbf{B}$ in (c) as the *inverse* of $\mathbf{A}$, and denote it by $\mathbf{A}^{-1}$. In particular, $\det(\mathbf{A}^{-1}) = 1/\det(\mathbf{A})$.

Definition A.105 A square matrix $\mathbf{A}$ is *positive (semidefinite)* if $\mathbf{x}'\mathbf{A}\mathbf{x} \geq 0$ for any $\mathbf{x}$. It is *positive definite* if in addition $\mathbf{x}'\mathbf{A}\mathbf{x} = 0$ implies $\mathbf{x} = \mathbf{0}$.

This is, of course, the matrix form of the notion of a positive map, as given in Definition A.82.[14] For matrices, Theorems A.83(a) and A.88 yield the following:

Theorem A.106 *Let* $\mathbf{A}$ *be a positive matrix. If* $\mathbf{A}$ *is positive definite then it is nonsingular, in which case* $\mathbf{A}^{-1}$ *is positive definite. Conversely, if* $\mathbf{A}$ *is symmetric and nonsingular then it is positive definite.*

Theorem A.90 gives us the following characterization:

Theorem A.107 *An* $n \times n$ *matrix* $\mathbf{P}$ *is the matrix of an orthogonal projection if and only if* $\mathbf{P}$ *is symmetric and idempotent* ($\mathbf{P}^2 = \mathbf{P}$).

A matrix $\mathbf{P}$ only satisfying $\mathbf{P}^2 = \mathbf{P}$ is a *projection matrix*. It is an *orthogonal projection matrix* if in addition $\mathbf{P}' = \mathbf{P}$.

Definition A.108 A square matrix $\mathbf{O}$ is *orthogonal* if its columns are orthonormal; equivalently, if $\mathbf{O}'\mathbf{O} = \mathbf{I}$.

Thus $\mathbf{O}' = \mathbf{O}^{-1}$, so we also have $\mathbf{O}\mathbf{O}' = \mathbf{I}$.

Remark A.109 The terminology of Definition A.108 is deficient, since the columns of $\mathbf{O}$ are more than simply orthogonal to each other: they also have unit length. Moreover, viewed as a linear transformation, $\mathbf{O}$ preserves more than orthogonality, as it also preserves length. However, this terminology is now standard. The term *unitary* is also used, although primarily when working over the complex numbers.

Let $\mathbf{A}$ be a square matrix. As with linear transformations, if $\mathbf{A}\mathbf{v} = \lambda\mathbf{v}$ for $\mathbf{v} \neq \mathbf{0}$ then we say that $\mathbf{v}$ is an *eigenvector of* $\mathbf{A}$ *belonging to the eigenvalue* λ. The set of eigenvectors belonging to λ is the *eigenspace* of λ.

[14] If $(\mathbf{x}, \mathbf{y}) = \mathbf{x}'\mathbf{y}$ then technically $(\mathbf{A}\mathbf{x}, \mathbf{x}) = \mathbf{x}'\mathbf{A}'\mathbf{x}$, not $\mathbf{x}'\mathbf{A}\mathbf{x}$. However, $\mathbf{x}'\mathbf{A}'\mathbf{x} = (\mathbf{x}'\mathbf{A}'\mathbf{x})' = \mathbf{x}'\mathbf{A}\mathbf{x}$, the first equality holding since these quantities are 1×1 matrices, and so Definition A.105 is consistent with Definition A.82.

If λ is an eigenvalue of $\mathbf{A}$, then $N(\mathbf{A} - \lambda\mathbf{I})$ is the eigenspace belonging to λ, and it must contain a nonzero vector. Therefore $\mathbf{A} - \lambda\mathbf{I}$ is singular.

Theorem A.110 *The eigenvalues of the square matrix* $\mathbf{A}$ *are the solutions* λ *to*

$$\det(\mathbf{A} - \lambda\mathbf{I}) = 0.$$

If λ *is an eigenvalue, then the eigenvectors* $\mathbf{v}$ *belonging to* λ *are the solutions to*

$$(\mathbf{A} - \lambda\mathbf{I})\mathbf{v} = \mathbf{0}.$$

Thus if an orthogonal basis of eigenvectors exists, it can be found in these steps: (1) Find the eigenvalues. (2) For each eigenvalue, find the eigenspace by solving a system of linear equations. (3) Using Gram-Schmidt if necessary, pick an orthogonal basis of the eigenspace. These steps are guaranteed to work in the following important case, a direct application of Theorem A.87:

Theorem A.111 (Spectral Theorem for Matrices) *If* $\mathbf{A}$ *is* $n \times n$ *and symmetric then* $\mathbb{R}^n$ *has an orthogonal basis consisting of eigenvectors of* $\mathbf{A}$.

Corollary A.112 *Let* $\mathbf{A}$ *be a symmetric* $n \times n$ *matrix, with eigenvalues* $\lambda_1, \ldots, \lambda_n$ *(not necessarily distinct). Then there is an orthogonal matrix* $\mathbf{O}$ *such that* $\mathbf{O}'\mathbf{A}\mathbf{O} = \operatorname{diag}(\lambda_1, \ldots, \lambda_n)$, *the diagonal matrix with the eigenvalues on the diagonal.*

Proof Let the columns of $\mathbf{O}$ be an orthonormal basis of eigenvectors. □

Corollary A.113 *If* $\mathbf{P}$ *is an* $n \times n$ *projection matrix of rank* r, *then there is an orthogonal matrix* $\mathbf{O}$ *such that*

$$\mathbf{O}'\mathbf{P}\mathbf{O} = \operatorname{diag}(\underbrace{1, \ldots, 1}_{r}, \underbrace{0, \ldots, 0}_{n-r}).$$

Proof Follows directly from Corollaries A.92 and A.112. □

Corollary A.114 *If* $\mathbf{A}$ *is a positive symmetric matrix, then it has a positive square root, i.e., a positive matrix* $\mathbf{B}$ *such that* $\mathbf{B}^2 = \mathbf{A}$. *The matrix* $\mathbf{B}$ *may be chosen to be symmetric. If* $\mathbf{A}$ *is positive definite, so is* $\mathbf{B}$.

Proof If λ_i are the eigenvalues of $\mathbf{A}$ then $\lambda_i \geq 0$ (Theorem A.83), and there is an orthogonal $\mathbf{O}$ such that $\mathbf{O}'\mathbf{A}\mathbf{O} = \mathbf{D}$ where $\mathbf{D} = \operatorname{diag}(\lambda_1, \ldots, \lambda_n)$. Then $\mathbf{A} = \mathbf{O}\mathbf{D}\mathbf{O}'$. Writing $\mathbf{D}^{1/2} = \operatorname{diag}(\lambda_1^{1/2}, \ldots, \lambda_n^{1/2})$, we see that $\mathbf{D}^{1/2}$ is positive and symmetric, and easy calculations show that $B = \mathbf{O}\mathbf{D}^{1/2}\mathbf{O}'$ has the properties we claim. □

Remark A.115 The matrix $\mathbf{B}$ in this corollary is often denoted $\mathbf{A}^{1/2}$. It is actually unique; see, e.g., [69, p. 166]. When $\mathbf{A}^{1/2}$ is positive definite, it is invertible (Theorem A.83), and its inverse may be denoted $\mathbf{A}^{-1/2}$.

Lemma A.116 (Maximization Lemma) *Let* $\mathbf{b} \in \mathbb{R}^n$ *be nonzero, and let* $\mathbf{A}$ *be positive definite and symmetric. Then*

$$\max_{\mathbf{z}} \frac{(\mathbf{z}'\mathbf{b})^2}{\mathbf{z}'\mathbf{A}\mathbf{z}} = \mathbf{b}'\mathbf{A}^{-1}\mathbf{b} \quad (\textit{maximizing over } \mathbf{z} \in \mathbb{R}^n, \mathbf{z} \neq \mathbf{0}),$$

the maximum attained iff $\mathbf{z} \propto \mathbf{A}^{-1}\mathbf{b}$.[15]

Proof The Cauchy-Schwarz inequality asserts that $(\mathbf{u}'\mathbf{v})^2 \leq (\mathbf{u}'\mathbf{u})(\mathbf{v}'\mathbf{v})$, with equality iff $\mathbf{u} \propto \mathbf{v}$, and we let $\mathbf{u} = \mathbf{A}^{1/2}\mathbf{z}$ and $\mathbf{v} = \mathbf{A}^{-1/2}\mathbf{b}$ to get what we want. □

Definition A.117 Let $\mathbf{A} = (a_{ij})$ be $m \times n$, and let $\mathbf{B}$ be a matrix. The *Kronecker product* of $\mathbf{A}$ and $\mathbf{B}$ is the block matrix

$$\mathbf{A} \otimes \mathbf{B} = \begin{pmatrix} a_{11}\mathbf{B} & \cdots & a_{1n}\mathbf{B} \\ \vdots & \ddots & \vdots \\ a_{m1}\mathbf{B} & \cdots & a_{mn}\mathbf{B} \end{pmatrix}.$$

That is, $\mathbf{A} \otimes \mathbf{B}$ consists of mn blocks in the above pattern, the ijth block being the matrix $a_{ij}\mathbf{B}$.

If $\mathbf{B}$ is $p \times q$, then it is evident that $\mathbf{A} \otimes \mathbf{B}$ is $mp \times nq$. In particular, the Kronecker product of two vectors of lengths m and p is a vector of length mp. In fact:

Lemma A.118 *If* $\mathbf{v} = (v_1, \ldots, v_m)'$ *and* $\mathbf{w} = (w_1, \ldots, w_p)'$, *then*

$$\mathbf{v} \otimes \mathbf{w} = (v_1 w_1, \ldots, v_1 w_p, v_2 w_1, \ldots, v_2 w_p, \ldots, v_m w_1, \ldots, v_m w_p)'.$$

Note that $\mathbf{v} \otimes \mathbf{w}$ lists the products $v_i w_j$ in *lexicographic order*. In similar fashion we have the following:

Lemma A.119 *Let* $\mathbf{A} = [\mathbf{a}_1 \cdots \mathbf{a}_n]$ *and* $\mathbf{B} = [\mathbf{b}_1 \cdots \mathbf{b}_q]$ *be matrices with columns as given. Then*

$$\mathbf{A} \otimes \mathbf{B} = [\mathbf{a}_i \otimes \mathbf{b}_j],$$

the matrix with (i, j)*-th column* $\mathbf{a}_i \otimes \mathbf{b}_j$ *(the pairs* (i, j) *ordered lexicographically).*

We conclude with some standard properties of the Kronecker product:

a. $\mathbf{A} \otimes (\mathbf{B} \otimes \mathbf{C}) = (\mathbf{A} \otimes \mathbf{B}) \otimes \mathbf{C}$.
b. $\mathbf{A} \otimes (\mathbf{B} + \mathbf{C}) = \mathbf{A} \otimes \mathbf{B} + \mathbf{A} \otimes \mathbf{C}$, and similarly for $(\mathbf{A} + \mathbf{B}) \otimes \mathbf{C}$ (distributivity)

[15] The symbol $\propto$ means "is proportional to".

c. $(c\mathbf{A}) \otimes \mathbf{B} = c(\mathbf{A} \otimes \mathbf{B}) = \mathbf{A} \otimes (c\mathbf{B})$ where c is a constant.
d. $(\mathbf{A} \otimes \mathbf{B})(\mathbf{C} \otimes \mathbf{D}) = (\mathbf{AC}) \otimes (\mathbf{BD})$ if the matrix products on the right are defined.
e. $(\mathbf{A} \otimes \mathbf{B})' = (\mathbf{A}' \otimes \mathbf{B}')$ and $(\mathbf{A} \otimes \mathbf{B})^{-1} = (\mathbf{A}^{-1} \otimes \mathbf{B}^{-1})$ (assuming inverses exist).
f. $\mathrm{tr}(\mathbf{A} \otimes \mathbf{B}) = \mathrm{tr}(\mathbf{A})\,\mathrm{tr}(\mathbf{B})$.

Properties (a) and (b) mean that the Kronecker product is associative, and is distributive over matrix addition. It is not commutative in general. Properties (b) and (c) together are known as *bilinearity*. Property (d) is sometimes called the *mixed-product* rule.

Some useful special cases are the following:

- $c\mathbf{A} = \mathbf{A} \otimes c = c \otimes \mathbf{A}$.
  Here $\mathbf{A} \otimes c$ means $\mathbf{A} \otimes [c]$, where $[c]$ is a 1×1 matrix.
- $\mathbf{1}_m \otimes \mathbf{1}_n = \mathbf{1}_{mn}, \quad \mathbf{I}_m \otimes \mathbf{I}_n = \mathbf{I}_{mn}, \quad \mathbf{J}_m \otimes \mathbf{J}_n = \mathbf{J}_{mn}.$
  Here $\mathbf{I}$ is an identity matrix, $\mathbf{1}$ is a vector of 1's, $\mathbf{J}$ is a square matrix of 1's, and subscripts denote dimensions.

Bibliography

1. A. Agresti, *Categorical Data Analysis*, 2nd edn. (Wiley, New York, 2002) [15]
2. M. Aigner, *Combinatorial Theory* (Springer, New York, 1979) [296]
3. A.A. Albert, R. Sandler, *An Introduction to Finite Projective Planes* (Holt, Rinehart and Winston, New York, 1968) [212]
4. I. Anderson, *Combinatorics of Finite Sets* (Oxford University Press, Oxford, 1987) [255, 296, 297]
5. T.W. Anderson, *An Introduction to Multivariate Statistical Analysis*, 3rd edn. (Wiley, New York, 2004) [13]
6. G.E. Andrews, *The Theory of Partitions*, volume 2 of Encyclopedia of Mathematics and Its Applications (Addison-Wesley Publishing Company, Reading, MA, 1976) [296]
7. R.A. Bailey, The decomposition of treatment degrees of freedom in quantitative factorial experiments. J. R. Stat. Soc. Ser. B **44**, 63–70 (1982) [203]
8. R.A. Bailey, *Association Schemes: Designed experiments, Algebra and Combinatorics* (Cambridge University Press, Cambridge, 2004) [155, 156, 157, 176, 296]
9. R.A. Bailey, F.H.L. Gilchrist, H.D. Patterson, Identification of effects and confounding patterns in factorial designs. Biometrika **64**, 347–354 (1977) [206]
10. M.M. Barnard, Enumeration of the confounded arrangements in the $2 \times 2 \times 2 \cdots$ factorial designs. Suppl. J. R. Stat. Soc. **3**, 195–202 (1936) [xii, 151, 166, 178, 179, 198, 203]
11. J.H. Beder, The problem of confounding in two-factor experiments. Commun. Stat. Theory Methods **A18**, 591–612 (1989). Reprinted more clearly on pages 2165–2188 of the same volume. Correction, **A23**, 2131–2132, 1994 [156, 213]
12. J.H. Beder, On Rao's inequalities for arrays of strength d. Utilitas Math. **54**, 85–109 (1998) [249, 256]
13. J.H. Beder, On the definition of effects in fractional factorial designs. Utilitas Math. **66**, 47–60 (2004) [249, 256, 258]
14. J.H. Beder, Main effects, in *Encyclopedia of Statistics in Quality and Reliability*, ed. by F. Ruggeri, R. Kenett, F.W. Faltin (Wiley, Chichester, 2007), pp. 990–993 [34]
15. J.H. Beder, J.S. Beder, Generalized wordlength patterns and strength. J. Stat. Plan. Inference **144**, 41–46 (2014) [278]
16. J.H. Beder, W.S. Diestelkamp, Box-Hunter resolution in nonregular fractional factorial designs. J. Stat. Theory Practice **3**, 879–889 (2009) [163, 249]
17. J.H. Beder, J.F. Willenbring, Invariance of generalized wordlength patterns. J. Stat. Plan. Inference **139**, 2706–2714 (2009) [278]
18. A. Ben-Israel, T.N.E. Greville, *Generalized Inverses: Theory and Applications*, 2nd edn. (Springer, New York, 2003) [65]

J. H. Beder, *Linear Models and Design*,
https://doi.org/10.1007/978-3-031-08176-7

19. S.K. Berberian, *Introduction to Hilbert Space*, 2nd edn. (Chelsea Publishing Company, New York, 1976) [314]
20. J. Bierbrauer, Bounds on orthogonal arrays and resilient functions. J. Comb. Des. **3**, 179–183 (1995) [256]
21. R.C. Bose, The fundamental theorem of linear estimation, in *Proceedings of the 31st Indian Scientific Congress* (1944), pp. 2–3 [69]
22. R.C. Bose, Mathematical theory of the symmetrical factorial design. Sankhyā **8**, 107–166 (1947) [xi, 33, 53, 157, 161]
23. R.C. Bose, K. Kishen, On the problem of confounding in the general symmetrical factorial design. Sankhyā **5**, 21–36 (1940) [xii, 179, 192]
24. R.C. Bose, S.S. Shrikhande, On the falsity of Euler's conjecture about the non-existence of two orthogonal Latin squares of order $4t+2$. Proc. Natl. Acad. Sci. **45**, 734–737 (1959) [212]
25. N. Bourbaki, *Elements of Mathematics: Algebra I, Chapters 1–3* (Hermann, Paris, 1974) [197]
26. J.F. Box, R. A. Fisher and the design of experiments, 1922–1926. Am. Stat. **34**, 1–7 (1980) [151]
27. G.E.P. Box, J.S. Hunter, The 2^{k-p} fractional factorial designs. Technometrics **3**, 311–351; 449–458 (1961) [xii, 238]
28. G. Box, J. Tyssedal, Projective properties of certain orthogonal arrays. Biometrika **83**, 950–955 (1996) [286]
29. G.E.P. Box, K.B. Wilson, On the experimental attainment of optimal conditions. J. R. Stat. Soc. Ser. B **13**, 1–45 (1951) [232, 265]
30. L. Breiman, *Probability* (Addison-Wesley, Reading, MA, 1968). Reissued by the Society for Industrial and Applied Mathematics in 1992 [1]
31. D.A. Bulutoglu, C.-S. Cheng, Hidden projection properties of some nonregular fractional factorial designs and their applications. Ann. Stat. **31**, 1012–1026 (2003) [287]
32. P.J. Cameron, *Combinatorics: Topics, Techniques, Algorithms* (Cambridge University Press, Cambridge, 1994) [213]
33. M.C. Chakrabarti, *Mathematics of Design and Analysis of Experiments* (Asia Publishing House, Bombay, 1962) [247]
34. H. Chen, Some projective properties of fractional factorial designs. Stat. Probab. Lett. **40**, 185–188 (1998) [285]
35. C.-S. Cheng, Some projection properties of orthogonal arrays. Ann. Stat. **23**, 1223–1233 (1995) [286]
36. C.-S. Cheng, Projection properties of factorial designs for factor screening, in *Screening: Methods for Experimentation in Industry, Drug Discovery, and Genetics*, ed. by A. Dean, S. Lewis, chapter 7 (Springer, 2006) [285, 287]
37. R. Christensen, *Plane Answers to Complex Questions: The Theory of Linear Models*, 2nd edn. (Springer, New York, 1996) [13, 65, 66, 101]
38. P. Crawley, R.P. Dilworth, *Algebraic Theory of Lattices* (Prentice-Hall, Englewood Cliffs, 1973) [296]
39. J.N. Darroch, S.D. Silvey, On testing more than one hypothesis. Ann. Math. Stat. **34**, 555–567 (1963) [25, 115]
40. B. A. Davey and H.A. Priestley, *Introduction to Lattices and Order* (Cambridge University Press, Cambridge, 1990) [293, 294]
41. A.M. Dean, J.A. John, Single replicate factorial experiments in generalized cyclic designs: II. Asymmetrical arrangements. J. R. Stat. Soc. Ser. B **37**, 72–76 (1975) [206]
42. A. Dean, S. Lewis, *Screening: Methods for Experimentation in Industry, Drug Discovery, and Genetics* (Springer, New York, 2006) [280]
43. A. Dean, D. Voss, D. Draguljić, *Design and Analysis of Experiments*, 2nd edn. (Springer, New York, 2017) [208, 209, 210]
44. L.Y. Deng, B. Tang, Generalized resolution and minimum aberration criteria for plackett-burman and other nonregular factorial designs. Stat. Sin. **9**, 1071–1082 (1999) [272]
45. A. Dey, R. Mukerjee, *Fractional Factorial Plans* (Wiley, New York, 1999) [247, 262]

46. W.S. Diestelkamp, The decomposability of simple orthogonal arrays on 3 symbols having $t+1$ rows and strength t. J. Comb. Des. **8**, 442–458 (2000) [286]
47. W.S. Diestelkamp, Parameter inequalities for orthogonal arrays with mixed levels. Des. Codes Cryptogr. **33**, 187–197 (2004) [256]
48. W.S. Diestelkamp, J.H. Beder, On the decomposition of orthogonal arrays. Utilitas Math. **61**, 65–86 (2002) [286, 289]
49. A.J. Dobson, A.G. Barnett, *Introduction to Generalized Linear Models*, 3rd edn. (Chapman and Hall/CRC, Boca Raton, 2008) [15]
50. P. Doubilet, On the foundations of combinatorial theory, VII: Symmetric functions through the theory of distribution and occupancy. Stud. Appl. Math. **51**, 377–396 (1972) [296]
51. N.R. Draper, H. Smith, *Applied Regression Analysis*, 3rd edn. (Wiley, New York, 1998) [40, 100, 101, 107, 124]
52. P. Erdős, C. Ko, R. Rado, Intersection theorems for systems of finite sets. Q. J. Math. **12**, 313–320 (1961) [255]
53. J.B.F. Field, F.E. Speed, T.P. Speed, J.M. Williams, Biometrics in the CSIR: 1930–1940. Aust. J. Stat. **30**(B), 54–76 (1988) [xiii, 152]
54. D.J. Finney, The fractional replication of factorial arrangements. Ann. Eugenics **12**, 291–301 (1945) [xii, 232]
55. R.A. Fisher, The correlation between relatives on the supposition of Mendelian inheritance. Trans. R. Soc. Edinb. **52**, 399–433 (1918) [58]
56. R.A. Fisher, The arrangement of field experiments. J. Ministry Agric. Great Britain **33**, 503–513, (1926). Reprinted in [60], Paper 17 [151, 203]
57. R.A. Fisher, *Design of Experiments* (Oliver & Boyd, Edinburgh, 1935). Ninth edition, 1971, published by Macmillan [151]
58. R.A. Fisher, The theory of confounding in factorial experiments in relation to the theory of groups. Ann. Eugenics **11**, 341–353 (1942). Reprinted in [60], Paper 39 [xii, 179, 192, 198, 232]
59. R.A. Fisher, Systems of confounding for factors with more than two alternatives, giving completely orthogonal cubes and higher powers. Ann. Eugenics **12**, 283–209 (1945). Reprinted in [60], Paper 40 [xii, 179, 192, 232]
60. R.A. Fisher, *Contributions to Mathematical Statistics* (Wiley, New York, 1951) [333]
61. M.F. Franklin, Constructing tables of minimum aberration p^{n-m} designs. *Technometrics* **26**, 225–232 (1984) [268]
62. A. Fries, W.G. Hunter, Minimum aberration 2^{k-p} designs. Technometrics **22**, 601–608 (1980) [245, 267, 268]
63. D.W. Gaylor, F.N. Hopper, Estimating the degrees of freedom for linear combinations of mean squares by Satterthwaite's formula. Technometrics **11**, 691–706 (1969) [145]
64. G. Grätzer, *General Lattice Theory*, 2nd edn. (Birkhäuser, Basel, 2003) [296]
65. F.A. Graybill, *Theory and Application of the Linear Model* (Wadsworth & Brooks/Cole, Monterey, 1976) [75]
66. U. Grenander, *Abstract Inference* (Wiley, New York, 1981) [8]
67. O.P. Hackney, Hypothesis testing in the general linear model, PhD thesis, Emory University, 1976 [111]
68. P.R. Halmos, *Introduction to Hilbert Space and the Theory of Spectral Multiplicity*, 2nd edn. (Chelsea Publishing Company, New York, 1957) [323]
69. P.R. Halmos, *Finite-Dimensional Vector Spaces* (Springer, New York, 1974) [327]
70. J.M. Hardin, B.M. Kurkjian, The calculus for factorial arrangements: a review and bibliography. Commun. Stat. Theory Methods **A18**, 1251–1277 (1989) [167]
71. A.S. Hedayat, J. Stufken, G. Su, On the construction and existence of orthogonal arrays with three levels and indexes 1 and 2. Ann. Stat. **25**, 2044–2053 (1997) [286]
72. A.S. Hedayat, N.J.A. Sloane, J. Stufken, *Orthogonal arrays: Theory and applications* (Springer, New York, 1999) [251, 256, 263, 271]
73. R.R. Hocking, *The Analysis of Linear Models* (Wadsworth & Brooks/Cole, Monterey, 1985) [46, 53, 58, 111, 145]

74. R.R. Hocking, F.M. Speed, A full rank analysis of some linear model problems. J. Am. Stat. Assoc. **70**, 706–712 (1975) [53]
75. R.R. Hocking, O.P. Hackney, F.M Speed, The analysis of linear models with unbalanced data, in *Contributions to Survey Sampling and Applied Statistics: Papers in Honor of H. O. Hartley*, ed. by H.A. David (Academic Press, New York, 1978) [111]
76. J.A. John, A.M. Dean, Single replicate factorial experiments in generalized cyclic designs: I. Symmetrical arrangements. J. R. Stat. Soc. Ser. B **37**, 63–71 (1975) [206]
77. I.M. Johnstone, D.M. Titterington, Statistical challenges of high-dimensional data. Philos. Trans. Math. Phys. Eng. Sci. **367**(1906), 4237–4253 (2009) [62]
78. O. Kempthorne, A simple approach to confounding and fractional replication in factorial experiments. Biometrika **34**, 255–272 (1947) [259]
79. O. Kempthorne, *The Design and Analysis of Experiments* (Robert E. Krieger Publishing Company, Malabar, 1983). Corrected reprint of the original 1952 edition by Wiley [208, 210, 212, 217, 259]
80. T.C. Koopmans, O. Reiersøl, The identification of structural characteristics. Ann. Math. Stat. **21**, 165–181 (1950) [8]
81. R.O. Kuehl, *Design of Experiments: Statistical Principles of Research Design and Analysis*, 2nd edn. (Brooks/Cole, Pacific Grove, 2000) [46, 59, 122, 133, 144, 176, 196]
82. B.M. Kurkjian, M. Zelen, A calculus for factorial arrangements. Ann. Math. Stat. **33**, 600–619 (1962) [167, 172, 203]
83. M.H. Kutner, C.J. Nachtshiem, J. Neter, W. Li, *Applied Linear Statistical Models*, 5th edn. (McGraw-Hill/Irwin, New York, 2005) [43, 46, 101]
84. C.W.H. Lam, L. Thiel, S. Swiercz, The non-existence of finite projective planes of order 10. Canad. J. Math. **41**, 1117–1123 (1989) [212]
85. S. Lang, *Linear Algebra*, 3rd edn. (Springer, New York, 1987) [39, 306, 307, 317]
86. S. Lang, *Algebra*, 3rd edn. (Springer, New York, 2002) [206, 299, 300, 306, 320]
87. J. Lawson, *Design and Analysis of Experiments with SAS* (CRC Press, Boca Raton, 2010) [53]
88. E.L. Lehmann, G. Casella, *Theory of Point Estimation*, 2nd edn. (Springer, New York, 1998) [8]
89. E.L. Lehmann, J.P. Romano, *Testing Statistical Hypotheses*, 3rd edn. (Springer, New York, 2005) [9, 82]
90. R. Lidl, H. Niederreiter, *Introduction to Finite Fields and Their Applications* (Cambridge University Press, Cambridge, 1994) [300]
91. P. Lin, Using the Chinese remainder theorem in constructing confounded designs for mixed factorial experiments. Commun. Stat. Theory Methods **15**, 1389–1398 (1986) [206, 212]
92. D.K.J. Lin, N.R. Draper, Projection properties of Plackett and Burman designs. Technometrics **34**, 423–428 (1992) [287]
93. D.K.J. Lin, N.R. Draper, Generating alias relationships for two-level Plackett and Burman designs. Comput. Stat. Data Anal. **15**, 147–157 (1993) [258, 266]
94. M.W. Loyer, Pairwise independent events in experimental designs. Am. Stat. **41**, 339–340 (1987) [157]
95. P. McCullagh, J. Nelder, *Generalized Linear Models*, 2nd edn. (Chapman and Hall/CRC, Boca Raton, 1989) [15]
96. D.C. Montgomery, *Design and Analysis of Experiments*, 8th edn. (Wiley, New York, 2012) [122, 144, 236]
97. D.C. Montgomery, C.L. Jennings, An overview of industrial screening experiments, in *Screening: Methods for Experimentation in Industry, Drug Discovery, and Genetics*, ed. by A. Dean, S. Lewis, chapter 1 (Springer, 2006) [285]
98. R. Mukerjee, C.F. Jeff Wu, *A Modern Theory of Factorial Designs* (Springer, New York, 2006) [xiii, 175, 225, 232, 241, 247, 262, 269, 270]
99. J.A. Nelder, R.W.M. Wedderburn, Generalized linear models. J. R. Stat. Soc. Ser. A **135**, 370–384 (1972) [15]

100. J. Neter, W. Wasserman, M.H. Kutner, *Applied Linear Statistical Models*, 3rd edn. (Richard D. Irwin, Homewood, IL, 1990) [46, 107, 144]
101. J. Neveu, *Processus Aléatoires Gaussiens*. Publications du Séminaire de Mathématiques Supérieurs (Les Presses de l'Université de Montréal, 1968) [170, 176]
102. J. Neyman, Existence of consistent estimates of the directional parameter in a linear structural relation between two variable. Ann. Math. Stat. **22**, 497–512 (1951) [8]
103. J. Ogawa, *Statistical Theory of the Analysis of Experimental Designs* (Marcel Dekker, New York, 1974) [197]
104. O. Ore, Theory of equivalence relations. Duke Math. J. **9**, 573–627 (1942) [296]
105. R.L. Plackett, A historical note on the method of least squares. Biometrika **36**, 458–460 (1949) [69]
106. R.L. Plackett, *Principles of Regression Analysis* (Oxford University Press, London, 1960) [124]
107. P. Pudlák, J. Tůma, Every finite lattice can be embedded in a finite partition lattice. Algebra Univers. **10**, 74–95 (1980) [296]
108. D. Raghavarao, *Constructions and Combinatorial Problems in Design of Experiments* (Wiley, New York, 1971). Reissued by Dover Publications in 1988 [176, 193, 196]
109. B.L. Raktoe, Combining elements from distinct finite fields in mixed factorials. Ann. Math. Stat. **40**, 498–504 (1969) [206]
110. B.L. Raktoe, A. Hedayat, W.T. Federer, *Factorial Designs* (Wiley, New York, 1981) [241, 262]
111. C.R. Rao, Factorial experiments derivable from combinatorial arrangements of arrays. Suppl. J. R. Stat. Soc. **9**, 128–139 (1947) [xii, 251, 253, 256]
112. C.R. Rao, On a class of arrangements. Proc. Edinb. Math. Soc. Ser. 2 **8**, 119–125 (1949) [256]
113. C.R. Rao, A note on a generalized inverse of a matrix, with applications to problems in mathematical statistics. J. R. Stat. Soc. Ser. B **24**, 152–158 (1962) [x, 65, 69]
114. C.R. Rao, Some combinatorial problems of arrays and applications to design of experiments, in *A Survey of Combinatorial Theory*, ed. by J.N. Srivastava, chapter 29 (North-Holland Publishing Company, 1973) [251, 253]
115. C.R. Rao, S.K. Mitra, *Generalized Inverse of matrices and its Applications* (Wiley, New York, 1971) [65]
116. V.K. Rohatgi, *An Introduction to Probability Theory and Mathematical Statistics* (Wiley, New York, 1976) [2]
117. E.J. Russell, Field experiments: How they are made and what they are. *J. Ministry Agric. Great Britain* **32**, 989–1001 (1926) [151]
118. H. Scheffé, A method for judging all contrasts in the analysis of variance. Biometrika **40**, 87–104 (1953) [130]
119. H. Scheffé, Alternative models for the analysis of variance. Ann. Math. Stat. **27**, 51–271 (1956) [54, 58]
120. H. Scheffé, A "mixed model" for the analysis of variance. Ann. Math. Stat. **27**, 23–36 (1956) [57]
121. H. Scheffé, *The Analysis of Variance* (Wiley, New York, 1959). Reissued in the Wiley Classics Library Edition, 1999 [xii, 45, 48, 49, 50, 53, 54, 57, 65, 82, 91, 108, 130, 133]
122. S.L. Sclove, Correlation, dependence, and normality. Unpublished, 2010 [5]
123. S.R. Searle, *Linear Models* (Wiley, New York, 1971) [45, 54, 65, 77, 100, 101, 106, 140, 141, 144]
124. S.R. Searle, *Linear Models for Unbalanced Data* (Wiley, New York, 1987) [xii, 85, 96, 106, 109]
125. S.R. Searle, G. Casella, C.E. McCulloch, *Variance Components* (Wiley, New York, 2006) [57, 58, 137, 141, 144, 145]
126. G.A.F. Seber, The linear hypothesis and idempotent matrices. J. R. Stat. Soc. Ser. B **26**, 261–266 (1964) [91]
127. G.A.F. Seber, *Linear Regression Analysis* (Wiley, New York, 1977) [124]

128. G.A.F. Seber, *The Linear Hypothesis: A General Theory*, 2nd edn. (Macmillan, New York, 1980) [xiii, 25, 73, 91, 113, 123]
129. E. Seiden, R. Zemach, On orthogonal arrays. Ann. Math. Stat. **37**, 1355–1370 (1966) [286]
130. B.V. Shah, On balancing in factorial experiments. Ann. Math. Stat. **29**, 766–779 (1958) [175]
131. J. Shao, X. Deng, Estimation in high-dimensional linear models with deterministic design matrices. Ann. Stat. **40**, 812–831 (2012) [10]
132. S.S. Sihota, K.S. Banerjee, On the algebraic structures in the construction of confounding plans in mixed factorial designs on the lines of White and Hultquist. J. Am. Stat. Assoc. **76**, 996–1001 (1981) [206]
133. J.H. Silverman, Rational points on, and the arithmetic of, elliptic curves: A tale of two books (and an article). Bull. Am. Math. Soc. **54**, 591–594 (2017) [xiv]
134. F.M. Speed, A new approach to the analysis of linear models. PhD thesis, Texas A&M University, 1969 [53]
135. R.P. Stanley, *Enumerative Combinatorics*, vol. I (Wadsworth & Brooks/Cole, Belmont, 1986) [296]
136. A.P. Street, D.J. Street, *Combinatorics of Experimental Design* (Oxford University Press, Oxford, 1987) [176, 196, 284]
137. A. Takemura, Tensor analysis of ANOVA decomposition. J. Am. Stat. Assoc. **78**, 894–900 (1983) [176]
138. B. Tang, The theory of J-characteristics for fractional factorial designs and projection justification of minimum G_2 aberration. Biometrika **88**, 401–407 (2001) [272, 273]
139. B. Tang, L.Y. Deng, Characterization of minimum aberration 2^{n-k} designs in terms of their complementary designs. Ann. Stat. **24**, 2549–2559 (1999) [272]
140. G. Tarry, Le problème des 36 officiers. C. R. Assoc. Française pour l'Avancement Sci. Secrétariat Assoc. **2**, 170–203 (1901) [212]
141. T. Tjur, Analysis of variance models in orthogonal designs. Int. Stat. Rev. **52**, 33–81 (1984). With discussion [155, 157, 296]
142. N.S. Urquhart, D.L. Weeks, C.R. Henderson, Estimation associated with linear models: a revisitation. Commun. Stat. **1**, 303–330 (1973) [53]
143. B.L. van der Waerden, *Modern Algebra*, vol. 1, 2nd edn. (Ungar, New York, 1953). Reissued by Springer in 2003 [197]
144. D.T. Voss, Confounding in single replicate factorial designs. PhD thesis, The Ohio State University, 1984 [xiii, 205, 210, 215]
145. D. T. Voss, A.M. Dean, A comparison of classes of single replicate factorial designs. Ann. Stat. **15**, 376–384 (1987) [206, 207, 211]
146. D.T. Voss, A.M. Dean, Comparing the classes of single replicate generalized cyclic factorial designs with and without pseudofactors. J. Stat. Plan. Inference **35**, 113–120 (1993) [211]
147. A. Wald, Tests of statistical hypotheses concerning several parameters when the number of observations is large. Trans. Am. Math. Soc. **54**, 426–482 (1943) [91]
148. W.P. Wardlaw, Row rank equals column rank. Math. Mag. **78**, 316–318 (2005) [325]
149. D. White, R.A. Hultquist, Construction of confounding plans for mixed factorial designs. Ann. Math. Stat. **36**, 1256–1271 (1965) [206, 212]
150. H. Working, H. Hotelling, Application of the theory of error to the interpretation of trends. J. Am. Stat. Assoc. **24**(165 Supplement), 73–85 (1929) [130, 136]
151. C.F.J. Wu, M. Hamada, *Experiments: Planning, Analysis, and Optimization*, 2nd edn. (Wiley, New York, 2009) [14, 40, 43, 59, 107, 122, 176, 235, 236, 241]
152. H. Xu, C.F.J. Wu, Generalized minimum aberration for asymmetrical fractional factorial designs. Ann. Stat. **29**, 1066–1077 (2001) [271, 277, 278]
153. F. Yates, Complex experiments. Suppl. J. R. Stat. Soc. **2**, 181–247 (1935) [12, 151]
154. F. Yates, The design and analysis of factorial experiments. Technical Report 35, Imperial Bureau of Soil Science, Harpenden, England, 1937 [209]

Index

J. H. Beder, *Linear Models and Design*,
https://doi.org/10.1007/978-3-031-08176-7

Printed in the United States
by Baker & Taylor Publisher Services

Printed in the United States
by Baker & Taylor Publisher Services